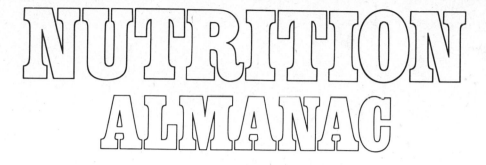

REVISED EDITION

Nutrition Search, Inc.

JOHN D. KIRSCHMANN,
Director

McGraw-Hill Book Company

NEW YORK	JOHANNESBURG	PARIS
ST. LOUIS	LONDON	SÃO PAULO
SAN FRANCISCO	MADRID	SINGAPORE
AUCKLAND	MEXICO	SYDNEY
BOGOTÁ	MONTREAL	TOKYO
DÜSSELDORF	NEW DELHI	TORONTO
	PANAMA	

First McGraw-Hill Paperback edition, 1975
Revised McGraw-Hill Paperback edition, 1979

1234567890 MUMU 7832109

Library of Congress Cataloging in Publication Data
Nutrition Search, Inc.
    Nutrition almanac.

    Bibliography: p.
    Includes index.
    1. Nutrition. 2. Health. 3. Food—Composition—
Tables. I. Kirschmann, John D. II. Title. [DNLM:
1. Nutrition. QU145.3 N9765n]
RA784.N848 1979   641.1   78-21072
ISBN 0-07-034849-9
ISBN 0-07-034848-0 pbk.

This book is dedicated to the purpose of increased harmony in the human body through a better understanding of nutrition. I wish to extend my appreciation to the many people who helped compile this book, especially to Jim Christianson for his editorial supervision and to Mona Holte and Deborah DuBois for their enthusiastic assistance. Also, a special thank you to my daughter Lavon for her diligent efforts in compiling research for the first edition as well as her continuing research resulting in this revised fourth edition.

JOHN D. KIRSCHMANN

Suggestions for Using This Book

The system presented in this book can be employed in two ways. It can help the reader work out a total plan for personal nutrition, or it can quickly answer simple questions regarding food, nutrition, and health.

Nutrients (p. 11). This section discusses over 40 vitamins and minerals in terms of description, absorption and storage, dosage and toxicity, deficiency effects and symptoms, beneficial effect on ailments, human tests, and animal tests. A list of ailments for which the nutrients may be beneficial follows the discussion of each vitamin or mineral. In order to obtain a more complete understanding of the function of nutrients in relation to total health, the reader should refer to related sections of the book.

Nutrients That Function Together (p. 93). Many vitamins and minerals prove to be more or less effective when taken simultaneously with other nutrients. This section provides an easy-to-follow guide for understanding which nutrients are compatable or antagonistic.

Available Forms of Nutrient Supplements (p. 100). This section may be of interest to persons who wish to determine which supplements are best suited to their needs. All types of nutrient supplements are explained in terms of available forms, source—natural or synthetic, and an explanation of the source.

Ailments (p. 107). It is a proven fact that many common ailments and weight problems are a result of unbalanced intake of nutrients. In this section, common ailments are discussed and explained in layman's language. The discussion of each ailment is accompanied by a list of nutrients that have proven beneficial in treatment of the ailment. When quantities for a particular nutrient are given, it must be remembered that these quantities are *not prescriptive* but merely represent research findings. This section can be best utilized when cross-referenced with the "Nutrients" and "Foods" sections.

Herbs (p. 175). Introducing the world of herbs with a brief commentary and a short summary of a number of common herbs.

Foods, Beverages and Supplementary Foods (p. 185). The discussions of foods and supplemental foods give valuable information about specific foods or classes of foods and supplements. The list of "Rich Sources of Nutrients," beginning on page 181, shows at a glance what foods are good sources of the vitamins and minerals.

Table of Food Composition (p. 199). The "Table of Food Composition" gives the complete nutrient analysis of over 600 foods. This simple guide makes it possible for the reader to compare food values and analyze and prepare meals balanced in nutrients and calories.

Essential Amino Acid Contents of Some Foods (p. 235). One of the most important breakthroughs in understanding the balance and value of foods in terms of the protein quality they provide, this table lists the essential amino acid content of many foods together with the percentage of protein Recommended Dietary Allowance for a man and a woman of average body size which the foods provide.

Nutrient Allowance Chart (p. 245). The "Nutrient Allowance Chart" gives a complete breakdown of the nutrient needs for each person in view of body size, metabolism, and calorie requirements.

Diet Analysis (p. 249). A sample form is provided so that individuals may examine their average daily consumption of food, and compare it to the Recommended Daily Allowance.

In summary, this "Almanac" is not the type of book that one would read from front cover to back cover as one would a novel, but it can be a very useful tool if a reader takes time to understand the importance of the various sections. Like the individual B-complex vitamins, each section of this book is important in its own right; when used simultaneously, *all* sections have a much more beneficial effect.

NOTE: The information contained in this book is not intended to be prescriptive. Any attempt to diagnose and treat an illness should come under the direction of a physician who is familiar with nutritional therapy. It is possible that some individuals may suffer allergic reactions from the use of various dietary supplement preparations or the media in which they are contained; if such reactions occur, consult your physician. Nutrition Search, Inc., and the publisher assume no responsibility.

Contents

Suggestions for Using This Book   v

I. Nutrition and Health   1

II. Sources of Calories: Carbohydrates, Fats, and Protein   7

III. Nutrients   11

  Vitamins   13

  Minerals   61

  Water   85

  Summary Chart of Nutrients   86

  Nutrients That Function Together   93

  Available Forms of Nutrient Supplements   100

IV. Ailments and Other Stressful Conditions   107

  Ailments   108

  Normal Life Cycle   169

V. Herbs   175

  Herbal Preparations   182
  Herb Glossary   182
  References   183

VI. Foods, Beverages, and Supplementary Foods   185

  Foods   186

  Beverages   193

  Supplementary Foods   194

  Some Rich Sources of Nutrients   196

VII. Table of Food Composition   199

VIII. Essential Amino Acid Contents of Some Foods   235

IX. Nutrient Allowance Chart   245

X.   Diet Analysis   249

Bibliography   253

Glossary   257

Index   261

Nutrition and Health

Nutrition is the relationship of foods to the health of the human body. Proper nutrition implies receiving adequate foods and supplements to convey the nutrients required for optimal health. Without proper nutrition and exercise, optimal health and well-being cannot be attained.

Proper nutrition means that all the essential nutrients—that is, carbohydrates, fats, protein, vitamins, minerals, and water—are supplied and utilized in adequate balance to maintain optimal health and well-being. Nutritional deficiencies result whenever inadequate amounts of essential nutrients are provided to tissues that must function normally over a long period of time. Good nutrition is essential for normal organ development and functioning; for normal reproduction, growth, and maintenance; for optimum activity level and working efficiency; for resistance to infection and disease; and for the ability to repair bodily damage or injury.

No single substance will maintain vibrant health. Although specific nutrients are known to be more important in the functions of certain parts of the body, even these nutrients are totally dependent upon the presence of other nutrients for their best effects. Every effort should therefore be made to attain and maintain an adequate, balanced daily intake of all the necessary nutrients throughout life.

Fasting and vegetarianism are two situations in which adequate daily intake of all essential nutrients may not be achieved if care is not taken to ensure the mainte- nance of good health. Fasting, whether for reasons of health, social protest, religion, or economic or environmental factors, may last from 1 to 70 days. Some persons advocate consuming only pure water during a fast, while others advocate drinking fruit and vegetable juices. Although many nutrients may not be as efficiently absorbed without the presence of solid food, one should consider taking nutrient supplements when fasting.

Vegetarianism is essentially the practice of eating a meatless diet, although there are several types of vegetarians. *Ovo-lacto vegetarians* include some animal products such as eggs, milk, and cheese, in their diet, but exclude all flesh foods, whether meat, poultry, or fish. *Pure*, or *strict*, *vegetarians* abstain from the use of all foods of animal origin. *Lacto-vegetarians* drink milk, eat cheese and other dairy products, but do not eat eggs. *Vegans* eat no meat or other animal-related foods.

The main concern in a vegetarian diet is the sufficient intake of protein. This can be achieved by the combination of nonflesh foods that are low in certain amino acids with other foods that have high concentrations of the same amino acids. This system of combining "complementary proteins" is described in detail in the section on protein (p. 9) and should be fully understood by anyone considering adopting a vegetarian diet. Amino acid contents of foods are listed in Section VIII—"Essential Amino Acid Contents of Some Foods" (pp. 235–243). Also of importance to vegans is the lack of vitamin B_{12} which is found only in animal products. The consequences of this deficiency include megaloblastic anemia and perhaps degeneration of the spinal cord. Most vegetarian diets also contain little vitamin D. The declining trace mineral content of edible plants results from soil exhaustion and overuse of nitrogen and phosphorus fertilizers. Important is zinc, which can be bound in the digestive system, along with other minerals, by foods that are rich in phytates (beans, legumes, and grains). This can become a problem if large quantities of these foods are consumed. The addition of yeast to grains in bread destroys the phytates by fermentation. Sprouting also neutralizes the phytates.[1] No one should attempt to vary from a standard diet for an extended period of time without first consulting a physician or naturopath knowledgeable in the field of nutrition and without studying the available literature on the subject.

The foods eaten by humans are chemically complex. They must be broken down by the body into simpler chemical forms so that they can be taken in through the intestinal walls and transported by the blood to the cells. There they provide energy and the correct building materials to maintain human life. These are the processes of digestion, absorption, and metabolism.

DIGESTION, ABSORPTION, AND METABOLISM

DIGESTION

Digestion is a series of physical and chemical changes by which food, taken into the body, is broken down in preparation for absorption from the intestinal tract into the bloodstream. These changes take place in the digestive tract, which includes the mouth, pharynx, esophagus, stomach, small intestine, and large intestine.

The active materials in the digestive juices which cause the chemical breakdown of food are called "enzymes," complex proteins that are capable of inducing chemical changes in other substances without themselves being changed. Each enzyme is capable of breaking down only a single specific substance. For example, an enzyme capable of breaking down fats cannot break down proteins or carbohydrates, or vice versa. Enzymatic action

[1]Pfeiffer, Ph.D., M.D.: *Mental and Elemental Nutrients* (New Canaan, Conn.: Keats Publishing, 1975), p. 103.

originates in four areas of the body: the salivary glands, the stomach, the pancreas, and the wall of the small intestine.

Digestion actually begins in the mouth, where chewing breaks large pieces of food into smaller pieces. The salivary glands in the mouth produce saliva, a fluid that moistens food for swallowing and which contains ptyalin, the enzyme necessary for carbohydrate breakdown. The masticated food mass passes back to the pharynx under voluntary control, but from there on and through the esophagus, the process of swallowing is carried on by peristalsis, a slow wavelike motion occurring along the entire digestive tract, which moves the food into the stomach.

Active chemical digestion begins in the middle portion of the stomach, where the food is mixed with gastric juices containing hydrochloric acid, water, and enzymes that break up protein and other substances.

After one to four hours, depending upon the combination of foods ingested by the system, peristalsis pushes the food, now in the liquid form of chyme, out of the stomach and into the small intestine. Foodstuffs leave the stomach and enter the small intestine in the following order: carbohydrates, protein, and fat—which takes the longest to digest.

When chyme enters the small intestine, the pancreas secretes its digestive juices. If fats are present in the food, bile, an enzyme produced by the liver and stored in the gallbladder, is also secreted. Bile separates the fat into small droplets so that the pancreatic enzymes can break it down. The pancreas also secretes a substance that neutralizes the digestive acids in the food, and it secretes additional enzymes that continue the breakdown of proteins and carbohydrates.

The remaining undigested products enter the large intestine and eventually are excreted. No digestive enzymes are secreted in the large intestine, and little change occurs there except for the absorption of water.

ABSORPTION

Absorption is the process by which nutrients in the form of glucose (from carbohydrates), amino acids (from protein), and fatty acids and glycerol (from fats) are taken up by the intestines and passed into the bloodstream to facilitate cell metabolism.

Absorption takes place primarily in the small intestine. The lining of the small intestine is covered with small fingerlike projections called "villi." These villi contain lymph channels and tiny blood vessels called "capillaries" that are the principal channels of absorption, depending upon the type of nutrient. Fats and fat-soluble vitamins move through the blood to the cells. Other nutrients are carried away from the villi by the capillaries, which funnel them into the portal vein leading to the liver.

In the liver, many different enzymes help change the nutrient molecules into new forms for specific purposes. Unlike earlier changes, which prepared nutrients for absorption and transport, the reactions in the liver produce the products needed by individual cells. Some of the products are used by the liver itself, but the rest are held in storage by the liver, to be released into the body as needed. The remainder go into the bloodstream, where they are picked up by the cells and put to work. Water-soluble vitamins and minerals are also absorbed into the bloodstream in the small intestine.

METABOLISM

At this point the handling of food within the body has reached its final stage. The process of metabolism involves all the chemical changes that nutrients undergo from the time they are absorbed until they become a part of the body or are excreted from the body. Metabolism is the conversion of the digested nutrients into building material for living tissue or energy to meet the body's needs.

Metabolism occurs in two general phases that occur simultaneously, *anabolism* and *catabolism*. Anabolism involves all the chemical reactions that the nutrients undergo in the construction or building up of body chemicals and tissues, such as blood, enzymes, hormones, glycogen, and others. Catabolism involves the reactions in which various compounds of the tissues are broken down to supply energy. Energy for the cells is derived from the metabolism of glucose, which combines with oxygen in a series of chemical reactions to form carbon dioxide, water, and cellular energy. The carbon dioxide and water are waste products, carried away from the cells by the bloodstream. Energy can also be derived from the metabolism of essential fatty acids and amino acids, although the primary effect of the metabolism of amino acids is to provide material for growth and the maintenance and repair of tissues. The waste products

of essential fatty acid and amino acid metabolism are also carried away from the cells by the bloodstream.

The process of metabolism requires that extensive systems of enzymes be maintained to facilitate the thousands of different chemical reactions and regulate the rate at which these reactions proceed. These enzymes often require the presence of specific vitamins and minerals to perform their functions.

FACTORS INHIBITING DIGESTION

The movements of the stomach are interfered with by nervousness and anxiety. Eating while agitated, fa-

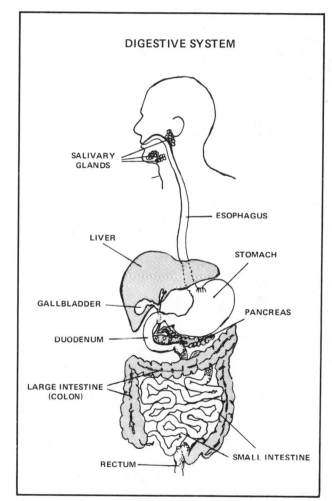

DIGESTIVE SYSTEM

SALIVARY GLANDS
ESOPHAGUS
LIVER
STOMACH
GALLBLADDER
PANCREAS
DUODENUM
LARGE INTESTINE (COLON)
SMALL INTESTINE
RECTUM

tigued, or worried may give rise to gastrointestinal disturbances. Hurried meals under tense conditions are not conducive to normal digestion. Weather variations and physical disorders such as diabetes or other illnesses may inhibit the proper digestion of foods.

EXERCISE

A healthy body is the result of proper nutrition combined with a regular pattern of physical exercise. Exercise imparts vigor and activity to all organs and secures and maintains healthful integrity of all their functions. Exercise improves the tone and quality of muscle tissue and stimulates the processes of digestion, absorption, metabolism, and elimination. It also strengthens blood vessels, lungs, and heart, resulting in improved transfer of oxygen to the cells and increased circulation of the blood and lymph systems. Exercise develops grace, poise, and symmetry of the body, helps in correcting defective development or injuries, and stimulates the mind.

The key to any type of exercise is a strong will and a sincere desire to improve one's physical condition. It is important to have a program that fits individual needs and capacities. A beginning exercise program should be light; it should increase in difficulty gradually as endurance increases. Exercise should not be done for at least an hour after eating because physical exertion may impede digestion. Exercise should be self-motivating and fun. An ideal exercise program may include many different forms of the following physical activities.

Calisthenics

Calisthenics consists of light exercises or gymnastics including sit-ups, push-ups, jumping jacks, etc., which promote grace and health. The emphasis of calisthenics is on building skeletal muscles.

Dancing

Dancing or rhythmic exercise is often an enjoyable way to exercise the body thoroughly and refresh the mind. Besides toning muscles, joints, glands, the respiratory system, and digestive organs, it gives everyday movements grace and poise.

Isometrics

Isometric exercise involves the pressure of a muscle or group of muscles against each other or against an immovable object. It is especially good for reducing because it can be applied to specific areas. Isometrics primarily tone and build the skeletal muscles.

Jogging

Jogging is a form of exercise that consists of alternately walking and running. It is an excellent exercise for improving the heart, lungs, and circulatory system by expanding their capacity to handle stress. It can help build muscle tone, reduce hips and thighs, redistribute weight, and flatten the abdomen.

Stretching

Stretching is natural exercise that should be practiced on a regular basis. A good habit to develop is stretching upon rising in the morning and throughout the day. Stretch exercises tend to increase both energy and endurance for all parts of the body. Stretching tends to

EXPENDITURE OF CALORIC ENERGY PER HOUR

Activity	Calories Expended per Hour
Ballroom dancing	330
Bed making	234
Bowling	264
Bricklaying	240
Carpentry	408
Desk work	132
Driving a car	168
Farm work in field	438
Golf	300
Handball	612
Horseback riding (trot)	480
Ironing (standing up)	252
Lawn mowing (hand mower)	462
Painting at an easel	120
Piano playing	150
Preparing a meal	198
Scrubbing of floors	216
Sitting and eating	84
Sitting and knitting	90
Sitting in a chair reading	72
Skiing	594
Sleeping (basal metabolism)	60
Standing up	138
Sweeping	102
Swimming (leisurely)	300
Walking (2.5 miles per hour)	216
Walking downstairs	312

relieve many aches and pains; loosen up ligaments, joints, and muscles; and increase coordination and suppleness. Stretching stimulates circulation and alleviates the stiffness of contracted muscles.

Walking

Walking is one of the best overall exercises and helps the entire system function better. The metabolism is increased while walking; thus fat is burned up and weight loss is promoted. Blood pressure, blood cholesterol, and sugar levels tend to fall. Walking builds up the heart muscle and keeps the arteries clear and elastic. Walking helps increase the oxygen supply to the blood, thus bringing more oxygen to the heart. It also increases the capacity of the lungs, making more oxygen available to the circulatory system.

Weight Lifting

Weight lifting is a form of exercise involving the lifting of weights and is often used by athletes to strengthen muscle tone.

Yoga

Yoga is a series of stretching movements that are performed slowly and methodically. Some postures are quite advanced and complicated for the average person, at least at first; however, there are simple yoga exercises that can be practiced by people of all ages with great benefit. The prime goal of yoga is to relieve the body of tension. Yoga, if practiced consistently, gives elasticity to the spine, firms the skin, tones flabby muscles, and improves poor posture. Many people feel that yoga increases their endurance and flexibility for participation in other more strenuous activities.

Above all, do not forget the recreational exercises, such as golf, tennis, riding, skating, skiing, etc. There are endless sports that can improve the functioning of the body. The important thing is to remember to exercise *regularly* and maintain a nutritionally balanced diet of good, healthy food.

Sources of Calories: Carbohydrates, Fats, and Protein

Carbohydrates, fats, and proteins are the primary sources of energy to the body because they supply fuel necessary for body heat and work. Their fuel potential is expressed in *calories*, a term that signifies the amount of chemical energy that may be released as heat when food is metabolized. Therefore foods that are high in energy value are high in calories, while foods that are low in energy value are low in calories. Fats yield approximately nine calories per gram, and carbohydrates and proteins yield approximately four calories per gram.

CARBOHYDRATES

Carbohydrates are the chief source of energy for all body functions and muscular exertion and are necessary to assist in the digestion and assimilation of other foods. Carbohydrates provide us with immediately available calories for energy by producing heat in the body when carbon in the system unites with oxygen in the bloodstream. Carbohydrates also help regulate protein and fat metabolism; fats require carbohydrates for their breakdown within the liver.

The principal carbohydrates present in foods are sugars, starches, and cellulose. Simple sugars, such as those in honey and fruits, are very easily digested. Double sugars, such as table sugar, require some digestive action, but they are not nearly as complex as starches, such as those found in whole grain. Starches require prolonged enzymatic action in order to be broken down into simple sugars (glucose) for digestion. Cellulose, commonly found in the skins of fruits and vegetables, is largely indigestible by humans and contributes little energy value to the diet. It does, however, provide the bulk necessary for intestinal action and aids elimination.

All sugars and starches are converted by the digestive juices to a simple sugar called "glucose." Some of this glucose, or "blood sugar," is used as fuel by tissues of the brain, nervous system, and muscles. A small portion of the glucose is converted to glycogen and stored by the liver and muscles; the excess is converted to fat and stored throughout the body as a reserve source of energy. When fat reserves are reconverted to glucose and used for body fuel, weight loss results.

Carbohydrate snacks containing sugars and starches provide the body with almost instant energy because they cause a sudden rise in the blood sugar level. However, the blood sugar level drops again rapidly, creating a craving for more sweet food and possibly fatigue, dizziness, nervousness, and headache.

Overindulgence in starchy and sweet foods may crowd out other essential foods from the diet and can therefore result in nutritional deficiency as well as in obesity and tooth decay. Diets high in refined carbohydrates are usually low in vitamins, minerals, and cellulose. Such foods as white flour, white sugar, and polished rice are lacking in the B vitamins and other nutrients. Excessive consumption of these foods will perpetuate any vitamin B deficiency an individual may have. If the B vitamins are absent, carbohydrate combustion cannot take place, and indigestion, symptoms of heartburn, and nausea can result. Research continues as to whether or not such problems as diabetes, heart disease, high blood pressure, anemia, kidney disorders, and cancer can be linked to an overabundance of refined carbohydrate foods in the diet.

Carbohydrates can be manufactured in the body from some amino acids and the glycerol component of fats; therefore the National Research Council lists no specific requirement for carbohydrates in the diet.[1]

Differences in basal metabolism, amount of activity, size, and weight will influence the amount of carbohydrates the body needs to get from an outside source. However, a total lack of carbohydrates may produce ketosis, loss of energy, depression, and breakdown of essential body protein.

FATS

Fats, or lipids, are the most concentrated source of energy in the diet. When oxidized, fats furnish more than twice the number of calories per gram furnished by carbohydrates or proteins. One gram of fat yields approximately nine calories to the body.

In addition to providing energy, fats act as carriers for the fat-soluble vitamins, A, D, E, and K. By aiding in the absorption of vitamin D, fats help make calcium available to body tissues, particularly to the bones and teeth. Fats are also important for the conversion of carotene to vitamin A. Fat deposits surround, protect, and hold in place organs, such as the kidneys, heart, and liver. A layer of fat insulates the body from environmental temperature changes and preserves body heat. This layer also rounds out the contours of the body. Fats prolong the process of digestion by slowing down the stomach's secretions of hydrochloric acid. Thus fats create a longer-lasting sensation of fullness after a meal.

The substances that give fats their different flavors, textures, and melting points are known as the "fatty acids." There are two types of fatty acids, saturated and unsaturated. Saturated fatty acids are those that are usually hard at room temperature and which, except for coconut oils, come primarily from animal sources. Unsaturated fatty acids, including polyunsaturates, are usually liquid at room temperature and are derived from vegetable, nut, or seed sources, such as corn, safflowers, sunflowers, and olives. Vegetable shortenings and margarines have undergone a process called "hydrogenation" in which unsaturated oils are converted to a more solid form of fat. Other sources of fat are milk products, eggs, and cheese.

There are three "essential" fatty acids: linoleic, arachidonic, and linolenic, collectively known as vitamin F. They are termed "essential" because the body cannot produce them. They are unsaturated fatty acids necessary for normal growth and healthy blood, arteries, and nerves. Also, they keep the skin and other tissues youthful and healthy by preventing dryness and scaliness. Essential fatty acids may be necessary for the transport and breakdown of cholesterol.[2]

Cholesterol is a lipid or fat-related substance necessary for good health. It is a normal component of most body tissues, especially those of the brain and nervous system, liver, and blood. It is needed to form sex and adrenal hormones, vitamin D, and bile, which is needed for the digestion of fats. Cholesterol also seems to play a part in lubricating the skin.

Although a cholesterol deficiency is unlikely to occur, abnormal amounts of cholesterol may be stored throughout the body if fats are eaten excessively. Research continues, although it is yet inconclusive, as to the relationship of increased cholesterol storage to the devel-

[1] National Research Council, *Recommended Dietary Allowances* (Washington, D.C.: National Academy of Science, 1974), p. 34.

[2] Helen S. Mitchel et al., *Copper's Nutrition in Health and Disease,* 15th ed. (Philadelphia: J. B. Lippincott Co., 1968), p. 318.

opment of arteriosclerosis. Lecithin has been found to decrease cholesterol levels in some individuals.

Fat and fat-containing foods should be stored in covered containers, away from direct light, in a cool place to prevent rancidity caused by oxidation. Some protection from rancidity will be provided by vitamin E, a fat-soluble vitamin that is a natural antioxidant and is present in most fat-containing foods.

Although a fat deficiency rarely occurs in man, such a deficiency would lead to a deficiency in the fat-soluble vitamins. A deficiency of fatty acids may produce eczema or other skin disorders. An extreme deficiency could lead to severely retarded growth.

Excessive amounts of fat in the diet may lead to abnormal weight gain and obesity if more calories are consumed than are needed by the body. In addition to obesity, excessive fat intake will cause abnormally slow digestion and absorption, resulting in indigestion. If a lack of carbohydrates is accompanied by a lack of water in the diet, or if there is a kidney malfunction, fats cannot be completely metabolized and may become toxic to the body.

The National Research Council sets no Recommended Dietary Allowance for fats because of the widely varying fat content of the diet among individuals. Linoleic acid, however, should provide about 2 percent of the calories in the diet.[3] Vegetable fats, such as corn, safflower, and soybean oils, are high in linoleic acid. Nutritionists suggest that an intake of fat providing 25 to 30 percent of the calories is compatible with good health.[4]

PROTEIN

Next to water, protein is the most plentiful substance in the body. Protein is one of the most important elements for the maintenance of good health and vitality and is of primary importance in the growth and development of all body tissues. It is the major source of building mate-

rial for muscles, blood, skin, hair, nails, and internal organs, including the heart and the brain.

Protein is needed for the formation of hormones, which control a variety of body functions such as growth, sexual development, and rate of metabolism. Protein also helps prevent the blood and tissues from becoming either too acid or too alkaline and helps regulate the body's water balance. Enzymes, substances necessary for basic life functions, and antibodies, which help fight foreign substances in the body, are also formed from protein. In addition, protein is important in the formation of milk during lactation and in the process of blood clotting.

As well as being the major source of building material for the body, protein may be used as a source of heat and energy, providing 4 calories per gram of protein. However, this energy function is spared when sufficient fats and carbohydrates are present in the diet. Excess protein that is not used for building tissue or energy can be converted by the liver and stored as fat in the body tissues.

During digestion the large molecules of proteins are decomposed into simpler units called "amino acids." Amino acids are necessary for the synthesis of body proteins and many other tissue constituents. They are the units from which proteins are constructed and are the end products of protein digestion.

The body requires approximately twenty-two amino acids in a specific pattern to make human protein. All but eight of these amino acids can be produced in the adult body. The eight that cannot be produced are called "essential amino acids" because they must be supplied in the diet. In order for the body to properly synthesize protein, all the essential amino acids must be present simultaneously and in the proper proportions. If just one essential amino acid is missing, even temporarily, protein synthesis will fall to a very low level or stop altogether.[5] The result is that *all* amino acids are reduced in the same proportion as the amino acid that is low or missing.

Foods containing protein may or may not contain all the essential amino acids. When a food contains all the essential amino acids, it is termed "complete protein." Foods that lack or are extremely low in any one of the essential amino acids are called "incomplete protein." Most meats and dairy products are complete-protein

[3]Helen Andrews Guthrie, *Introductory Nutrition*, 2d ed. (St. Louis: C. V. Mosby Co., 1971), p. 46.
[4]Guthrie, *Introductory Nutrition*, p. 46.

[5]A. M. Altschul, *Proteins, Their Chemistry and Politics* (New York: Basic Books, 1965), p. 118.

foods, while most vegetables and fruits are incomplete-protein foods. To obtain a complete-protein meal from incomplete proteins, one must combine foods carefully so that those weak in an essential amino acid will be balanced by those adequate in the same amino acid.

The minimum daily protein requirement, the smallest amino acid intake that can maintain optimum growth and good health in man, is difficult to determine. Protein requirements differ according to the nutritional status, body size, and activity of the individual. Dietary calculations are usually based on the National Research Council's Recommended Dietary Allowances. The protein recommendations are considered to cover individual variations among most persons living in the United States under usual environmental stress. The National Research Council recommends that 0.42 gram of protein per day be consumed for each pound of body weight. To figure out individual protein requirements, simply divide body weight by 2, and the result will indicate the approximate number of grams of protein required each day. For example, a person weighing 120 pounds requires approximately 60 grams of protein daily. However, total daily protein needs in grams per pound will be reduced if the daily limited amino acid requirements are met. (See "Essential Amino Acid Contents of Some Foods," pp. 235–243.)

Protein deficiency may lead to abnormalities of growth and tissue development. The hair, nails, and skin especially will be affected, and muscle tone will be poor. A child whose diet is deficient in protein may not attain his potential physical stature. Extreme protein deficiency in children results in kwashiorkor, a disease characterized by stunted mental and physical growth, loss of hair pigment, and swelling of the joints. It is often fatal. In adults, protein deficiency may result in lack of vigor and stamina, mental depression, weakness, poor resistance to infection, impaired healing of wounds, and slow recovery from disease.

Loss of body protein occurs as a result of particular bodily stresses, such as surgery, hemorrhage, wounds, or prolonged illness. At times of stress, it is necessary to consume extra protein in order to rebuild or replace used or worn out tissues. However, excessive intake of protein may cause fluid imbalance.

Nutrients

Knowledge of the nutrients and their functions in the body is necessary for understanding the importance of good nutrition. The six nutrients—carbohydrates, fats, protein, vitamins, minerals, and water—are present in the foods we eat and contain chemical substances that function in one or more of three ways: they furnish the body with heat and energy, they provide material for growth and repair of body tissues, and they assist in the regulation of body processes.

Each nutrient has its own specific functions and relationship to the body, but no nutrient acts independently of other nutrients. All of the nutrients must be present in the diet in varying quantities in order for the body to maintain basic life processes. Although all persons have need for the same nutrients, the amounts of the nutrients required by an individual are influenced by age, sex, body size, environment, level of activity, and nutritional status. Processing, storage, and preparation of food may influence the nutritional value of food. Proper understanding of the nutrients and the means of balancing a diet of the foods that contain them will result in optimum health for the body and mind.

VITAMINS

All natural vitamins are organic food substances found only in living things, that is, plants and animals. There are about twenty substances that are believed to be active as vitamins in human nutrition. Each of these vitamins is present in varying quantities in specific foods, and each is absolutely necessary for proper growth and maintenance of health. With a few exceptions, the body cannot synthesize vitamins; they must be supplied in the diet or in dietary supplements.

Vitamins have no caloric or energy value but are important to the body as constituents of enzymes, which function as catalysts in nearly all metabolic reactions. As such, vitamins help regulate metabolism, help convert fat and carbohydrates into energy, and assist in forming bone and tissues. Vitamins are not components of major body structures but aid in the building of these structures.

Much work has been done to determine requirements of vitamins for various age groups and in circumstances of additional needs, such as pregnancy and lactation. The Recommended Dietary Allowances (RDA) of the nutrients mentioned in this book are based on the standards established by the Food and Nutrition Board of the National Research Council. Desirable levels for those vitamins whose requirements are known to be essential to healthy humans are based upon available scientific knowledge and are considered adequate to meet the known nutritional needs of practically all healthy persons. These levels are intended to apply to persons whose physical activity is considered "light" and who live in temperate climates, and they provide a safety margin for each vitamin above the minimum level that will maintain health.

To ensure that as yet unrecognized nutritional needs

are met, one should obtain one's RDA from as varied a selection of foods as is practical: present knowledge of nutritional needs is incomplete. The human requirement for many nutrients has not been established. There is no way of actually predicting the requirements of specific individuals because of the variables of climate, sex, age, state of health, body size, genetic makeup, and amount of activity.

Where there is doubt that the requirements for certain nutrients are being met through the diet alone, supplements may be ingested to offset any deficiency. Vitamins taken in excess of the finite amount utilized in the metabolic processes are valueless and will be either excreted in the urine or stored in the body. Excessive ingestion of some nutrients may result in toxicity, and risks associated with ingestion of excessive quantities of nutrients are mentioned at appropriate points in the text.

Vitamins are usually distinguished as being water-soluble or fat-soluble. The water-soluble vitamins, B-complex vitamins, vitamin C, and the compounds termed "bioflavonoids," are usually measured in milligrams. The fat-soluble vitamins, A, D, E, and K, are measured in units of activity known as "International Units" (IU) or "United States Pharmacopoeia Units" (USP). (Vitamins A, D, E, and K are expressed in International Units (IU) throughout this book.) Generally, each unit represents the amount of any form of the vitamin needed to produce a specific change in the nutritional health of a laboratory animal.

MINERALS

Minerals are nutrients that exist in the body and in food in organic and inorganic combinations. Approximately seventeen minerals are essential in human nutrition. Although only 4 or 5 percent of the human body weight is mineral matter, minerals are vital to overall mental and physical well-being. All tissues and internal fluids of living things contain varying quantities of minerals. Minerals are constituents of the bones, teeth, soft tissue, muscle, blood, and nerve cells. They are important factors in maintaining physiological processes, strengthening skeletal structures, and preserving the vigor of the heart and brain as well as all muscle and nerve systems.

Minerals act as catalysts for many biological reactions within the human body, including muscle response, the transmission of messages through the nervous system, digestion, and metabolism or utilization of nutrients in foods. They are important in the production of hormones.

Minerals help to maintain the delicate water balance essential to the proper functioning of mental and physical processes. They keep blood and tissue fluids from becoming either too acid or too alkaline and permit other nutrients to pass into the bloodstream. They also help draw chemical substances in and out of the cells and aid in the creation of antibodies.

All of the minerals known to be needed by the human body must be supplied in the diet. No RDAs have been established for minerals other than calcium, phosphorus, iodine, and iron. However, a varied and mixed diet of animal and vegetable origin which meets the energy and protein needs of healthy persons will also furnish adequate minerals.

Calcium, chlorine, phosphorus, potassium, magnesium, sodium, and sulfur are known as the "macro-minerals" because they are present in relatively high amounts in body tissues. They are measured in milligrams. Other minerals, termed "trace minerals," are present in the body only in the most minute quantities but are essential for proper body functioning. Trace minerals are measured in micrograms.

Although the minerals are discussed separately, it is important to note that their actions within the body are interrelated; no one mineral can function without affecting others. Physical and emotional stress causes a strain on the body's supply of minerals. A mineral deficiency often results in illness, which may be checked by the addition of the missing mineral to the diet.

HOW VITAMINS AND MINERALS ARE EXPLAINED IN THIS BOOK

Vitamins and minerals are explained in this book in terms of description, absorption and storage, dosage and toxicity, deficiency effects and symptoms, and beneficial effect on ailments. Human and animal tests are described at the end of some listed nutrients. A chart listing the ailments that are associated with a specific nutrient follows the discussion of each nutrient.

Description

The description of the vitamin or mineral defines the nutrient—whether or not it is water- or fat-soluble (if it is a vitamin) and its function in the body—and lists the major foods in which it is contained.

Absorption and Storage

The section on absorption and storage explains the places where the nutrient is absorbed and stored in the body, the synthesis of body processes, and if possible, the time factor involved. Any variables that may stimulate or interfere with absorption and storage of the nutrient are also mentioned together with the way the nutrient is excreted.

Dosage and Toxicity

Dosage is given in accordance with the Recommended Dietary Allowances as suggested by the National Research Council's Food and Nutrition Board. Symptoms and effects are given for those nutrients that may be toxic.

Deficiency Effects and Symptoms

If nutrient intake is insufficient to meet requirements for a prolonged period of time, the ability to respond to stress is lessened and depletion and deterioration eventually occur, despite the effectiveness of the various mechanisms that prolong survival. The effects and symptoms of a deficiency are stated for each nutrient.

Beneficial Effect on Ailments

Those ailments that have been successfully treated with a specific nutrient are mentioned here. Additional information, including dosages, is provided in the section "Ailments and Other Stressful Conditions." Dosages listed in the "Ailments" section should not be taken as prescriptive but merely as representations of research findings. In many instances, nutrients should not be taken alone: they are more beneficial when accompanied by other nutrients.

Human Tests

Examples of tests on humans, in clinical situations, are those involving nutritional therapy. Dosages used in these tests should not be taken as prescriptive but merely as examples of how specific nutrients affect some people. Nutritional therapy applied to one individual may not work as well on others. Sources of further information are provided.

Animal Tests

Before results are applied to humans, extensive animal tests are done. There are, however, many biological similarities between humans and animals in nutritional therapy.

Chart of Beneficial Effects on Ailments

A chart listing the ailments that are associated with a specific vitamin or mineral follows the discussion of each nutrient. These include ailments for which, according to nutritional studies, this particular nutrient may be beneficial.

VITAMINS

VITAMIN A

Description

Vitamin A is a fat-soluble nutrient that occurs in nature in two forms: preformed vitamin A and provitamin A, or carotene. Preformed vitamin A is concentrated only in certain tissues of animal products in which the animal has metabolized the carotene contained in its food into vitamin A.[1] One of the richest natural sources of preformed vitamin A is fish-liver oil, which is classified as a food supplement. Some animal products, such as cream and butter, may contain both preformed vitamin A and carotene.

Carotene is a substance that must be converted into vitamin A before it can be utilized by the body. Carotene is abundant in carrots, from which its name is derived, but it is present in even higher concentrations in certain green leafy vegetables, such as beet greens, spinach, and broccoli. If, due to any disorder, the body is unable to use carotene, a vitamin A deficiency may arise.

Vitamin A aids in the growth and repair of body tissues and helps maintain smooth, soft, disease-free skin. Internally it helps protect the mucous membranes of the mouth, nose, throat, and lungs, thereby reducing susceptibility to infection. This protection also aids the mucous membranes in combating the effects of various

[1] Helen Andrews Guthrie, *Introductory Nutrition*, 2d ed. (St. Louis: C. V. Mosby Co., 1971), p. 196.

air pollutants. The soft tissue and all linings of the digestive tract, kidneys, and bladder are also protected. In addition, vitamin A prompts the secretion of gastric juices necessary for proper digestion of proteins. Other important functions of vitamin A include the building of strong bones and teeth, the formation of rich blood, and the maintenance of good eyesight. It is essential in the formation of visual purple, a substance in the eye which is necessary for proper night vision.

Through recent studies at the University of Oklahoma School of Medicine, a definite relationship has been found between vitamin A and the synthesis of RNA. RNA (ribonucleic acid) is a nucleic acid that transmits to each cell of the body instructions on how to perform so that life, health, and proper function can be maintained. Using laboratory animals, the researchers found that vitamin A facilitated the absorption of RNA in the liver and also in the nucleus of the individual cells in other parts of the body. One of the best sources of RNA is yeast. (*Complete Book of Vitamins*, 1977 ed., p. 139.)

Absorption and Storage

The upper intestinal tract is the primary area of absorption of vitamin A; it is here that the fat-splitting enzymes and bile salts convert carotene into a usable nutrient. This conversion is stimulated by thyroxine, an amino acid obtained from the thyroid gland. Once converted into vitamin A, carotene is absorbed in the same way as is the preformed vitamin. Vitamin A is carried through the bloodstream, readily accessible to tissues throughout the body. Preformed vitamin A as found in fish-liver oil or other animal products is absorbed by the body three to five hours after ingestion, whereas the conversion and absorption of carotene takes six to seven hours.[2]

The conversion of carotene into vitamin A is not 100 percent complete; approximately one-third of the carotene in food is converted into vitamin A. Less than one-fourth of the carotene in carrots and root vegetables undergoes conversion, and about one-half of the carotene in leafy green vegetables undergoes conversion.[3] Some unchanged carotene is absorbed into the circulatory system and stored in the fat tissues rather than in the liver. Unabsorbed carotene is excreted in the feces.

The ability of the body to utilize carotene varies with the food and the form in which the food is in-

gested. Cooking, pureeing, or mashing of vegetables ruptures the cell membranes and therefore makes the carotene more available for absorption.

Factors interfering with absorption of vitamin A and carotene include strenuous physical activity performed within four hours of consumption, intake of mineral oil, excessive consumption of alcohol, excessive consumption of iron, and the use of cortisone and other drugs. The intake of polyunsaturated fatty acids with carotene results in rapid destruction of carotene unless antioxidants also are present.[4] Even cold weather can hinder the transport and metabolism of both vitamin A and carotene. Diabetics cannot convert carotene into vitamin A.

Approximately 90 percent of the body's vitamin A is stored in the liver, with small amounts deposited in the fat tissues, lungs, kidneys, and retinas of the eyes. Under stressful conditions the body will use this reserve supply if it is not receiving enough vitamin A from the diet. Gastrointestinal and liver disorders, infections of any kind, or any condition in which the bile duct is obstructed may limit the body's capacity to retain and use vitamin A. Factors affecting absorption of vitamin A include the quantity given, influence of other substances present in the intestines, and amount of the vitamin stored in the body. For these reasons, the recommended dietary amounts vary for each individual.

Dosage and Toxicity

Recommended Dietary Allowances of vitamin A, as established by the National Research Council, are 1,500 International Units (IU) for infants, 3,000 IU for children one to eleven years of age, and 5,000 IU for adults. These amounts increase during disease, trauma, pregnancy, and lactation. Requirements vary for people who smoke, those who live in highly polluted areas, people who easily absorb vitamin A, and those who have had their stored supply of vitamin A depleted by pneumonia or nephritis. Increased intake of vitamins C and E will help prevent excessive oxidation of stored vitamin A.

Research indicates that no more than 50,000 IU per day can be utilized by the body except in therapeutic cases, where up to 100,000 IU is recommended. It has been suggested that the best level is somewhere between 25,000 and 50,000 IU.[5] If there is no vitamin defi-

---

[2] J. I. Rodale, *The Health Builder* (Emmaus, Pa.: Rodale Books, 1957), pp. 273-274.

[3] Rodale, *The Health Builder*, p. 196.

[4] Rodale, *The Health Builder*, p. 196.

[5] Paavo Airola, *How to Get Well* (Phoenix, Ariz.: Health Plus Pub., 1974), p. 260.

ciency, daily administration of 50,000 IU may be toxic. Dosages of 18,500 IU given daily for one to three months have been reported toxic for infants. Recommended amounts may be supplied through food sources; e.g., ½ pound of calf's liver contains approximately 74,000 IU preformed vitamin A, whereas a carrot contains 11,000 IU of carotene.

Toxicity symptoms include nausea, vomiting, diarrhea, dry skin, hair loss, headaches, appetite loss, sore lips, and flaky, itchy skin. Bone fragility, thickening of long bones, deep bone pain, enlargement of the liver and spleen, blurred vision, and skin rashes are symptoms of prolonged excessive intake. Excessive daily use of massive dosages of vitamin A also may lead to reduced thyroid activity and abnormalities in the skin, eyes, and mucous membranes. Vitamin A toxicity can occur when a person takes 100,000 IU of straight vitamin A daily for many months. If toxicity is detected, the symptoms will disappear in a few days if the vitamin is withdrawn. Vitamin C can help prevent the harmful effects of vitamin A toxicity.

Deficiency Effects and Symptoms

The eyes are well-known indicators of vitamin A deficiency. One of the first symptoms is night blindness, an inability of the eyes to adjust to darkness. Another eye-related deficiency symptom is xerosis, a disease in which the eyeball loses luster, it becomes dry and inflamed, and visual acuity is reduced.

Other signs of deficiency include rough, dry, or prematurely aged skin; loss of sense of smell; loss of appetite; frequent fatigue; skin blemishes; sties in the eye; and diarrhea. More severe symptoms are corneal ulcers and softening of bones and teeth. Deficiency of vitamin A leads to the rapid loss of vitamin C.

Vitamin A deficiency may occur when an inadequate dietary supply exists; when the body is unable to absorb or store the vitamin (as in ulcerative colitis, cirrhosis of the liver, and obstruction of the bile ducts); when an ailment interferes with the conversion of carotene to vitamin A (as in diabetes mellitus and hypothyroidism); and when any rapid bodily loss of the vitamin occurs (as in pneumonia, hyperthyroidism, chronic nephritis, scarlet fever, and some respiratory infections).

Beneficial Effect on Ailments

Many people are unaware of the importance of vitamin A in fighting infections. By giving strength to cell walls,

it helps protect the mucous membranes against invading bacteria. People who live in environments with high air-pollution counts are more susceptible to infections and colds than are people who live in environments with cleaner air. If infection has already occurred, therapeutic doses of vitamin A will help keep it from spreading.

Vitamin A can be used successfully in treating several eye disorders, such as Bitot's spots (white, elevated, sharply outlined patches on the white of the eye), blurred vision, night blindness, cataracts, crossed eyes, and nearsightedness. Therapeutic dosages of vitamin A are necessary for treatment of glaucoma and conjunctivitis, an inflammation of the mucous membrane that lines the eyelids.

Administration of vitamin A has helped shorten the duration of communicable diseases—measles, scarlet fever, the common cold, and infections of the eye, middle ear, intestines, ovaries, uterus, and vagina. It also has been effective in reducing high cholesterol levels and atheroma, fatty degeneration or thickening of the wall of the larger arteries.

Vitamin A has proved successful in treating cases of bronchial asthma, chronic rhinitis, and dermatitis. Vitamin A has also been helpful in treating patients suffering from tuberculosis, cirrhosis of the liver, emphysema, gastritis, and hyperthyroidism. Patients with nephritis (inflammation of the kidney), migraine headaches, and tinnitus (ringing in the ear) have benefited from vitamin A therapy.

Externally, vitamin A is used in treating acne; when applied locally, it can clear up impetigo, boils, carbuncles, and open ulcers. Vitamin A applied directly to open wounds hastens the healing process in cases where healing has been retarded because cortisone has been used. It also stimulates the production of mucus, which in turn prevents scarring. A treatment using injections of vitamin A has proved effective in the removal of planter's warts.[6]

Human Tests

1. Vitamin A and Stress Ulcers. Dr. Merril S. Chernov and his associates, Dr. Harry W. Hale, Jr., and Dr. Mac-Donald Wood, did a two-part study of severely injured patients to determine whether administration of vitamin A would prevent formation of stress ulcers. According

[6]J. I. Rodale and Staff, *The Health Seeker* (Emmaus, Pa.: Rodale Books, 1967), p. 897.

to Chernov, serum vitamin A levels dropped "sharply and profoundly" in severely injured patients. (*Medical World News*, January 7, 1972.)

The first part of the study involved 35 patients suffering from burns covering more than 25 percent of their bodies or major injuries to two or more organs. Vitamin A levels in the serum fell dramatically in 29 of the patients within 24 to 72 hours after hospitalization.

In the second part of the study, 14 of 36 similarly stressed patients received 10,000 to 400,000 IU of water-soluble vitamin A daily. Their care was the same as that of the other 22 patients.

Results. Evidence of stress ulcers was seen in 15 of the 22 untreated patients in the second group (69 percent). Massive intestinal bleeding developed in seven of these patients, and serious intestinal bleeding developed in another seven. Of the fourteen patients treated with massive doses of vitamin A, upper gastrointestinal bleeding occurred in only two.

Dr. Chernov stated, "The sudden and marked depletion of vitamin A is directly related to the corresponding depression of the serum protein, and particularly that fragment of the serum protein involved in transport of vitamin A. This results initially in the development of superficial mucosal erosions followed later by frank ulceration and hemorrhage." The results of Dr. Chernov's study suggest that treatment with high doses of vitamin A reduced the risk of gastroduodenal ulceration in these severely stressed patients. (J. I. Rodale, ed., *Prevention*, April 1972.)

2. Vitamin A and Acne. 100 acne patients were given oral doses of 100,000 IU of vitamin A (halibut-liver oil) at bedtime.

Results. 36 patients were completely relieved of acne, and 43 were relieved except for an occasional pustule. In most cases, responses occurred in less than nine months. (Jon V. Straumfjord, M.D., Astoria, Oregon, reported in Rodale, ed., *Prevention*, November 1968.)

3. Vitamin A and Acne Lesions. 75 patients who failed to respond to other forms of treatment were given 100,000 IU of vitamin A per day.

Results. Disappearance of the lesions occurred for 30 patients in two and one-half months, for another 30 in three months, and for 10 more in five and one-half

months. All could be regarded as cured at the end of three months. Drawbacks stated: (1) treatment could take up to a year; (2) dosage given was very high and could have toxic effects. (Dr. K. D. Larharl, *Journal of the Indian Medical Association*, March 1954; reported in Rodale, ed., *Prevention*, November 1968.)

4. Vitamin A and Asthma. 5,000 cases suffering from bronchial dermatitis, bronchial asthma, and chronic rhinitis were treated with vitamins A and D and bone meal.

Results. There was success in relieving the symptoms of 75 percent of the patients, including 1,000 patients suffering from bronchial asthma. (Dr. Carl J. Reich, 1972; reported in Rodale, ed., *Prevention*, September 1970.)

5. Vitamin A and Premenstrual Symptoms. 24 patients were given large doses of vitamin A.

Results. There were improvements in premenstrual symptoms. Seventeen patients were partially relieved of symptoms, and all breast tenderness was eliminated. Three more noticed considerable improvement but had some distress. Four patients did not respond to the therapy. (Dr. Alexander Pou, *American Journal of Obstetrics and Gynecology*, June 1951.)

Animal Tests

1. Vitamin A and Tumors. Hamsters given high doses of vitamin A before being subjected to benzpyrene (a carcinogen in smoke) were protected against the appearance of squamous tumors on the lung. Hamsters given a similar high dosage after the development of lung cancer showed a complete block of the cancer process.

Results. Of the 60 treated animals, 5 developed tumors and 4 of these were noncancerous. Of the 53 untreated animals, 16 developed lung cancer. (Dr. Umberto Saffioto of the National Cancer Institute, Bethesda, Maryland, as reported in Rodale, ed., *Prevention*, December 1969.)

2. Vitamin A and Reproductive Processes. Bulls deficient in vitamin A suffered degeneration of their seminiferous tubules. They reportedly regained full potency after receiving strong doses of vitamin A. (J. L. Madsen, *Journal of Animal Science*, reported in Rodale, ed., *Prevention*, January 1971.)

VITAMIN A MAY BE BENEFICIAL FOR THE FOLLOWING AILMENTS*:

Body Member	Ailment or Other Stressful Condition*
Bladder	Cystitis
Blood/Circulatory system	Angina pectoris
	Arteriosclerosis
	Atherosclerosis
	Diabetes
	Hemophilia
	Jaundice
	Mononucleosis
	Stroke (cerebrovascular accident)
Bones	Fracture
	Osteomalacia
	Rickets
Bowel	Celiac disease
	Colitis
	Diarrhea
Brain/Nervous system	Alcoholism
	Epilepsy
	Meningitis
Ear	Ear infection
Eye	Amblyopia
	Bitot spots
	Cataracts
	Conjunctivitis
	Eyestrain
	Glaucoma
	Night blindness
Gallbladder	Gallstones
Glands	Cystic fibrosis
	Diabetes
	Goiter
	Hyperthyroidism
	Prostatitis
	Swollen glands
Hair/Scalp	Hair problems
Head	Fever
	Headache
	Sinusitis
Heart	Angina pectoris
	Arteriosclerosis
	Atherosclerosis

Body Member	Ailment or Other Stressful Condition*
	Congestive heart failure
	Myocardial infarction
Intestine	Celiac disease
	Constipation
	Hemorrhoids
	Worms
Joints	Arthritis
	Gout
Kidney	Kidney stones (renal calculi)
	Nephritis
Leg	Varicose veins
Liver	Cirrhosis of liver
	Hepatitis
	Jaundice
Lungs/Respiratory system	Allergies
	Asthma
	Bronchitis
	Common cold
	Croup
	Emphysema
	Hay fever (allergic rhinitis)
	Influenza
	Sinusitis
	Tuberculosis
Mouth	Canker sore
	Halitosis
Muscles	Muscular dystrophy
Nails	Nail problems
Reproductive system	Prostatitis
	Vaginitis
Skin	Abscess
	Acne
	Athlete's foot
	Bedsores
	Boil (furuncle)
	Burns
	Carbuncle
	Dandruff
	Dermatitis
	Dry skin
	Eczema
	Impetigo
	Psoriasis
	Shingles (herpes zoster)

*The word "ailment" used in subsequent tables of beneficial effects of nutrients is intended to include other stressful conditions.

Body Member	Ailment or Other Stressful Condition*
	Ulcers
	Warts
Stomach	Gastritis
	Gastroenteritis
	Stomach ulcer (peptic)
Teeth/Gums	Pyorrhea
	Tooth and gum disorders
General	Alcoholism
	Chicken pox
	Fatigue
	Fever
	Infection
	Kwashiorkor
	Measles
	Pregnancy
	Rheumatic fever
	Rhinitis
	Scurvy
	Stress

VITAMIN B COMPLEX

Description

All B vitamins are water-soluble substances that can be cultivated from bacteria, yeasts, fungi, or molds. *The known B-complex vitamins* are B_1 (thiamine), B_2 (riboflavin), B_3 (niacin), B_6 (pyridoxine), B_{12} (cyanocobalamin), B_{13} (orotic acid), pangamic acid, biotin, choline, folic acid, inositol, and PABA (para-aminobenzoic acid). The grouping of these water-soluble compounds under the term "B complex" is based upon their common source distribution, their close relationship in vegetable and animal tissues, and their functional relationships.

The B-complex vitamins are active in providing the body with energy, basically by converting carbohydrates into glucose, which the body "burns" to produce energy. They are vital in the metabolism of fats and protein. In addition, the B vitamins are necessary for normal functioning of the nervous system and may be the single most important factor for health of the nerves. They are essential for maintenance of muscle tone in the gas-

trointestinal tract and for the health of skin, hair, eyes, mouth, and liver.

All the B vitamins except B_{17} are natural constituents of brewer's yeast, liver, or whole-grain cereals. Brewer's yeast is the richest natural source of the B-complex group. Another important source of the B vitamins is production by the intestinal bacteria. These bacteria grow best on milk sugar and small amounts of fat in the diet. Maintaining milk-free diets or taking sulfonamides and other antibiotics may destroy these valuable bacteria.

Absorption and Storage

Because of the water-solubility of the B-complex vitamins, any excess is excreted and not stored. Therefore, they must be continually replaced. All B vitamins mixed with salve absorb readily.

Sulfa drugs, sleeping pills, insecticides, and estrogen create a condition in the digestive tract which can destroy the B vitamins. Certain B vitamins are lost through perspiration.

Dosage and Toxicity

The most important thing to remember is that all the B vitamins should be taken together. They are so interrelated in function that large doses of any one of them may be therapeutically valueless or may cause a deficiency of others. For example, if extra B_6 is taken in 50-milligram potencies, it is important that a complete B complex accompany it. In nature, we find the B-complex vitamins in yeast, green vegetables, etc., but nowhere do we find a single B vitamin isolated from the rest. Natural forms of the B vitamins are preferable to the synthetic forms since the natural forms have all of the B factors, even those not yet known, plus valuable enzymes. Most preparations of single B vitamins are synthetic or, at least, no longer in their natural form. These synthetic B vitamins are used primarily to overcome severe deficiencies or serious physical conditions in which rapid results are needed. When taking supplements, it is very important to remember that the B vitamins exert many different effects upon each other; therefore excesses and insufficiencies may be harmful.

The need for the B-complex vitamins increases during infection or stress. Alcoholics and individuals who consume excessive amounts of carbohydrates require a higher intake of B vitamins for proper metabolism. Coffee uses up the B vitamins. Children and pregnant women need extra B vitamins for normal growth.

Deficiency Effects and Symptoms

The 13 or more B vitamins are so meagerly supplied in the American diet that almost every American lacks some of them. If a person is tired, irritable, nervous, depressed, or even suicidal, suspect a vitamin B deficiency. Gray hair, falling hair, baldness, acne, or other skin troubles indicate a lack of B vitamins. A poor appetite, insomnia, neuritis, anemia, constipation, or high cholesterol level is also an indicator of a vitamin B deficiency. Having an enlarged tongue (including the buds on each side) that is shiny, bright red, and full of grooves means B vitamins are needed. One reason there is so much B-vitamin deficiency in the American population is that Americans eat so many processed foods from which the B vitamins have often been removed. Another reason for widespread deficiency is the high amount of sugar consumed. *Sugar and alcohol destroy the B-complex vitamins.*

Beneficial Effect on Ailments

The B vitamins have been used in the treatment of barbiturate overdosage, alcoholic psychoses, and drug-induced delirium. An adequate dose has been found to control migraine headaches and attacks of Ménière's syndrome. Some heart abnormalities have responded to use of B complex because the nerves affecting the heart need the B-complex vitamins for smooth, quiet functioning. Massive dosages of the B-complex vitamins have been used to cure polio, to improve the condition of hypersensitive children who fail to respond favorably to drugs such as Ritalin, and to improve cases of shingles. Nervous individuals and persons working under tension can greatly benefit from taking larger than normal doses of B vitamins.

Postoperative nausea and vomiting, resulting from anesthesia, can be successfully treated with B vitamins. The amount of B vitamins needed seems to be related to the amount of female sex hormones available. Menstrual difficulty is often relieved with small doses. The B vitamins may also help these ailments: beriberi, pellagra, constipation, burning feet, tender gums, burning and drying eyes, fatigue, lack of appetite, skin disorders, cracks at the corner of the mouth, and anemia.

Human Tests

1. B Vitamins and Ménière's Syndrome. A person testified that the therapy of Dr. Mills Atkinson, which consisted of heavy intakes of the B-complex vitamins four times daily, reversed his case of Ménière's syndrome (see "Ailments," p. 149), which had lasted almost four months.

Results. Within two months the B-vitamin treatment relieved the dizziness, double vision, nausea, and inability to concentrate associated with this ailment. ("Migraine, Ménière's and Mealtime," Rodale, ed., *Prevention*, August 1971.)

2. B Vitamins and Senile Dementia (Deteriorative Mental State of the Aged). Patients in mental hospitals and convalescent homes who were suffering from senile dementia exhibited a dramatic improvement in their mental condition 24 to 48 hours after large doses of B vitamins were administered. (Bicknell and Prescott, *Vitamins in Medicine*, as reported in Linda Clark, *Know Your Nutrition*, 1973, p. 67.)

Animal Tests

1. B Complex; Natural versus Synthetic. Silver foxes were fed a synthetic diet so that each component of the diet could be known. The foxes were fed all of the known synthetic B vitamins as part of their rations, but the animals did not grow; their fur quality deteriorated, and finally they died. This condition was reversed with only one change in the diet fed to another group of foxes: B-complex foods—yeast and liver—were added.

Results. The animals in the second group grew normally, and the quality of the fur improved. (*Scandinavian Veterinary*, vol. 30, pp. 1121-1143, 1940, as reported in J. I. Rodale, ed., *The* Prevention *Method for Better Health*, Rodale Books, Emmaus, Pa., 1968, p. 568.)

2. B-Complex Vitamins and Hair. A group of mice were placed on a synthetic diet that included all necessary nutrients. They grew for a few days and then became stationary in weight. After 20 to 30 days they began to lose their hair and developed hunched backs. A similar group were placed on the same diet, with whole yeast added.

Results. When the natural products were added to their diet, the second group did not show the symptoms shown by the first group. (*Journal of Nutrition*, vol. 21, p. 609, 1941.)

3. B-Complex Vitamins and Fatigue. Three groups of rats were fed three different diets for 12 weeks. The first group ate a basic diet, fortified with nine synthetic and two natural vitamins. The second group was fed the same diet, vitamins and all, with a plentiful supply of vitamin B complex added. The third group was fed the original fortified diet, but instead of vitamin B complex, 10 percent desiccated liver was added to their ration.

Results. The first group showed the least amount of growth in 12 weeks. The second group experienced a little higher rate of growth in that 12-week period. The third group grew about 15 percent faster than the first group. (B. H. Ershoff, M.D., *Proceedings of the Society of Experimental Biology and Medicine*, July 1951, as reported in Rodale, ed., *The* Prevention *Method for Better Health*, p. 610.)

4. B-Complex Vitamins and Fatigue. This experiment is based on the same rats and their diets used in Test 3. These same rats were placed one by one into a drum of water from which they could not climb out.

Results. The rats on the original diet swam for an average of 13.3 minutes before they gave up. The second group of rats swam for 13.4 minutes before giving up. Of the third group, three swam for 63, 83, and 87 minutes, respectively. The rest of the rats in the third group were swimming vigorously at the end of two hours, when testing terminated. The rats that received desiccated liver (those in the third group) swam almost six times as long as did the others. (Rodale, ed., *The* Prevention *Method for Better Health*, p. 611.)

VITAMIN B COMPLEX MAY BE BENEFICIAL FOR THE FOLLOWING AILMENTS:

Body Member	Ailment
Bladder	Cystitis
Blood/Circulatory system	Anemia
	Angina pectoris
	Arteriosclerosis
	Atherosclerosis
	Cholesterol level, high
	Diabetes
	Hypertension
	Hypoglycemia
	Leukemia
	Stroke (cerebrovascular accident)
Bowel	Diarrhea
Brain/Nervous system	Alcoholism

Body Member	Ailment
	Bell's palsy
	Epilepsy
	Insomnia
	Meningitis
	Mental illness
	Multiple sclerosis
	Neuritis
	Parkinson's disease
	Stroke (cerebrovascular accident)
	Vertigo
Ear	Ménière's syndrome
Eye	Amblyopia
	Cataracts
	Conjunctivitis
	Eyestrain
	Glaucoma
	Night blindness
Gallbladder	Gallstones
Glands	Adrenal exhaustion
	Cystic fibrosis
	Hyperthyroidism
	Prostatitis
	Swollen glands
Hair/Scalp	Baldness
	Dandruff
	Hair problems
Head	Fever
	Headache
Heart	Angina pectoris
	Arteriosclerosis
	Atherosclerosis
	Congestive heart failure
	Hypertension
	Myocardial infarction
Intestine	Celiac disease
	Constipation
	Diverticulitis
	Hemorrhoids
	Indigestion (dyspepsia)
	Worms
Joints	Arthritis
	Bursitis
	Gout
Kidney	Nephritis

Body Member	Ailment
Leg	Leg cramp
	Phlebitis
	Sciatica
	Varicose veins
Liver	Cirrhosis of liver
	Hepatitis
Lungs/Respiratory system	Common cold
	Emphysema
	Hay fever (allergic rhinitis)
	Influenza
	Pneumonia
Mouth	Canker sore
	Halitosis
Muscles	Parkinson's disease
Nails	Nail growth
Reproductive system	Prostatitis
	Vaginitis
Skin	Abscess
	Acne
	Bedsores
	Bruises
	Burns
	Dandruff
	Dermatitis
	Eczema
	Psoriasis
	Shingles (herpes zoster)
	Ulcers
Stomach	Gastritis
	Gastroenteritis
	Indigestion (dyspepsia)
	Stomach ulcer (peptic)
Teeth/Gums	Pyorrhea
General	Aging
	Alcoholism
	Arthritis
	Backache
	Beriberi
	Cancer
	Edema
	Fatigue
	Fever
	Hypoxia
	Infection

Body Member	Ailment
	Overweight and obesity
	Pellagra
	Pregnancy
	Stress
	Stroke (cerebrovascular accident)

VITAMIN B$_1$ (THIAMINE)

Description

Thiamine or vitamin B$_1$ is a water-soluble vitamin that combines with pyruvic acid to form a coenzyme necessary for the breakdown of carbohydrates into glucose, or simple sugar, which is oxidized by the body to produce energy. Thiamine is vulnerable to heat, air, and water in cooking. Thiamine is a component of the germ and bran of wheat, the husk of rice, and that portion of all grains which is commercially milled away to give the grain a lighter color and finer texture.[7]

Known as the "morale vitamin" because of its relation to a healthy nervous system and its beneficial effect on mental attitude (see Human Test 4), thiamine is also linked with improving individual learning capacity.[8] It is necessary for consistent growth in children and for the improvement of muscle tone in the stomach, the intestines, and the heart. Thiamine is essential for stabilizing the appetite by improving food assimilation and digestion, particularly that of starches, sugars, and alcohol.

A diet rich in brewer's yeast, wheat germ, blackstrap molasses, and bran will provide the body with adequate thiamine and will help prevent undue accumulation of fatty deposits in the artery walls.

Absorption and Storage

Thiamine is rapidly absorbed in the upper and lower small intestine. It is then carried by the circulatory system to the liver, kidneys, and heart, where it may combine further with manganese and specific proteins to become active enzymes. These are the enzymes that break down carbohydrates into simple sugars.

Thiamine is not stored in the body in any great quantity and therefore must be supplied daily. It is excreted in the urine in amounts that reflect the intake and the quantity stored. Eating excessive amounts of sugar will

[7]J. I. Rodale, *The Complete Book of Vitamins* (Emmaus, Pa.: Rodale Books, 1968), pp. 179-184.
[8]Rodale, *The Complete Book of Vitamins*, p. 84.

cause a thiamine depletion, as will smoking and drinking alcohol. Thiamine can be destroyed by an enzyme present in raw clams and oysters.

Dosage and Toxicity

Individual thiamine needs are determined by body weight, the quantity of the vitamin synthesized in the intestinal tract, and daily calorie intake. As the calorie intake, especially of carbohydrates, increases, the proportion of thiamine ingested increases. The National Research Council recommends 0.5 milligram of thiamine per 1000 calories daily for all ages.[9] A thiamine intake of 1.4 milligrams daily is recommended during pregnancy and lactation. The need for additional B_1 increases during severe diarrhea, fever, stress, and surgery. There are no known toxic effects with thiamine.

Deficiency Effects and Symptoms

A deficiency of thiamine not only makes it difficult for a person to digest carbohydrates but also leaves too much pyruvic acid in the blood. This causes an oxygen deficiency that results in loss of mental alertness, labored breathing, and cardiac damage. First signs of a thiamine deficiency include easy fatigue, loss of appetite, irritability, and emotional instability. If the deficiency is not arrested, confusion and loss of memory appear, followed closely by gastric distress, abdominal pains, and constipation. Heart irregularities crop up, and finally, prickling sensations in the lower extremities, impaired vibratory sense, and tenderness of calf muscles will occur. A thiamine deficiency can also lead to inflammation of the optic nerve. Without thiamine, the function of the central nervous system, which depends upon glucose for energy, is impaired.

A thiamine deficiency affects the cardiovascular system as well. The heart muscles are weakened, and cardiac failure may occur. The gastrointestinal tract is also affected, and symptoms such as indigestion, severe constipation, anorexia (a loss of appetite), and gastric atony (loss of muscle tone in the stomach) may occur. "Some researchers believe that the lack of thiamine may be the first link in a chain leading by way of the liver and female hormones to cancer of the uterus."[10]

Beneficial Effect on Ailments

Thiamine is used in the treatment of beriberi, a deficiency disease associated with malnutrition.[11] Thiamine intake has improved the excretion of fluid stored in the body, decreased rapid heart rate, shrunken enlarged hearts, and normalized electrocardiograms.

Nutrients such as thiamine and niacin have been used together to treat multiple sclerosis patients. Dr. George Schumacher tells of his use of thiamine hydrochloride given intraspinally to two multiple sclerosis patients with noted improvement. Dr. Fredrick Klenner used large doses (100 milligrams) of B_1, B_3, and B_6 with reported success.[12]

Many other ailments have been aided by the administration of thiamine. Thiamine is essential in the manufacture of hydrochloric acid, which aids in digestion. It helps in eliminating nausea, especially that caused by air or sea sickness. It has improved people's dispositions by alleviating fatigue. Thiamine helps improve muscle tone in the stomach and intestines, which in turn relieves constipation. Herpes zoster, a painful clustering of blisters behind the ear, has been successfully treated with thiamine.[13]

Dentists have found B_1 useful. Dental postoperative pain is promptly and completely relieved in many patients by the administration of thiamine. Pain can often be prevented before the operation by administration of B_1 to the patient. Thiamine therapy has reduced the healing time of dry tooth sockets. Evidence shows that replacement of thiamine to injured and diseased nerves not only restores proper functioning but also relieves pain.[14]

Human Tests

1. Vitamin B_1 and Morale. Over several years, Horwitt and coworkers studied the psychological effects of thiamine deficiency on psychiatric patients in an institution. The subjects received varying amounts of thiamine in an adequate diet. They were tested for various deficiency effects.

[9]Marie V. Krause and Martha A. Hunscher, *Food, Nutrition and Diet Therapy* (Philadelphia: W. B. Saunders Co., 1972), p. 132.
[10]Ernest Ayre and W. A. G. Gauld, *Science*, April 12, 1946; also J. I. Rodale, *The Encyclopedia for Healthful Living* (Emmaus, Pa.: Rodale Books, 1970), p. 117.
[11]See "Beriberi," p. 117.
[12]J. I. Rodale and Staff, *Encyclopedia of Common Diseases* (Emmaus, Pa.: Rodale Books, 1969), pp. 786-787.
[13]Betty Lee Morales (ed.), *Cancer Control Journal,* vol. 2, no. 3, p. 13, June 1974.
[14]J. L. O. Bock, *U.S. Armed Forces Medical Journal,* March 1953.

Results. When approximately four-tenths milligram of thiamine was administered, specific conditions, including loss of inhibitory emotional control, paranoid trends, manic-depressive features, and confusion, were helped. (M. K. Horwitt et al., "Investigations of Human Requirements of B-Complex Vitamins," *National Research Council Bull.* 116, 1948.)

2. Vitamin B₁ and Herpes Zoster. 25 patients were given intramuscular injections of 200 milligrams of thiamine hydrochloride daily.

Results. Herpes zoster, a stubborn, painful clustering of small blisters near the ear, was successfully treated. (A. L. Oriz, *Medical World*, November 1958.)

3. Vitamin B₁ and Mental Ability. An experiment was conducted by Dr. Ruth Linn Harrell which involved 104 children from nine to nineteen years of age. Half of the children were given a vitamin B₁ pill each day, and the other half received a placebo. The test lasted six weeks.

Results. It was found by a series of tests that the group that was given the vitamin gained one-fourth more in learning ability than did the other group. (Dr. Ruth Flinn Harrell, "Effect of Added Thiamine on Learning," as reported in Rodale and Staff, *The Health Seeker*, pp. 18 and 19.)

VITAMIN B₁ MAY BE BENEFICIAL FOR THE FOLLOWING AILMENTS:

Body Member	Ailment
Blood/Circulatory system	Anemia
	Diabetes
Bowel	Constipation
	Diarrhea
Brain/Nervous system	Alcoholism
	Bell's palsy
	Mental illness
	Multiple sclerosis
	Neuritis
Ear	Ménière's syndrome
Eye	Amblyopia
	Night blindness
Head	Fever
	Headache
Heart	Congestive heart failure
Intestine	Worms
Leg	Leg cramp
	Sciatica
Lungs/Respiratory system	Influenza
Skin	Shingles (herpes zoster)
Stomach	Indigestion (dyspepsia)
General	Alcoholism
	Beriberi
	Pellagra
	Stress

VITAMIN B₂ (RIBOFLAVIN)

Description

Vitamin B₂, also known as riboflavin, is a water-soluble vitamin occurring naturally in those foods in which the other B vitamins exist. Riboflavin is stable to heat, oxidation, and acid although it disintegrates in the presence of alkali or light, especially ultraviolet light.

Riboflavin functions as part of a group of enzymes that are involved in the breakdown and utilization of carbohydrates, fats, and proteins. Riboflavin is necessary for cell respiration because it works with enzymes in the utilization of cell oxygen. It also is necessary for the maintenance of good vision, skin, nails, and hair.

The amount of B₂ found in most foods is so little that it normally is quite difficult to obtain a sufficient supply without supplementing the diet. Good sources of riboflavin are liver, tongue, and other organ meats. The richest natural source is brewer's yeast.

Absorption and Storage

Riboflavin is easily absorbed through the walls of the small intestine. It is then carried by the blood to the tissues of the body and excreted in the urine. The amount excreted depends upon the intake and relative need of the tissues and may be accompanied by a loss of protein from the body. Small amounts of riboflavin are found in the liver and kidneys, but it is not stored to any great degree in the body and therefore must be supplied regularly in the diet.[15]

[15] Krause and Hunscher, *Food, Nutrition and Diet Therapy*, p. 134.

Dosage and Toxicity

According to the National Research Council, the daily riboflavin requirements are related to body size, metabolic rate, and rate of growth. These factors are directly related to the protein and calorie intake of the individual. The Recommended Dietary Allowance is 1.6 milligrams for the adult male and 1.2 milligrams for the female. Pregnancy and lactation requirements are 1.5 and 1.7 milligrams, respectively.

There is no known toxicity of riboflavin. However, prolonged ingestion of large doses of any one of the B-complex vitamins, including riboflavin, may result in high urinary losses of other B vitamins. Therefore, it is important to take a complete B complex with any single B vitamin.

Deficiency Effects and Symptoms

Riboflavin deficiency is the most common vitamin deficiency in America. Deficiency may result from one or several of these factors: (1) long-established faulty dietary habits; (2) food idiosyncrasies ("I won't eat liver!"); (3) alcoholism; (4) arbitrarily selected diets for relief of symptoms of digestive trouble; and (5) prolonged following of a restricted diet in the treatment of a disease such as peptic ulcer or diabetes.[16]

The most common symptoms of a lack of B_2 are cracks and sores in the corners of the mouth; a red, sore tongue; a feeling of grit and sand on the insides of the eyelids; burning of the eyes; eye fatigue; dilation of the pupil; changes in the cornea; sensitivity to light; lesions of the lips; scaling around the nose, mouth, forehead, and ears; trembling; sluggishness; dizziness; dropsy; inability to urinate; vaginal itching; oily skin; and baldness. A vitamin B_2 deficiency can cause some types of cataracts.[17] Experimental studies have shown that some forms of cancer may be related to B_2 deficiency.[18]

A lack of stamina and vigor, retarded growth, digestive disturbances, impaired lactation, and pellagra are results of a riboflavin deficiency. Hair and weight losses also frequently result.

[16]Rodale and Staff, *The Complete Book of Vitamins*, pp. 194-195.
[17]Linda Clark, *Know Your Nutrition* (New Canaan, Conn.: Keats Publ., 1973), p. 78.
[18]Boris Sokoloff, *Cancer: New Approaches, New Hope* (New York: Devin-Adair).

Beneficial Effect on Ailments

Riboflavin plays an important role in the prevention of some visual disturbances, especially cataracts. Undernourished women during the end of pregnancy often suffer from conditions such as visual disturbances, burning sensations in the eyes, excessive watering of eyes, and failing vision. These conditions can be helped by supplementing the diet with large doses of B_2. Riboflavin has brought relief to children suffering from eczema.

Human Test

1. B_2 (Riboflavin) and Visual Disturbances. 47 patients suffered from a variety of visual disturbances. They were sensitive to light; they suffered from eyestrain, burning sensations in their eyes, and visual fatigue; and their eyes watered easily. Six of them had cataracts.

Results. Within 24 hours after the administration of riboflavin, symptoms began to improve. After two days, the burning sensations and other symptoms began to disappear. All disorders were gradually cured. When riboflavin was removed, the symptoms gradually appeared again and once again were cured with administration of riboflavin. (Dr. Syndensticker, as reported in Rodale, ed., *Prevention*, November 1970.)

VITAMIN B_2 MAY BE BENEFICIAL FOR THE FOLLOWING AILMENTS:

Body Member	Ailment
Blood/Circulatory system	Diabetes
Bowel	Diarrhea
Brain/Nervous system	Multiple sclerosis
	Neuritis
	Parkinson's disease
	Vertigo
Ear	Ménière's syndrome
Eye	Cataracts
	Conjunctivitis
	Glaucoma
	Night blindness
Glands	Adrenal exhaustion
Hair/Scalp	Baldness
Intestine	Worms
Joints	Arthritis

Body Member	Ailment
Kidney	Nephritis
Leg	Leg cramp
Lungs/Respiratory system	Influenza
Reproductive system	Vaginitis
Skin	Acne
	Bedsores
	Dermatitis
	Ulcers
Stomach	Indigestion (dyspepsia)
	Stomach ulcer (peptic)
General	Alcoholism
	Cancer
	Pellagra
	Retarded growth
	Stress

VITAMIN B_6 (PYRIDOXINE)

Description

Vitamin B_6 is a water-soluble vitamin consisting of three related compounds: pyridoxine, pyridoxinal, and pyridoxamine. It is required for the proper absorption of vitamin B_{12} and for the production of hydrochloric acid and magnesium. It also helps linoleic acid function better in the body. Pyridoxine plays an important role as a coenzyme in the breakdown and utilization of carbohydrates, fats, and proteins. It must be present for the production of antibodies and red blood cells. The release of glycogen for energy from the liver and muscles is facilitated by vitamin B_6. It also aids in the conversion of tryptophan, an essential amino acid, to niacin and is necessary for the synthesis and proper action of DNA and RNA.

Vitamin B_6 helps maintain the balance of sodium and potassium which regulates body fluids and promotes the normal functioning of the nervous and musculoskeletal systems. The best sources of vitamin B_6 are meats and whole grains. Desiccated liver and brewer's yeast are the recommended supplemental sources.

Absorption and Storage

A daily supply of vitamin B_6, together with the other B-complex vitamins, is necessary because it is excreted in the urine within eight hours after ingestion and is not stored in the liver. Fasting and reducing diets can deplete the body's supply of vitamin B_6 if proper supplements are not taken.

Dosage and Toxicity

Vitamin B_6 seems to be another B vitamin that, if administered alone, can cause an imbalance or deficiency of other B vitamins. The Recommended Dietary Allowance of vitamin B_6 is determined by an individual's daily protein intake. Adults need 2 milligrams of pyridoxine per 100 grams of protein per day, and children need 0.6 to 1.2 milligrams per 100 grams of protein per day. The need for vitamin B_6 increases during pregnancy, lactation, exposure to radiation, cardiac failure, aging, and use of oral contraceptives. Intravenous doses of 200 milligrams have proved nontoxic, and daily oral doses of 100 to 300 milligrams have been administered to alleviate drug-induced neuritis without side effects.[19]

Deficiency Effects and Symptoms

In cases of B_6 deficiency there is low blood sugar and low glucose tolerance, resulting in a sensitivity to insulin. Deficiency may also cause loss of hair, water retention during pregnancy, cracks around the mouth and eyes, numbness and cramps in arms and legs, slow learning, visual disturbances, neuritis, arthritis, heart disorders involving nerves, temporary paralysis of a limb, and an increase in urination.

If a vitamin B_6 deficiency is allowed to continue through late pregnancy, stillbirths or postdelivery infant mortality may result. Certain types of anemia may also be related to a B_6 deficiency.

Symptoms of a B_6 deficiency are similar to those seen in niacin and riboflavin deficiencies and may include muscular weakness, nervousness, irritability, depression, and dermatitis. Tingling hands, shoulder-hand syndrome, wrist-hand syndromes and arthritis associated with menopause also may be present.

Beneficial Effect on Ailments

There is evidence that suggests a relationship between vitamin B_6 and cholesterol metabolism; therefore B_6

[19] National Academy of Sciences, *Toxicants Occurring Naturally in Foods* (Washington, D.C.: National Research Council, 1973), p. 246.

may be involved in the control of atherosclerosis. Vitamin B_6 has been used in the treatment of nervous disorders and in the control of nausea and vomiting during pregnancy.

Vitamin B_6 has been successfully used to help treat a form of anemia in which red blood cells are too small; also male sexual disorders, eczema, thinning and loss of hair, elevated cholesterol level, diarrhea, hemorrhoids, pancreatitis, ulcers, muscular weakness, some types of heart disturbances, burning feet, some types of kidney stones, acne, tooth decay, and diabetes. It is needed to prevent and treat shoulder-hand syndrome. Administration of B_6 to mentally retarded children has helped relieve convulsize seizures. It also appears to be beneficial in treating stress.

As a natural diuretic, vitamin B_6 aids in the prevention of water buildup in the tissues. It has helped women who suffer from temporary premenstrual changes such as edema and may be effective in helping problems of overweight caused by water retention.

Human Tests

1. Vitamin B_6 and Parkinson's Disease. It was found that Parkinson's disease, a nervous disorder that causes trembling hands, responded to B_6 treatments. A case of the disease which had existed for 25 years responded to B_6 injections within 2 months. This is one of the unexpected results of B_6—whereas it may take a long time to derive benefits from some vitamins, B_6 seems to bring results quickly and dramatically. (Dr. Douw G. Stern, University of South Africa, as reported in Clark, *Know Your Nutrition*, p. 91.)

2. Vitamin B_6 and Painful Finger Joints. Vitamin B_6 was given to women and men near the age of menopause who had developed painful spurs or knots on the sides of their finger joints.

Results. There was a dramatic change after the administration of B_6. Finger joints ceased to be painful, and finger sensitivity and hand flexion improved within six weeks. (John M. Ellis, "The Doctor Who Looked at Hands," as reported in Clark, *Know Your Nutrition*, p. 91.)

Animal Tests

1. Vitamin B_6 and Cleft Palates. Cleft palates developed in 85 percent of the offspring of mice injected with cortisone four times daily during pregnancy.

Results. When pyridoxine was injected along with the cortisone, such abnormalities were reduced to 45 percent, and the addition of folic acid reduced the occurrence of cleft palate to 20 percent. On the basis of these experiments, folic acid and pyridoxine were given to human mothers who had previously borne cleft palate children, and all children subsequently born to these mothers were normal. (Dr. Lyndon A. Peer, 22d Annual Meeting of International College of Surgeons, as reported in Rodale, *The Health Seeker*, p. 194.)

VITAMIN B_6 MAY BE BENEFICIAL FOR THE FOLLOWING AILMENTS:

Body Member	Ailment
Blood/Circulatory system	Anemia
	Cholesterol level, high
	Diabetes
	Hypoglycemia
	Jaundice
	Pernicious anemia
Bladder	Cystitis
Bowel	Colitis
	Diarrhea
Brain/Nervous system	Bell's palsy
	Epilepsy
	Insomnia
	Mental illness
	Multiple sclerosis
	Neuritis
	Parkinson's disease
Ear	Dizziness
Eye	Conjunctivitis
Glands	Prostatitis
Hair/Scalp	Baldness
	Dandruff
Head	Headache
Intestine	Celiac disease
	Hemorrhoids
	Worms

Body Member	Ailment
Joints	Arthritis
Kidney	Kidney stones (renal calculi)
Lungs/Respiratory system	Asthma
	Common cold
	Influenza
	Tuberculosis
Mouth	Halitosis
Muscles	Muscular dystrophy
	Rheumatism
Reproductive system	Prostatitis
	Vaginitis
Skin	Acne
	Dandruff
	Dermatitis
	Eczema
	Psoriasis
	Shingles (herpes zoster)
Stomach	Gastritis
	Indigestion (dyspepsia)
	Nausea of pregnancy
Teeth/Gums	Pyorrhea
General	Alcoholism
	Edema
	Overweight and obesity
	Stress

VITAMIN B_{12}

Description

Vitamin B_{12}, a water-soluble vitamin, is unique in being the first cobalt-containing substance found to be essential for longevity, and it is the only vitamin that contains essential mineral elements. It cannot be made synthetically but must be grown, like penicillin, in bacteria or molds. Animal protein is almost the only source in which B_{12} occurs naturally in foods in substantial amounts. Liver is the best source; kidney, muscle meats, fish and dairy products are other good sources.

Vitamin B_{12} is necessary for normal metabolism of nerve tissue and is involved in protein, fat, and carbohydrate metabolism. B_{12} is closely related to the actions of four amino acids, pantothenic acid, and vitamin C. It also helps iron function better in the body and aids folic acid in the synthesis of choline.

Absorption and Storage

Vitamin B_{12} is prepared for absorption by two gastric secretions. It is poorly absorbed from the gastrointestinal tract unless the "intrinsic factor," a mucoprotein enzyme, is present. B_{12} needs to be combined with calcium during absorption to benefit the body properly. The presence of hydrochloric acid aids in the absorption of B_{12} given orally, and a properly functioning thyroid gland also helps B_{12} to be better absorbed.

After absorption, B_{12} is bound to serum protein (globulins) and is transported in the bloodstream to various tissues. The highest concentrations of B_{12} are found in the liver, kidneys, heart, pancreas, testes, brain, blood, and bone marrow. These body members are all related to red blood cell formation.

People deficient in B_{12} usually lack one or more gastric secretions necessary for its absorption. Many people lack the ability to absorb it at all.

Absorption of B_{12} appears to decrease with age and with iron, calcium, and B_6 deficiencies; absorption increases during pregnancy. The use of laxatives depletes the storage of B_{12}.

Dosage and Toxicity

Human requirements are minute but essential. The Recommended Dietary Allowance of vitamin B_{12} is 3 micrograms for adults and 4 micrograms for pregnant and lactating women. Infants require a daily intake of 3 micrograms, and growing children need 1 to 2 micrograms. A vegetarian diet frequently is low in vitamin B_1 and high in folic acid, which may mask a vitamin B_{12} deficiency. No cases of vitamin B_{12} toxicity have been reported, even with large doses.

Deficiency Effects and Symptoms

Symptoms of a vitamin B_{12} deficiency may take five or six years to appear, after the body's supply from natural sources has been restricted.[20] A deficiency of vitamin B_{12} is usually due to an absorption problem caused by a lack of the intrinsic factor. A deficiency begins with changes in the nervous system such as soreness and weakness in the legs and arms, diminished reflex re-

[20]Krause and Hunscher, *Food, Nutrition and Diet Therapy*, p. 141.

sponse and sensory perception, difficulty in walking and speaking (stammering), and jerking of limbs.

Lack of B_{12} has been found to cause a type of brain damage resembling schizophrenia. This brain damage may be detected by the following symptoms: sore mouth, numbness or stiffness, a feeling of deadness, shooting pains, needles-and-pins, or hot-and-cold sensations. The *British Medical Journal* (March 26, 1966) stated editorially, "It is true that vitamin B_{12} deficiency may cause severe psychotic symptoms which may vary in severity from mild disorders of mood, mental slowness, and memory defect to severe psychotic symptoms . . . occasionally, these mental disturbances may be the first manifestations of B_{12} deficiency. . . ."

Vitamin B_{12} deficiency also manifests itself in nervousness, neuritis, unpleasant body odor, menstrual disturbances, and difficulty in walking. If a deficiency is not detected in early stages, it *may* result in permanent mental deterioration and paralysis. When symptoms become serious, do not try to treat them yourself. Consult a doctor.

Beneficial Effect on Ailments

Injections of B_{12} can be used to treat patients suffering from pernicious anemia, an ailment characterized by insufficient red blood cells in the bone marrow. Injections rather than oral doses of B_{12} are used to bypass the absorption defect in pernicious anemic patients. B_{12} helps the red blood cells to mature up to a certain point, and, after that, protein, iron, vitamin C, and folic acid help to finish the development of the cells so that they can mature.[21] Like folic acid, vitamin B_{12} has been effective in the treatment of the intestinal syndrome sprue.

The *Medical Press* reported remarkable results in the treatment of osteoarthritis, a degenerative joint disease, and osteroporosis, a softening of the bone, with vitamin B_{12} (see Human Tests). The condition known as "tobacco amblyopia," a dimness of vision or a loss of vision due to poisoning by tobacco, has been improved with injections of vitamin B_{12} whether or not the patient stopped smoking. Symptoms are blackouts, headaches, and farsightedness.

B_{12} has provided relief of the following symptoms: fatigue, increased nervous irritability, mild impairment in memory, inability to concentrate, mental depression, insomnia, and lack of balance.[22] B_{12} also has been used

[21] Rodale and Staff, *The Encyclopedia of Common Diseases*, p. 451.
[22] Rodale and Staff, *The Complete Book of Vitamins*, p. 101.

successfully in the treatment of hepatitis, bursitis, and asthma.

Human Tests

1. Vitamin B_{12} and Cancer. Cancerous children were treated with B_{12} so that it could be shown that B_{12} could reduce the growth rate of cancer of the nervous system in children.

Results. Among 82 children who were treated with B_{12}, 32 (39 percent) survived up to 12 years. With conventional treatment, 8 out of 25 (32 percent) survived. (*Archives of Disease in Childhood*, December 1963, as reported in *Cancer*, March 28, 1964.)

2. Vitamin B_{12} and Osteoarthritis and Osteoporosis. 33 cases of osteoarthritis and two cases of osteoporosis were treated with vitamin B_{12}. The injected dosages varied between 30 and 900 micrograms, but the optimum dose was 100 micrograms per week.

Results. 20 patients benefited from the treatment within the first week; 7 obtained complete relief. At the end of the second week, four more showed partial relief. By the end of the third week, all but three of the patients showed some benefit. Three cases of rheumatoid arthritis did not react at all to the vitamin. (*Medical Press*, March 12, 1952, as reported in Rodale, *The Encyclopedia for Healthful Living*, p. 942.)

3. Vitamin B_{12} and Mental Confusion. A seventy-six-year-old patient was suffering from ailments relating to a poor system of blood vessels and heart. He was unable to walk without pain in his legs, and he showed signs of extreme depression and mental confusion. Finally he came down with a siege of pneumonia and sciatica, severe pain leg. Dr. Grabner prescribed 400 micrograms daily of injected vitamin B_{12}.

Results. After the fourth injection the patient exhibited a more pleasant attitude, and his state of confusion had improved. After two weeks, the dosage was reduced to 200 micrograms daily; then that was cut to every other day; and finally the patient was receiving 200 micrograms twice weekly. The doctor described his condition as healthy and completely normal mentally. (Dr. Grabner, *"Munchener Medizenische Wochenschrift,"* Munich Medical Weekly, October 31, 1958, as reported in Rodale, *The Encyclopedia for Healthful Living*, 1970, p. 946.)

4. Vitamin B$_{12}$ and Bursitis. Injections of 1,000 micrograms of vitamin B$_{12}$ were given to subjects suffering from all types of bursitis. They were given the doses daily for three weeks, then once or twice a week for two or three weeks depending upon clinical observations.

Results. Rapid relief was achieved in all cases. Calcium deposits, if present, were absorbed, and there were no side effects or toxicity. Dr. Klemes reported that over a five-year period, only three patients failed to respond to vitamin B$_{12}$ therapy for treatment of bursitis. (Dr. I. S. Klemes, *Industrial Medicine and Surgery*, June 1957, as reported in Rodale, *The Encyclopedia for Healthful Living*, pp. 108-110.)

VITAMIN B$_{12}$ MAY BE BENEFICIAL FOR THE FOLLOWING AILMENTS:

Body Member	Ailment
Blood/Circulatory system	Anemia
	Angina pectoris
	Arteriosclerosis
	Atherosclerosis
	Diabetes
	Hypoglycemia
	Pernicious anemia
Bones	Osteoporosis
Brain/Nervous system	Epilepsy
	Insomnia
	Multiple sclerosis
	Neuritis
	Vertigo
Glands	Adrenal exhaustion
Heart	Angina pectoris
	Arteriosclerosis
	Atherosclerosis
Intestine	Celiac disease
	Worms
Joints	Arthritis
	Bursitis
Liver	Cirrhosis of liver
Lungs/Respiratory system	Allergies
	Asthma
	Tuberculosis
Muscles	Muscular dystrophy
Skin	Pellagra
	Psoriasis
	Shingles (herpes zoster)
	Ulcers

Body Member	Ailment
Stomach	Gastritis
	Stomach ulcer (peptic)
General	Alcoholism
	Overweight and obesity

VITAMIN B$_{13}$ (OROTIC ACID)

Description

Vitamin B$_{13}$, orotic acid, is not yet available in the United States but has been synthesized in Europe and used to treat multiple sclerosis. Orotic acid is found in natural sources such as organically grown root vegetables and whey, the liquid portion of soured or curdled milk.

Orotic acid is utilized by the body in the metabolism of folic acid and vitamin B$_{12}$. Orotic acid is also vital for aiding the replacement or restoration of some cells.[23]

Absorption and Storage

No available information.

Dosage and Toxicity

Dietary requirements are not known. This nutrient is available in supplemental form as calcium orotate.

Deficiency Effects and Symptoms

Deficiency symptoms are not known, but is believed that a deficiency may lead to liver disorders, cell degeneration, and premature aging.[24] A deficiency of vitamin B$_{13}$ also may lead to degenerative symptoms in multiple sclerosis patients.

Beneficial Effects on Ailments

Dr. J. Evers, from West Germany, has produced successful results in treating multiple sclerosis patients with vitamin B$_{13}$.[25]

VITAMIN B$_{13}$ MAY BE BENEFICIAL FOR THE FOLLOWING AILMENT:

Body Member	Ailment
Brain/Nervous system	Multiple sclerosis

[23] Airola, *How to Get Well*, p. 267.
[24] Airola, *How to Get Well*, p. 267.
[25] "Multiple Sclerosis," *Cancer Control Journal*, vol. 2, no. 3, p. 8, May-June 1971.

BIOTIN

Description

Biotin is a water-soluble B-complex vitamin. As a co-enzyme, it assists in the making of fatty acids and in the oxidation of fatty acids and carbohydrates. Without biotin the body's fat production is impaired. Biotin also aids in the utilization of protein, folic acid, pantothenic acid, and vitamin B_{12}.

Biotin is an essential nutrient that appears in trace amounts in all animal and plant tissue. Some rich sources of biotin are egg yolk, beef liver, unpolished rice, and brewer's yeast.

Absorption and Storage

Biotin is synthesized by the intestinal bacteria; thus, man is not dependent upon dietary sources to ensure an adequate supply. Raw egg white contains the protein avidin, which binds with biotin in the intestine and prevents its absorption by the body. However, since eggs are usually eaten in a cooked form and avidin is inactivated by heat, there is no real danger of a deficiency resulting from the ingestion of a cooked egg.

Dosage and Toxicity

The National Research Council indicates that 150 to 300 micrograms of biotin will meet the body's daily needs. Additional amounts are required during pregnancy and lactation. There are no known toxic effects of this nutrient.

Deficiency Effects and Symptoms

Deficiency states have been reported in man only when the diet contained large amounts of raw egg white. A deficiency of biotin in man causes muscular pain, poor appetite, dry skin, lack of energy, sleeplessness, and a disturbed nervous system. Dermatitis, grayish skin color, and depression are other symptoms of a biotin deficiency. In severe deficiency there may be impairment of the body's fat metabolism.

Beneficial Effect on Ailments

Dermatitis has shown improvement when treated with biotin. The use of biotin has been beneficial in treating baldness.

Human Tests

1. Biotin and Seborrheic Dermatitis and Leiner's Disease. Nine cases of seborrheic dermatitis and two cases of Leiner's disease in infants were given 5 milligrams of biotin injected intramuscularly daily for seven to fourteen days. Milder cases were given 2 to 4 milligrams orally for two to three weeks.

Results. Both ailments showed marked improvement when treated with biotin. (*Journal of Pediatrics*, November 1957.)

2. Biotin and Biotin Deficiency Symptoms. Persons who were suffering from dermatitis, a grayish pallor of the skin and mucous membranes, diminution of hemoglobin, a striking rise in serum cholesterol, depression, and muscle pain were given 150 or more milligrams of biotin, injected intravenously daily. The excretion of biotin in the urine was much below that of a person on a normal diet.

Results. After the injections the symptoms became less evident. The ashy pallor disappeared in four days, serum cholesterol was reduced, and urinary excretion of biotin increased. (Margaret S. Chaney and Margaret L. Ross, *Nutrition*, Houghton Mifflin Co., Boston, 1971, p. 307.)

BIOTIN MAY BE BENEFICIAL FOR THE FOLLOWING AILMENTS:

Body Member	Ailment
Hair/Scalp	Baldness
Muscles	Muscle pains
Skin	Dermatitis
	Eczema
	Infant dermatitis
General	Depression

CHOLINE

Description

Choline is considered one of the B-complex vitamins. It functions with inositol as a basic constituent of lecithin. It is present in the body of all living cells and is widely distributed in animal and plant tissues. The richest source of choline is lecithin, but other rich dietary sources include egg yolk, liver, brewer's yeast, and wheat germ.

Choline appears to be associated primarily with the utilization of fats and cholesterol in the body. It prevents fats from accumulating in the liver and facilitates the movement of fats into the cells. Choline combines with fatty acids and phosphoric acid within the liver to form lecithin. It is essential for the health of the liver and kidneys.

Choline is also essential for the health of the myelin sheaths of the nerves; the myelin sheaths are the principal component of the nerve fibers. It plays an important role in the transmission of the nerve impulses.[26] It also helps to regulate and improve liver and gallbladder functioning[27] and aids in the prevention of gallstones.

Absorption and Storage

Choline is synthesized by the interaction of B_{12} and folic acid with the amino acid methionine.

Dosage and Toxicity

Daily requirements for choline are not known. The average diet has been estimated to contain 500 to 900 milligrams of choline per day, according to the 1968 revision of the *Recommended Dietary Allowances.*[28] Dr. Paavo Airola has estimated the daily dietary intake to be 1,000 or more milligrams.[29] Usual therapeutic daily doses range from 500 to 6,000 milligrams; prolonged ingestion of massive doses of isolated choline may induce a deficiency of vitamin B_6.[30] It is important to remember that the B-complex vitamins function better when all are taken together.

Deficiency Effects and Symptoms

A choline deficiency is associated with fatty deposits in the liver, resulting in bleeding stomach ulcers, heart trouble, and blocking of the tubes of the kidneys. Insufficient supplies of choline may cause hemorrhaging of the kidneys. A deficiency can also result when too little protein is in the diet.[31] Prolonged deficiencies may cause high blood pressure, cirrhosis and fatty degeneration of the liver, atherosclerosis, and hardening of the arteries.[32]

Beneficial Effect on Ailments

Choline has been successful in reducing high blood pressure because it strengthens weak capillary walls.[33] Symptoms such as heart palpitation, dizziness, headaches, ear noises, and constipation have been relieved or removed entirely within five to ten days after administration of choline treatments. Insomnia, visual disturbances, and blood flow to the eyes have also benefited from choline therapy.

Because choline is a fat and cholesterol dissolver, it is used to treat atherosclerosis and hardening of the arteries. It can be used to treat fatty livers, liver damage, cirrhosis of the liver, and hepatitis. Choline is also used in kidney damage, hemorrhaging of the kidneys, and nephritis, as well as for eye conditions such as glaucoma.

Human Tests

1. Choline and Atherosclerosis. 230 patients were hospitalized for atherosclerosis. Half the patients were given conventional medication but no choline after discharge from the hospital; the other half received choline daily for one to three years.

Results. Among the untreated patients, the three-year death rate was nearly 30 percent. Only 12 percent of the choline-treated patients died. (Dr. L. M. Morrison and W. F. Gonzalez, *Proceedings of the Society of Biology and Medicine*, vol. 73, pp. 37-38, 1950, as reported in Rodale, *The Encyclopedia for Healthful Living*, pp. 457 and 458.)

CHOLINE MAY BE BENEFICIAL FOR THE FOLLOWING AILMENTS:

Body Member	Ailment
Blood/Circulatory system	Angina pectoris
	Cholesterol level, high
	Hepatitis

[26]Krause and Hunscher, *Food, Nutrition and Diet Therapy,* p. 144.
[27]Airola, *How to Get Well,* p. 266.
[28]Krause and Hunscher, *Food, Nutrition and Diet Therapy,* p. 145.
[29]Airola, *How to Get Well,* p. 266.
[30]Airola, *How to Get Well,* p. 266.
[31]*The Vitamins Explained Simply* (Melbourne: Science of Life Books, PTY., 1972), p. 32.
[32]Airola, *How to Get Well,* p. 266.
[33]Clark, *Know Your Nutrition,* p. 110.

Body Member	Ailment
	Hypoglycemia
	Stroke (cerebrovascular accident)
Brain/Nervous system	Dizziness
	Multiple sclerosis
Eye	Glaucoma
Glands	Hyperthyroidism
Hair/Scalp	Hair problems
Heart	Arteriosclerosis
	Atherosclerosis
	Hypertension
Intestine	Constipation
Liver	Cirrhosis of liver
Lungs/Respiratory system	Asthma
Muscles	Muscular dystrophy
Skin	Eczema
General	Alcoholism

FOLIC ACID (FOLACIN)

Description

Folic acid is part of the water-soluble vitamin B complex and functions as a coenzyme, together with vitamins B_{12} and C, in the breakdown and utilization of proteins. Folic acid performs its basic role as a carbon carrier in the formation of heme, the iron-containing protein found in hemoglobin, necessary for the formation of red blood cells. It also is needed for the formation of nucleic acid, which is essential for the processes of growth and reproduction of all body cells. It also increases the appetite and stimulates the production of hydrochloric acid, which helps prevent intestinal parasites and food poisoning. In addition, it aids in performance of the liver. Folic acid is easily destroyed by high temperature, exposure to light, and being left at room temperature for long periods of time. The best sources of folic acid are green leafy vegetables, liver, and brewer's yeast.

Absorption and Storage

Folic acid is absorbed in the gastrointestinal tract by active transport and diffusion and is stored primarily in the liver. Sulfa drugs may interfere with the bacteria in the intestine which manufacture folic acid. Aminoperin and streptomycin destroy folic acid.

Dosage and Toxicity

The Recommended Dietary Allowance of folic acid is 400 micrograms for adults, 800 micrograms during pregnancy, and 600 micrograms during lactation. Stress and disease increase the body's need for folic acid, as does the consumption of alcohol. There is no known toxicity of this vitamin, although an excessive intake of folic acid can mask a vitamin B_{12} deficiency. A prescription is required for dosages higher than 400 micrograms per tablet.

Deficiency Effects and Symptoms

Deficiency of folic acid results in poor growth, graying hair, glossitis (tongue inflammation), and gastrointestinal-tract disturbances arising from inadequate dietary intake, impaired absorption, excessive demands by tissues of the body, and metabolic disturbances. Because of the role folic acid plays in the formation of red blood cells, a deficiency could lead to anemia that cannot be corrected by supplementary iron.[34] In the past few years there have been a number of studies implicating folic acid deficiency as a contributing factor in mental illness. Almost any interference with the metabolism of folic acid in the fetus encourages deformities such as cleft palate, brain damage, or slow development and poor learning ability in the child.[35] In addition, deficiency of folic acid may lead to toxemia, premature birth, after-birth hemorrhaging, and megaloblastic anemia in both mother and child.

Beneficial Effect on Ailments

Folic acid is not limited to treatment of anemia. It is beneficial in treating diarrhea, sprue, dropsy, stomach ulcers, menstrual problems, leg ulcers, and glossitis. Circulation may be improved in patients suffering from atherosclerosis. Folic acid may prevent the graying of hair when used with PABA and pantothenic acid.[36] During pregnancy, folacin-rich foods should be stressed in the diet so that the fetal and maternal needs are met and megaloblastic anemia is prevented.

Human Tests

1. Folic Acid and Toxicity. 20 healthy young adults were given 15 milligrams of folic acid daily for one month and were matched with a control group given placebos.

[34] Clark, *Know Your Nutrition*, p. 103.
[35] Rodale Press Editors, *Be a Healthy Mother, Have a Healthy Baby* (Emmaus, Pa.: Rodale Press, 1973), p. 29.
[36] Adelle Davis, *Let's Get Well* (New York: Harcourt, Brace & World, 1965), p. 166.

Results. No ill effects were detected. Physicians have given 150 milligrams of folic acid to children and 450 milligrams to adults, both daily, with no report of toxicity. (Davis, *Let's Get Well.*)

2. Folic Acid and Megaloblastic Anemia. A sixty-nine-year-old woman was suffering from megaloblastic anemia. She was brought to the hospital with a history of pallor, fatigue, forgetfulness, and lack of energy. According to tests, she lacked vitamin B_{12}, and some was administered before she came to the hospital. She was then given folic acid.

Results. Her condition improved immediately, and she was soon discharged from the hospital. Tests six months later showed her in good health; all symptoms of megaloblastic anemia had disappeared. (*Journal of the American Medical Association*, July 31, 1972.)

3. Folic Acid and Atherosclerosis. 17 elderly patients were treated with 5 to 7.5 milligrams of folic acid daily.

Results. 15 patients responded with increased capillary blood flow, resulting in improved vision due to better blood supply to the retina. In many cases there was increased skin temperature. (Roger J. Williams, *Nutrition Against Disease,* Pitman Publ., New York, 1971, pp. 75–76.)

Animal Tests

1. Folic Acid and Cleft Palate. Pregnant mice were first injected with cortisone, which can cause interference with vital life chemistry, four times daily. Cleft palates developed in 85 percent of their offspring. Pyridoxine and folic acid were separately injected with the cortisone.

Results. When pyridoxine was injected, the abnormalities were reduced to 45 percent; the folic acid in the combination reduced the cleft palate cases to 20 percent. (Dr. Lyndon A. Peer, *Chicago Daily Tribune*, September 11, 1957.)

FOLIC ACID MAY BE BENEFICIAL FOR THE FOLLOWING AILMENTS:

Body Member	Ailment
Blood/Circulatory system	Anemia
	Leukemia
	Pernicious anemia
Bowel	Diarrhea
Brain/Nervous system	Alcoholism
	Mental illness
Glands	Adrenal exhaustion
Hair/Scalp	Baldness
Heart	Arteriosclerosis
	Atherosclerosis
Intestine	Celiac disease
	Diverticulitis
Joints	Arthritis
Lungs/Respiratory system	Emphysema
Nails	Nail problems
Skin	Psoriasis
	Ulcers
Stomach	Gastritis
	Indigestion (dyspepsia)
General	Alcoholism
	Anemia
	Bruises
	Fatigue
	Kwashiorkor
	Pellagra
	Scurvy
	Stress
	Tonsilitis

INOSITOL

Description

Inositol is recognized as part of the vitamin B complex and is closely associated with choline and biotin. Like choline, inositol is found in high concentrations in lecithin.

Both animal and plant tissues contain inositol. In animal tissues it occurs as a component of phospholipids, substances containing phosphorus, fatty acids, and nitrogenous bases. In plant cells it is found as phytic acid, an organic acid that binds calcium and iron in an insoluble complex and interferes with their absorption.[37] Inositol is found in unprocessed whole grains, citrus fruits, brewer's yeast, crude unrefined molasses, and liver.

Inositol is effective in promoting the body's production of lecithin. Fats are moved from the liver to the

[37]Guthrie, *Introductory Nutrition*, p. 276.

cells with the aid of lecithin; therefore inositol aids in the metabolism of fats and helps reduce blood cholesterol.[38] In combination with choline, it prevents the fatty hardening of arteries and protects the liver, kidneys, and heart.

Inositol is also found to be helpful in brain cell nutrition. It is needed for the growth and survival of cells in bone marrow, eye membranes, and the intestines.[39] It is vital for hair growth and can prevent thinning hair and baldness.

Absorption and Storage

The body is able to synthesize sufficient amounts of inositol from glucose to meet its needs.[40] About seven percent of ingested inositol is converted to glucose; inositol is only one-third as effective as glucose in alleviating ketosis, the complete metabolism of fatty acids.[41]

There is some disagreement as to whether inositol is synthesized by the intestinal flora. One reliable source indicates it is,[42] while another claims that synthesis occurs within the individual cell rather than by intestinal organisms.[43] The amount the body excretes daily in the urine is small, averaging 37 milligrams. The diabetic excretes more inositol than does the nondiabetic.[44] Large amounts of coffee may deplete the body's storage of inositol.

Dosage and Toxicity

The Recommended Dietary Allowance has not yet been established, but most authorities recommend consuming the same amount of inositol as choline. The daily consumption of inositol in food is about one gram. The human body contains more inositol than any other vitamin except niacin. One tablespoon of yeast provides approximately forty milligrams each of choline and inositol. Therapeutic doses range from 500 to 1,000 milligrams daily.[45] There is no known toxicity of inositol.

[38] Airola, How to Get Well, p. 266.
[39] Clark, Know Your Nutrition, p. 113.
[40] Guthrie, Introductory Nutrition, p. 276.
[41] Robert Goodhart and Maurice Shils, Modern Nutrition in Health and Disease (Philadelphia: Lea and Febiger, 1973), p. 264.
[42] Rodale and Staff, The Health Seeker, p. 869.
[43] John Hoover (ed.), Remington's Pharmaceutical Sciences (Easton, Pa.: Mack Pub. Co., 1970), p. 1029.
[44] Krause and Hunscher, Food, Nutrition and Diet Therapy, p. 145.
[45] Airola, How to Get Well, p. 266.

Deficiency Effects and Symptoms

Caffeine may create an inositol shortage in the body. An inositol deficiency may cause constipation, eczema, and abnormalities of the eyes. The deficiency contributes to hair loss and a high blood cholesterol level, which may result in artery and heart disease.

Beneficial Effect on Ailments

Inositol is beneficial in the treatment of constipation because it has a stimulating effect on the muscular action of the alimentary canal. It also is recommended for men who are becoming bald and is vital in helping to lower cholesterol levels in the blood. Inositol aids in eliminating liver fats from patients about to be operated on for stomach cancer.

Animal Tests

1. Inositol and Cholesterol. Two groups of rabbits were fed a capsule of cholesterol daily. One group of rabbits received just cholesterol and a regulation diet. The other group of rabbits received a capsule of inositol in addition to the cholesterol.

Results. At the end of the feeding period, the first group of rabbits showed an increase of 337 percent in the cholesterol content in their blood. Those who had received inositol showed a cholesterol increase of only 181 percent. (Newsweek, September 11, 1950, Dr. Louis B. Potte, Dr. William C. Felch, and Stephanie J. Ilka of St. Luke's Hospital, New York; reported in Rodale, The Encyclopedia for Healthful Living.)

INOSITOL MAY BE BENEFICIAL FOR THE FOLLOWING AILMENTS:

Body Member	Ailment
Blood/Circulatory system	Arteriosclerosis
	Atherosclerosis
	Cholesterol level, high
	Stroke (cerebrovascular accident)
Bowel	Constipation
Brain/Nervous system	Dizziness
Eye	Glaucoma
Hair/Scalp	Baldness
Intestine	Constipation
Liver	Cirrhosis of the liver
Lungs/Respiratory system	Asthma

Body Member	Ailment
Stomach	Gastritis
General	Overweight and obesity

LAETRILE
(AMYGDALIN, NITRILOSIDES)

Description

Laetrile is an amygdalin, a simple chemical compound consisting of two molecules of sugar, one molecule of benzaldehyde, and one molecule of cyanide. Nitrilosides are known as "laetrile" when used in medical dosage form.

Laetrile is a natural substance made from apricot pits and is claimed by its developers to have a specific cancer preventive and controlling effect. Dr. Ernest Krebs, Sr., who was the first to use laetrile therapeutically in this country, considered laetrile to be an essential vitamin and named it B_{17}.

Laetrile has been legalized in several states in the United States; however, many doctors in the medical community reject its use in human cancer patients on the grounds that it is ineffective and may be poisonous because of its cyanide content. This view is not held by Dr. Dean Burk, chief cytologist of the National Cancer Institute, who has conducted extensive tests including the use of laetrile and states that "Laetrile is remarkably non-toxic . . . compared with virtually all cancer chemotherapeutic agents currently studied."[46] Other scientists claim that cyanide occurring naturally in food is not dangerous. Laetrile is manufactured and used legally in over 17 countries throughout the world, including Mexico, Germany, Italy, Belgium, and the Philippines.

Natural cyanide is locked in a sugar molecule. It is normally found in over 2,000 known unrefined foods and grasses. A concentration of about 2 or 3 percent laetrile is found in the whole kernels of most fruits, including apricots, apples, cherries, peaches, plums, and nectarines, and in some 70 plants commonly fed to animals for fodder. A sprouting seed produces from 10 to 30 times as much laetrile as does the mature plant. Few citrus fruits contain laetrile. Shelled and unshelled apricot kernels contain 2 to 3 percent amygdalin and are also excellent sources of protein, unsaturated fatty acids, and minerals.

[46]"Laetrile—An Answer to Cancer?" *Prevention*, December 1971, p. 162.

According to its advocates, laetrile is a highly selective substance that attacks only the cancerous cells. When laetrile is eaten and absorbed by normal cells, an enzyme called rhodanese detoxifies the cyanide, which is then excreted through the urine. But because cancer cells are completely deficient in rhodanese and are instead surrounded by another enzyme, beta-glucosidase, which releases the bound cyanide from the laetrile at the site of malignancy, laetrile is believed to attack only the malignant areas.

Absorption and Storage

Oral doses of laetrile are not affected by the action of the acid medium of the stomach but pass directly into the intestine, where the substance is acted upon by bacterial enzymes. The bacterial enzymes in the intestine decompose the amygdalin into four components, which are then absorbed into the lymph and portal systems and circulated throughout the body.

A Loyola University biologist has conducted laboratory tests on mice indicating that laetrile in conjunction with various vitamins and enzymes is more effective in causing a remission of cancer than laetrile administered alone. (*Los Angeles Times*, Sept. 7, 1977.)

Dosage and Toxicity

Although much research on laetrile is still needed, the usual dosage is 0.25 to 1.0 gram taken with meals. Cumulative amounts of more than 3.0 grams are sometimes taken, but *more than 1.0 gram is never taken at any one time*. Dosages as high as 20 grams daily of combined oral and intravenous administration have been used on patients whose detoxification and elimination levels of laetrile were adequate.

Five to thirty apricot kernels eaten through the day may be a sufficient preventive amount, but they should never be taken all at one time. It is not considered desirable to prepare a slurry of ground up kernels (as in a solution of water, milk, or orange juice) and then let it stand for long periods of time before consumption.

Toxicity levels have not been established, and one should exercise extreme caution in order to avoid ingesting excessive amounts all at one time.

Deficiency Effects and Symptoms

Prolonged deficiency may lead to diminished resistance to malignancies.

Beneficial Effect on Ailments

Amygdalin may reduce the size of cancer tumors, ease accompanying pain, and inhibit the growth of cancer cells. In addition, it favorably regulates blood pressure and may have an antirheumatic and esthesizing effect.

LAETRILE MAY BE BENEFICIAL FOR THE FOLLOWING AILMENT:

Body Member	Ailment
General	Cancer

NIACIN (NICOTINIC ACID, NIACINAMIDE, NICOTINAMIDE)

Description

Niacin, a member of the vitamin B complex, is water-soluble. It is more stable than thiamine or riboflavin and is remarkably resistant to heat, light, air, acids, and alkalies. There are also three synthetic forms of niacin: niacinamide, nicotinic acid, and nicotinamide. As a co-enzyme, niacin assists enzymes in the breakdown and utilization of proteins, fats, and carbohydrates. Niacin is effective in improving circulation and reducing the cholesterol level in the blood. It is vital to the proper activity of the nervous system and for formation and maintenance of healthy skin, tongue, and digestive-system tissues. Niacin is necessary for the synthesis of sex hormones.

Relatively small amounts of pure niacin are present in most foods. The niacin "equivalent" listed in dietary tables means either pure niacin or adequate supply of tryptophan, an amino acid that can be converted into niacin by the body. Lean meats, poultry, fish, and peanuts are rich daily sources of both niacin and tryptophan, as are such dietary supplements as brewer's yeast, wheat germ, and desiccated liver. Niacin is difficult to obtain except from these foods.

Absorption and Storage

Niacin is absorbed in the intestine and is stored primarily in the liver. Any excess is eliminated through the urine. Excessive consumption of sugar and starches will deplete the body's supply of niacin, as will certain antibiotics.

Dosage and Toxicity

The National Research Council suggests that daily allowances of niacin be based on caloric intake; 6.6 milli-grams of niacin per 1000 calories is recommended. Tryptophan may provide part or all of the daily niacin requirements; 60 milligrams of tryptophan yield 1 milligram of niacin. The Recommended Dietary Allowance is 18 milligrams for men, 13 milligrams for women, and 9 to 16 milligrams for children. During pregnancy, lactation, illness, tissue trauma, and growth periods and after physical exercise, daily requirements are increased.

No real toxic effects are known, but large doses, usually 100 or more milligrams, may cause passing side effects such as tingling and itching sensations, intense flushing of the skin, and throbbing in the head due to a dilation of the lumen in the blood vessels. The flush is not considered dangerous. It lasts for approximately fifteen minutes and then disappears. By taking a synthetic form of niacin, niacinamide, a person gets all the benefits of niacin but avoids the above side effects. Acne and migraine headaches are two disturbances that do not respond as well to the synthetic forms as they do to the natural form.

Deficiency Effects and Symptoms

The symptoms of niacin deficiency are many. In the early stages, muscular weakness, general fatigue, loss of appetite, indigestion, and various skin eruptions occur. A niacin deficiency may also cause bad breath, small ulcers, canker sores, insomnia, irritability, nausea, vomiting, recurring headaches, tender gums, strain, tension, and deep depression. Severe niacin deficiency results in pellagra, which is characterized by dermatitis; dementia; diarrhea; rough, inflamed skin; tremors; and nervous disorders. Many digestive abnormalities causing irritation and inflammation of mucous membranes in the mouth and gastrointestinal tract develop from a niacin deficiency.

Beneficial Effect on Ailments

The amazing thing about niacin is the speed with which it can reverse disorders. Diarrhea has been cleared up in two days. Atherosclerosis, attacks of Ménière's syndrome (vertigo), and some cases of progressive deafness have improved or even disappeared. Niacin is often used to reduce high blood pressure and increase circulation in cramped, painful legs of the elderly. It also helps to stimulate the production of hydrochloric acid to aid impaired digestion. Acne has been successfully treated with niacin.

Lewis J. Silvers, M.D., writes: "Many a migraine headache can be prevented from developing into the excruciating painful stage by taking niacin at the first sign of attack."[47] Large doses of niacin have effectively cured schizophrenia and have helped elderly patients who are mentally confused.

Drs. Richard M. Halpern and Robert A. Smith have reported research indicating that the flushless nicotinamide may be a factor in preventing cancer, due to enzyme regulation that protects normal cells and prevents them from becoming malignant. Investigators have found niacin able to cure pellagra, a disease that affects the skin, intestinal tract, and nervous system. When given in high doses, niacin may bring complete relief from delirium within 24 to 48 hours.

Human Tests

1. Niacin and Acne. 20 cases of acne were treated with 100 milligrams three times daily. This treatment continued for two or three weeks or until the patients experienced regular flushing.

Results. The niacin treatment provided definite relief in all 20 cases. (Lewis J. Silvers, M.D., as reported in Clark, *Know Your Nutrition*, pp. 83-84.)

2. Niacin and Cancer. Drs. Richard M. Halpern and Robert A. Smith reported that malignancy is, in some way, associated with a deficiency of niacin. To prove that niacin could help prevent cancer, they exposed isolated malignant cells in their laboratory to nicotinamide and watched the vitamin suppress the malignancy. The doctors did not state dosages since individual needs vary so greatly. (Drs. Richard M. Halpern and Robert A. Smith, Molecular Biology Institute, as reported in Clark, *Know Your Nutrition*, p. 84.)

NIACIN MAY BE BENEFICIAL FOR THE FOLLOWING AILMENTS:

Body Member	Ailment
Blood/Circulatory system	Arteriosclerosis
	Atherosclerosis
	Cholesterol level, high
	Diabetes
	Hemophilia
	Hypertension
	Phlebitis
Bowel	Diarrhea
Brain/Nervous system	Dizziness
	Epilepsy
	Headache
	Insomnia
	Mental illness
	Multiple sclerosis
	Neuritis
	Parkinson's disease
Ear	Ménière's syndrome
Eye	Conjunctivitis
	Night blindness
Hair/Scalp	Baldness
Heart	Arteriosclerosis
	Atherosclerosis
	Hypertension
Intestine	Constipation
Joints	Arthritis
Leg	Phlebitis
Lungs/Respiratory system	Tuberculosis
Mouth	Canker sore
	Halitosis
Skin	Acne
	Bedsores
	Dermatitis
Stomach	Indigestion (dyspepsia)
Teeth/Gums	Pyorrhea
General	Alcoholism
	Cancer
	Stress

PARA-AMINOBENZOIC ACID (PABA)

Description

Para-aminobenzoic acid, an integral part of the vitamin B complex, is water-soluble and is considered unique in that it is a "vitamin within a vitamin," occurring in combination with folic acid.[48] PABA is found in liver, yeast, wheat germ, and molasses.

PABA stimulates the intestinal bacteria, enabling them to produce folic acid, which in turn aids in the production of pantothenic acid. As a coenzyme, PABA func-

[47]Clark, *Know Your Nutrition*, pp. 83-84.

[48]Krause and Hunscher, *Food, Nutrition and Diet Therapy*, p. 140.

tions in the breakdown and utilization of proteins and in the formation of blood cells, especially red blood cells. PABA plays an important role in determining skin health, hair pigmentation, and health of the intestines.[49] PABA acts as a sunscreen and is incorporated into some sunscreen ointments.[50]

Absorption and Storage

PABA is stored in the tissues but is synthesized by friendly bacteria in the intestines. This means that the body will manufacture its own PABA if conditions in the intestines are favorable.

Dosage and Toxicity

The need for PABA in human nutrition has not yet been established. PABA is available in supplements in potencies higher than 30 milligrams, but these higher doses (up to 100 milligrams) are used for therapeutic purposes. Continued ingestion of high doses of PABA is not recommended and can be toxic to the liver, heart, and kidneys.

Symptoms of toxicity are nausea and vomiting. Careful study must be done before any serious recommendations can be made for the use of PABA in dermatological conditions.[51]

Deficiency Effects and Symptoms

A deficiency of PABA may result from the use of sulfa drugs, which reduce the capacity of PABA to function properly in the intestines. Deficiency symptoms include fatigue, irritability, depression, nervousness, headache, constipation, and other digestive disorders.

Beneficial Effect on Ailments

PABA is used in treating vitiligo, a condition characterized by depigmentation of some areas of the skin. (Vitiligo may also be caused by a deficiency of hydrochloric acid in the stomach, by a lack of vitamin C, or by a lack of pantothenic acid.) PABA is used in treating some parasitic diseases, including Rocky Mountain spotted fever. In certain laboratory animals, PABA, when combined with pantothenic acid, has helped restore color to hair that was turning gray and has prevented further gray-

ing. Research continues as to whether PABA has this effect on human hair.

According to Adelle Davis, the administration of PABA and folic acid has restored graying or white hair to its natural color. A daily intake of folic acid and PABA should be continued so that the restored hair is prevented from returning to its previous color.

PABA often soothes the pain of burns even more effectively than vitamin E.[52] PABA ointment has been effective in preventing and treating sunburn. Persons normally susceptible to sunburn have been able to remain many hours in the sun after applying PABA ointment. PABA alleviates the pain of sunburn and other burns immediately.[53] Adelle Davis has stated that PABA ointment may delay old-age skin changes such as wrinkles, dry skin, and dark spots.

Human Tests

1. PABA and Lupus Erythematosus (a Severe Skin Disorder). 33 patients with lupus erythematosus were given one to four grams of para-aminobenzoic acid at two- to three-hour intervals.

Results. Two of ten with chronic discord lupus showed no improvement, one patient had a poor response, and seven showed good to excellent responses. Improvement occurred in all of seven patients with scleroderma, a skin disorder; the sclerodermatous areas gradually softened and became thinner and more pliable. (*Zarafonetis: Ann. Intern. Med.*, vol. 30, p. 1188, 1949.)

PABA MAY BE BENEFICIAL FOR THE FOLLOWING AILMENTS:

Body Member	Ailment
Blood/Circulatory system	Anemia
Bowel	Constipation
Hair/Scalp	Baldness
Head	Headache
Skin	Burns
	Sunburn
	Vitiligo

---

[49] *The Vitamins Explained Simply*, p. 28.
[50] Hoover (ed.), *Remington's Pharmaceutical Sciences*, p. 1041.
[51] Goodhart and Shils, *Modern Nutrition in Health and Disease*, pp. 946-947.
[52] Davis, *Let's Get Well*, p. 37.
[53] Davis, *Let's Get Well*, p. 154.

PANGAMIC ACID

Description

Pangamic acid is a water-soluble nutrient that was originally isolated in extracted apricot kernels and later was obtained in crystalline form from rice bran, rice polish, whole-grain cereals, brewer's yeast, steer blood, and horse liver.[54] Pangamic acid promotes oxidation processes and cell respiration and stimulates glucose oxidation.[55] The chief merit of pangamic acid is its ability to eliminate the phenomena of hypoxia, an insufficient supply of oxygen in living tissue.[56] This is especially true in the cardiac and other muscles.

Pangamic acid is essential in promoting protein metabolism, particularly in the muscles of the heart. It regulates fat and sugar metabolism, which partly accounts for its effects on atherosclerosis and diabetes.[57] In some treatments, the action of pangamic acid is improved by the addition of vitamins A and E.

Pangamic acid is helpful in stimulating the glandular and nervous system and is helpful in treating high blood cholesterol levels, impaired circulation, and premature aging.[58] It can help protect against the damaging effect of carbon monoxide poisoning.

Little is actually known about pangamic acid, and only small quantities are used in the United States although it is used widely in Russia and other European countries. Pharmaceutical pangamic acid is derived from ground apricot pits. Good natural sources of pangamic acid are brewer's yeast, whole brown rice, whole grains, pumpkin seeds, and sesame seeds.

Absorption and Storage

Little is known about the absorption and storage of pangamic acid, but excessive amounts are excreted through the kidneys and bowels and in perspiration.[59]

Dosage and Toxicity

The Recommended Dietary Allowance has not been established. According to Dr. Ernest T. Krebs, Jr., pangamic acid has no undesirable effects and its toxic level for man is 100,000 times the therapeutic dose.[60] Clinical tests in which intramuscular injections of pangamic acid were given in doses of 2.5 to 10 milligrams daily proved completely nontoxic. After injections, some patients experienced a flushing of the skin. Similar effects were noted with niacin, but no laboratory changes were reported.[61] The valuable quality of the substance is its nontoxicity.

Deficiency Effects and Symptoms

A deficiency of pangamic acid may cause diminished oxygenation of cells, hypoxia, heart disease, and glandular and nervous disorders.[62]

Beneficial Effect on Ailments

Many claims have been made concerning the therapeutic value of pangamic acid. In widespread Soviet clinical tests, over one-half of hospitalized sclerosis patients responded to pangamic acid therapy.[63] Even patients who have had serious heart attacks have been restored to good health with treatments of pangamic acid.[64] Most tests on pangamic acid have been conducted in the USSR.

People complaining of headaches, chest pains, shortness of breath, tension, insomnia, and other common symptoms of advancing atherosclerosis have benefited from additional pangamic acid. Pangamic acid has been found to alleviate hypoxia and has been used in cases of coronary artery insufficiency. It has been shown to relieve symptoms of angina, cyanosis (a discoloration of skin due to poor oxidation), and asthma.[65]

Good results have been obtained in the treatment of rheumatism, rheumatic heart disease, and acute and chronic cases of alcoholism.[66] Some alcoholics have lost their craving for alcohol when treated with pangamic

[54]Clark, *Know Your Nutrition*, p. 129.
[55]Ya. Yu. Shpirt, *Vitamin B15 (Pangamic Acid) Indications for Use and Efficacy in Internal Disease* (Moscow: V/O Medexport, 1968), p. 7.
[56]"The Life-Saving Banned Vitamin," Rodale (ed.), *Prevention*, May 1968.
[57]*Northern Neighbors*, November 1969, p. 6.
[58]Airola, *How to Get Well*, p. 268.
[59]"The Life-Saving Banned Vitamin," *Prevention*, May 1968.

[60]Shpirt, *Vitamin B15 (Pangamic Acid) Indications*, p. 7.
[61]"The Life-Saving Banned Vitamin," *Prevention*, May 1968.
[62]Airola, *How to Get Well*, p. 268.
[63]*Northern Neighbors*, November 1969, p. 6.
[64]*Northern Neighbors*, November 1969, p. 6.
[65]"The Life-Saving Banned Vitamin," *Prevention*, May 1968.
[66]"The Life-Saving Banned Vitamin," *Prevention*, May 1968.

acid.[67]   Pangamic acid has been helpful in treating chronic hepatitis and early stages of liver cirrhosis.[68]

Betty Lee Morales, a pangamic acid researcher, has had success using pangamic acid in treating conditions such as circulatory problems, emphysema, and premature aging.[69] Dr. Ya. Yu. Shpirt, a Russian, developed a combination of vitamins A and E (AEVIT) which has proved to be therapeutically successful in treating severe cases of atherosclerosis of the lower limbs.[70]

There are indications that pangamic acid may be a preventive substance in the treatment of cancer. Dr. Felix Warburg states, "The primary cause of cancer is the replacement of the respiration of oxygen in normal body cells by a fermentation of sugar. All normal body cells meet their energy needs by respiration of oxygen, whereas cancer cells meet their energy needs in great part by fermentation, an oxidative decomposition of complex substances through the action of enzymes. All normal cells require oxygen and cancer cells can thrive without oxygen."[71] According to Warburg's theory, because of the lack of oxygen, the cell is faced with death. The cells without oxygen are able to change their metabolism and to derive their energy from glucose fermentation. These cells may become malignant. Thus a preventive treatment against deoxidation of cells is inclusion of sufficient pangamic acid in the diet.

Human Tests

1. Pangamic Acid and Circulatory Disturbance. 42 patients suffering from circulatory problems were given pangamic acid in the form of calcium pangamate. They were given 30 milligrams three times daily orally, for a total of 90 milligrams daily. The treatment lasted 20 days.

Results. All patients showed improvement in their clinical conditions. The pains in the heart subsided or disappeared. (Clark, *Know Your Nutrition*, pp. 127 and 128.)

2. Pangamic Acid and Cholesterol Level. A study was conducted on the general cholesterol levels of the same

[67]Clark, *Know Your Nutrition*, p. 128.
[68]Clark, *Know Your Nutrition*, p. 128.
[69]Clark, *Know Your Nutrition*, p. 127.
[70]"The Life-Saving Banned Vitamin," *Prevention*, May 1968.
[71]"The Life-Saving Banned Vitamin," *Prevention*, May 1968.

42 cases mentioned in Test 1. They were measured before treatment, after 10 days of treatment, and at the end of 20 days of treatment.

Results. In most cases a drop of the cholesterol was noticed as early as 10 days after the treatment began and continued over the following period. Ten days after the end of treatment with pangamic acid, the general level of cholesterol was greatly reduced. (Clark, *Know Your Nutrition*, p. 128.)

3. Pangamic Acid and Coronary Sclerosis. 118 patients, all over fifty years of age, having coronary sclerosis, were observed after being treated with calcium pangamate. Both subjective symptoms and objective characteristics (EGG, biochemical analysis of the blood, and oscillation findings) were taken as criteria of the effectiveness of the treatment.

Results. Of all 118 cases, good results were obtained in 49 and satisfactory results in 55; in 11 cases the treatment had no effect; deterioration was noted in 3 cases. [Shpirt, *Vitamin B_{15} (Pangamic Acid) Indications*, p. 10.]

4. Pangamic Acid and Muscles of Injured Legs. Groups of athletes were given various amounts of substances to stimulate energy in muscular activity. Then they were given 300 milligrams of pangamic acid on successive days.

Results. The pangamic acid was effective in early healing of muscles of injured legs. (Clark, *Know Your Nutrition*, p. 129.)

5. Pangamic Acid and Cardiopulmonary Insufficiency. 16 patients suffering from cardiopulmonary insufficiency due to pneumosclerosis and bronchial asthma were treated with calcium pangamate. It was administered for 20 to 30 days orally in a dosage of 120 to 160 milligrams per day and as an aerosol in a dosage of 80 milligrams per day.

Results. 4 patients obtained good results, 10 obtained satisfactory results, and 2 showed no effects of the treatment. [Shpirt, *Vitamin B_{15} (Pangamic Acid) Indications*, pp. 24 and 25.]

6. Pangamic Acid and Atherosclerosis. 27 patients were receiving calcium pangamate for treatment of atherosclerosis. They were given 120 to 150 milligrams daily for 15 to 30 days.

Results. 15 patients showed good results, 8 showed satisfactory results, 2 showed no effects of treatment, and 2 showed relapse. [Shpirt, *Vitamin B₁₅ (Pangamic Acid) Indications*, p. 25.]

PANGAMIC ACID MAY BE BENEFICIAL FOR THE FOLLOWING AILMENTS:

Body Member	Ailment
Blood/Circulatory system	Angina pectoris
	Atherosclerosis
	Cholesterol level, high
	Hypertension
Brain/Nervous system	Hypertension
	Multiple sclerosis
Head	Headache
Heart	Angina pectoris
	Atherosclerosis
	Hypertension
Liver	Cirrhosis of liver
Lungs/Respiratory system	Asthma
	Emphysema
General	Alcoholism
	Autism
	Cancer
	Hepatitis
	Hypoxia
	Rheumatic fever
	Rheumatism

PANTOTHENIC ACID

Description

Pantothenic acid, a part of the vitamin B complex, is water-soluble. It occurs in all living cells, being widely distributed in yeasts, molds, bacteria, and individual cells of all animals and plants. Organ meats, brewer's yeast, egg yolks, and whole-grain cereals are the richest sources. Pantothenic acid is synthesized in the body by the bacterial flora of the intestines.[72]

There is a close correlation between pantothenic acid tissue levels and functioning of the adrenal cortex. Pantothenic acid stimulates the adrenal glands and in-

creases production of cortisone and other adrenal hormones important for healthy skin and nerves.

Pantothenic acid plays a vital role in cellular metabolism. As a coenzyme it participates in the release of energy from carbohydrates, fats, and proteins and in the utilization of other vitamins, especially riboflavin. Pantothenic acid is an essential constituent of the enzyme COA, which forms active acetate and, as such, acts as an activating agent in metabolism. Pantothenic acid is essential for the synthesis of cholesterol, steroids (fat-soluble organic compounds), and fatty acids.[73] It is important in maintaining a healthy digestive tract.

Pantothenic acid can improve the body's ability to withstand stressful conditions. Adequate intake of pantothenic acid reduces the toxicity effects of many antibiotics. It aids in the prevention of premature aging and wrinkles. It also protects against cellular damage caused by excessive radiation.[74]

Absorption and Storage

Pantothenic acid is found in the blood, particularly in the plasma, which is the liquid part of the lymph. Pantothenic acid is excreted daily in the urine.

Approximately thirty-three percent of the pantothenic acid content of meat is lost during cooking and about fifty percent is lost by the milling of flour.[75] It is easily destroyed by acid, such as vinegar, or alkali, such as baking soda.

Dosage and Toxicity

Individual needs for pantothenic acid vary according to periods of stress, daily food intake, and urinary excretion levels. Several sources, including the National Research Council, suggest 5 to 10 milligrams daily for adults and children, respectively.[76] The Heinz Handbook of Nutrition suggests daily requirements to be 10 to 15 milligrams. Dr. Paavo Airola has estimated the optimum daily intake to be between 30 and 50 milligrams per day.

Therapeutic dosages usually range from 50 to 200 milligrams per day. In some studies, 1,000 and more milligrams were given daily for six months without side

---

[72]Hoover (ed.), *Remington's Pharmaceutical Sciences*, p. 1030.

[73]Chaney and Ross, *Nutrition*, p. 304.
[74]Airola, *How to Get Well*, p. 265.
[75]Krause and Hunscher, *Food, Nutrition and Diet Therapy*, p. 138.
[76]Goodhart and Shils, *Modern Nutrition in Health and Disease*, p. 207.

effects.[77] It is presumed that folic acid aids in the assimilation of pantothenic acid. There are no known toxic effects with pantothenic acid.

Deficiency Effects and Symptoms

Pantothenic acid is so widely distributed in foods that an occurrence of deficiency is rare. The means of detecting deficiencies are limited, although low intakes may slow down many metabolic processes.[78]

Symptoms of a deficiency may include vomiting, restlessness, abdominal pains, burning feet, muscle cramps, sensitivity to insulin, decreased antibody formation, gastrointestinal disturbances, and upper respiratory infections. A deficiency may lead to skin disorders, adrenal exhaustion, and low blood sugar (hypoglycemia).[79] The list of deficiency symptoms reflects impaired health of cells in many tissues. A lack of pantothenic acid may result in duodenal ulcers. Deficiencies may occur when the body lacks the intestinal flora needed to synthesize pantothenic acid. The function of the adrenal gland is diminished, which may lead to physical and mental depression, insufficient secretions of hydrochloric acid in the stomach, and disturbances of the motor nerves.

Beneficial Effect on Ailments

Pantothenic acid has been used successfully to treat paralysis of the gastrointestinal tract after surgery.[80] It appears to stimulate gastrointestinal movement and aids in the prevention of nerve degeneration due to a deficiency. Nerve degeneration includes peripheral neuritis, nerve disorders, and epilepsy.

Blood pantothenic acid levels decrease during rheumatoid arthritis; the more severe the symptoms, the lower the acid level. Daily injections of pantothenic acid may lead to a rise in blood pantothenic acid levels. Pantothenic acid is important in the prevention of arthritis.[81] It is probably the greatest defense against stress and fatigue, and it also helps build antibodies for fighting infection.

Animal Tests

1. Pantothenic Acid and Duodenal Ulcers. Rats were kept on a diet deficient in pantothenic acid.

[77]Airola, *How to Get Well*, p. 265.
[78]Guthrie, *Introductory Nutrition*, p. 261.
[79]Airola, *How to Get Well*, p. 265.
[80]Guthrie, *Introductory Nutrition*, p. 262.
[81]Williams, *Nutrition against Disease*, p. 126.

Results. Increased hormonal activity was shown to cause ulcers in 11 to 14 weeks. The same hormonal activity in rats that had been fed pantothenic acid did not produce any ulcers. (*Drug Trade News*, March 11, 1957, as reported in J. I. Rodale, ed., *Best Health Articles from Prevention Magazine*, pp. 231 and 232.)

2. Pantothenic Acid and Infection. Rats were divided into two groups: one with a diet containing pantothenic acid and one without any. They were then exposed to an infection source.

Results. Spontaneous infections were widespread in the rats whose diet did not contain pantothenic acid. No infections were seen in the rats whose diet was complete. In the rats (deficient in pantothenic acid) that were inoculated with the infection source, 100 percent infection was noted. The rats whose diet included this vitamin showed an infection incidence of only 1 in 45 when given the same inoculation. (*Nutrition Review*, February 1957, as reported in Rodale, *Encyclopedia for Healthful Living*, p. 951.)

3. Pantothenic Acid and Life-Span. Mice were divided into two groups. They were treated alike except that each animal in the control group received 0.3 milligram of extra pantothenate per day in its drinking water. This amount was several times the amount that mice supposedly require.

Results. The 41 mice on the regular diet lived an average of 550 days. The 33 mice who received extra pantothenate lived an average of 653 days. (550 days is equivalent to 75 years for humans, and 653 days is equivalent to 89 years.) (Williams, *Nutrition against Disease*, pp. 141 and 142.)

PANTOTHENIC ACID MAY BE BENEFICIAL FOR THE FOLLOWING AILMENTS:

Body Member	Ailment
Blood/Circulatory system	Anemia
	Hypoglycemia
Bladder	Cystitis
Bones	Fracture
Bowel	Diarrhea
Brain/Nervous system	Epilepsy
	Fainting spells
	Insomnia

Body Member	Ailment
	Mental illness
	Multiple sclerosis
	Neuritis
Eye	Cataracts
Foot	Burning and tingling sensations
Glands	Adrenal exhaustion
Hair/Scalp	Baldness
Head	Headache
Intestine	Worms
Joints	Arthritis
	Gout
Leg	Leg cramp
	Phlebitis
Lungs/Respiratory system	Allergies
	Asthma
	Tuberculosis
Muscles	Muscular dystrophy
Skin	Acne
	Psoriasis
Stomach	Gastritis
	Indigestion (dyspepsia)
	Nausea
General	Alcoholism
	Cancer
	Depression
	Fatigue
	Infection
	Retarded growth
	Stress

VITAMIN C (ASCORBIC ACID)

Description

Vitamin C, also known as ascorbic acid, is a water-soluble nutrient. Although fairly stable in acid solution, it is normally the least stable of vitamins and is very sensitive to oxygen. Its potency can be lost through exposure to light, heat, and air, which stimulate the activity of oxidative enzymes.

A primary function of vitamin C is maintaining collagen, a protein necessary for the formation of connective tissue in skin, ligaments, and bones. Vitamin C plays a role in healing wounds and burns because it facilitates the formation of connective tissue in the scar. Vitamin C also aids in forming red blood cells and preventing hemorrhaging. In addition, vitamin C fights bacterial infections and reduces the effects on the body of some allergy-producing substances. For these reasons, vitamin C is frequently used in preventing and treating the common cold.

Vitamin C has significant relationships with other nutrients. It aids in the metabolism of the amino acids phenylalanine and tyrosine. Vitamin C converts the inactive form of folic acid to the active form, folinic acid, and may have a role in calcium metabolism.[82] In addition, vitamin C protects thiamine, riboflavin, folic acid, pantothenic acid, and vitamins A and E against oxidation.

Vitamin C is present in most fresh fruits and vegetables. Natural vitamin C dietary supplements are prepared from rose hips, acerola cherries, green peppers, and citrus fruits.

Absorption and Storage

The level of ascorbic acid in the blood reaches a maximum in two or three hours after ingestion of a moderate quantity, then decreases as it is eliminated in the urine and through perspiration.[83] Most vitamin C is out of the body in three or four hours. Because vitamin C is a "stress vitamin," it is used up even more rapidly under stressful conditions. Man, apes, and guinea pigs are the only animals that need vitamin C in their foodstuffs because they are unable to meet body needs by synthesis and must rely upon a dietary source. Ascorbic acid is readily absorbed from the gastrointestinal tract into the bloodstream. Two factors influencing absorption are the manner in which the vitamin is administered and the presence of other substances in the intestinal tract. The normal human body when fully saturated contains about 5,000 milligrams of vitamin C, of which 30 milligrams are found in the adrenal glands, 200 milligrams in the extracellular fluids, and the rest distributed in varying concentrations throughout the cells of the body. The body's ability to absorb vitamin C is reduced by smoking, stress, high fever, prolonged administration of antibiotics or cortisone, inhalation of DDT or fumes of petroleum, and ingestion of aspirin or other pain killers. Sulfa drugs increase urinary excretion of vitamin C by two or three times the normal amount. Baking soda

[82]Henrietta Fleck, *Introduction to Nutrition* (London: The Macmillan Co., 1971), p. 147.
[83]Linus C. Pauling, *Vitamin C and the Common Cold* (New York: Bantam Books, 1971), pp. 63 and 64.

creates an alkaline medium that destroys vitamin C. In addition, drinking excessive amounts of water will deplete the body's vitamin C. Cooking in copper utensils will destroy the vitamin C content of foods.

Dosage and Toxicity

The National Research Council recommends 45 milligrams of vitamin C for adults. According to Dr. Linus C. Pauling, Nobel Laureate Professor of Chemistry, University of California, Stanford, the optimum daily intake of vitamin C for most human adults is from 2,300 to 9,000 milligrams. The variation is caused by differences in weight, amount of activity, rate of metabolism, ailments, and age. Periods of stress, such as anxiety, infection, injury, surgery, burns, or fatigue, increase the body's need for this vitamin. It is better to take frequent small doses of the vitamin instead of a single large dose, because the body can absorb only a certain amount during a given period of time. For example, it is preferable to take one 250-milligram tablet of vitamin C six times daily rather than one or two gram tablets during the day. When megavitamin doses of vitamin C are given for colds, it is important that calcium intake be increased.

Toxicity symptoms usually do not occur with high intakes of vitamin C, because the body simply discharges whatever it cannot use. However, daily intake of between 5,000 and 15,000 milligrams may have side effects in some persons. Toxicity symptoms can be a slight burning sensation during urination, loose bowels, and/or skin rashes. When any symptom occurs, dosage should be reduced.

Deficiency Effects and Symptoms

Signs of deficiency are shortness of breath, impaired digestion, poor lactation, bleeding gums, weakened enamel or dentine, tendency to bruising, swollen or painful joints, nosebleeds, anemia, lowered resistance to infections, and slow healing of wounds and fractures. Severe deficiency results in scurvy. Breaks in the capillary walls are signs of vitamin C deficiency, and clots usually form at the point of the break. Therefore a lack of vitamin C is a probable cause of heart attacks and strokes initiated by clots. The blood level of ascorbic acid is known to be lowered by smoking. Nicotine added to a sample of human blood of known ascorbic acid content decreased the ascorbic acid content of the blood by 24 to 31 percent.[84]

[84] Rodale, *The Encyclopedia for Healthful Living*, p. 953.

Beneficial Effect on Ailments

Vitamin C plays an important role in preventing and relieving scurvy. Vitamin C promotes fine bone and tooth formation while protecting the dentine and pulp. Some types of viral and bacterial infections are prevented or cured by vitamin C, and it reduces the effects on the body of some allergy-producing substances. Vitamin C is frequently used in the prevention and treatment of the common cold.

The lubricating fluid of joints (synovial fluid) becomes thinner (allowing freer movement) when the serum levels of ascorbic acid are high. Therefore arthritic patients given vitamin C may find some relief of pain. It is an important nutrient in treating wounds because it speeds up the healing process. Ascorbic acid may lower blood cholesterol content of patients with artereosclerosis.

The need for vitamin C increases with age due to a greater need to regenerate collagen. With age, the sex glands develop a greater need for vitamin C and will draw it from other tissues, leaving these tissues vulnerable to disease. Therefore proper supplementation will help reduce depletion. Vitamin C is important in all stressful conditions. The tissue requirements for ascorbic acid are increased under conditions of increased metabolism.

For more than 25 years, Dr. Frederick Klenner of Reidsville, North Carolina, has been using vitamin C to treat viral diseases, including hepatitis, viral pneumonia, herpes simplex, measles, and mononucleosis. His treatment involves administration, either intravenously or by mouth, of 20 to 40 grams vitamin C daily.

Massive doses of vitamin C have been used to cure drug addicts, including users of heroin, methadone, and barbiturates. Chiropractor Alfred F. Libby of Santa Ana, California, has successfully administered 25 to 85 grams of sodium ascorbate, a buffered version of vitamin C, for four days, then reduced the dose to 5 grams of sodium ascorbate and 5 grams of ascorbic acid. The treatment eases heroin withdrawal, helps to restore proper appetite and restfulness, and helps to eliminate abnormal thought patterns.

Vitamin C has been found to be of value in minimizing the effects of environmental pollution, including carbon monoxide, cadmium, and mercury, and lead poisoning.

Human Tests

1. Vitamin C and Whooping Cough. 90 children with whooping cough were given vitamin C orally or were injected with 5,000 milligrams daily for seven days, with the dosage being gradually reduced until a daily level of 100 milligrams was reached. A control group was given whooping cough vaccine.

Results. The duration of the disease in the children receiving ascorbic acid was 15 to 20 days, while the average duration for the children receiving vaccine was 34 days. When ascorbic acid therapy was started during the catarrhal stage, the spasmodic stage was prevented in 75 percent of the cases. (*Journal of the American Medical Association*, November 4, 1950, as reported in Rodale, *The Encyclopedia for Healthful Living*, p. 956.)

2. Vitamin C and Prickly Heat. 30 children were divided into two groups of 15. One group was given vitamin C in proportion to body weight; the other group was given placebos, in this case, sugar pills. Only the pharmacist knew who had which. After two weeks, Dr. Hindson and the pharmacist compared their notes:

Vitamin C Group	Placebo Group
1 same	9 same
4 improved	4 improved
10 free from lesions	2 worse

The 15 patients given the placebos were then given vitamin C following the first comparison. Within two months, no lesions were seen on any of the 30 children. (Dosage: Child of 38 pounds = 250 milligrams a day.) (Dr. C. Hindson, as reported in Rodale, ed., *Prevention*, July 1972.)

3. Vitamin C and Iron Deficiency. 30 females ages fourteen to forty-two were suffering from iron deficiency. They were given one tablet of 200 milligrams of ascorbic acid daily.

Results. After 60 days of treatment, the iron deficiency was alleviated. A chronic deficiency of iron is often complicated by the side effect of scurvy. In order to influence absorption of iron, a vitamin C intake of at least 200 to 500 milligrams per day is needed. (Enil Margo Schleicher, Director of Hematology at St. Barnabas Hospital, Minneapolis, as reported in Rodale, ed., *Prevention*, August 1970.)

4. Vitamin C and Nicotine. 14 smokers and 14 non-smokers having similar characteristics and dietary habits

were placed on vitamin C-deficient diets. Blood samples of all were taken. Then the subjects were given 1.1 grams of vitamin C and high doses of water-soluble vitamins to facilitate absorption. This process continued for five days, until the subjects' bodies were saturated with vitamin C. For three days vitamin C intakes were carefully limited, and the urine was closely examined.

Results. Blood tests showed that the smokers had about 30 percent less vitamin C in their blood than the non-smokers. (Omar Pelletier of the Nutrition Research Division of the Food and Drug Directorate in Ottawa, Canada, as reported in Rodale, ed., *Prevention*, July 1969.)

5. Vitamin C and Inflammation of the Urethra. 12 men were suffering from painful inflammation of the urethra. The patients were examined, and each was given 3 grams of vitamin C daily for four days. The irritation was caused by phosphatic crystals formed in the urine due to insufficient acidity.

Results. The large doses of vitamin C proved to be a safe way of introducing enough acidity to force the crystals back into solution. What cured the patients was the "wasted" vitamin C, the part not stored in the body and spilled into the urine. The excess vitamin C in the urine proved to be 100 percent effective in relieving the symptoms. (Rodale, ed., *Prevention*, July 1973.)

Animal Tests

1. Vitamin C and Tooth Formation. In vitamin C-deficient guinea pigs, the dentine near the developing teeth ceased to form and the pulp was separated from the dentine by liquid. Either dentine ceased being manufactured, or it was of inferior quality. The pulp itself shrunk and once free from the dentine, was apparently floating in a liquid.

Results. Rapid repair followed the administration of vitamin C. (*Journal of Dentistry for Children*, Third Quarter, 1943, as reported in Rodale, *The Encyclopedia for Healthful Living*, pp. 953 and 954.)

2. Vitamin C and Mercury Poisoning. 20 guinea pigs were given 200 milligrams of vitamin C daily for six days (equivalent to 14 grams per day for humans). On the sixth day, each pig was given what should have been a fatal dosage of mercury. After the poisoning, they were put back on their regular diet, which included 200 milligrams of vitamin C daily.

Results. After two days, they lost weight but ate and behaved normally. The experiment was finally terminated. After 20 days the animals were considered saved. (Momcilo Mokranjae and Ceda Petrovic in the *C. R. Acad. Sc. Paris*, 1964, as reported in Rodale, ed., *Prevention*, July 1972, p. 82.)

3. Storage of Ascorbic Acid. Experimental guinea pigs supplied with natural sources of vitamin C had better storage in their tissues than when supplied with synthetic ascorbic acid. (Estelle E. Hawley, "The Effect of the Administration of Acid Content of Guinea Pigs Tissues," *Journal of Nutrition*, 1937, as reported in Rodale, ed., *Prevention*, July 1972.)

4. Vitamin C and Oxygen Starvation. 42 rats were placed in a decompression chamber until the atmospheric pressure equaled that at an altitude of 33,000 feet. All died within 13 minutes. A second group of rats were injected with vitamin C before being placed in the decompression chamber. The dosage given was equivalent to a human dosage of 7 grams.

Results. Three rats did not die; the others stayed alive for an average of 23.7 minutes. A third group of 44 rats were injected with double the vitamin C dosage of the second group (equivalent to a human dosage of 14 grams) and then were put in the decompression chamber.

Results. 21 rats did not die, and the others stayed alive for nearly an hour. The investigators admitted that they did not know why the vitamin C had this effect. (Kazuo Asahina and Katsumi Asano, Toho University School of Medicine, Tokyo, as reported in Rodale, ed., *Prevention*, July 1972.)

VITAMIN C MAY BE BENEFICIAL FOR THE FOLLOWING AILMENTS:

Body Member	Ailment
Bladder	Cystitis
Blood/Circulatory system	Alcoholism
	Anemia
	Angina pectoris
	Arteriosclerosis
	Bruising
	Cholesterol level, high
	Diabetes
	Hemophilia
	Hypertension
	Hypoglycemia
	Jaundice
	Leukemia
	Mononucleosis
	Pernicious anemia
	Phlebitis
	Stroke (cerebrovascular accident)
	Varicose veins
Bones	Fracture
	Osteomalacia
	Osteoporosis
	Rickets
Bowel	Celiac disease
	Colitis
	Cystic fibrosis
	Diarrhea
	Worms
Brain/Nervous system	Dizziness
	Epilepsy
	Fatigue
	Hypertension
	Hypoxia
	Insomnia
	Meningitis
	Mental illness
	Multiple sclerosis
	Parkinson's disease
	Shingles (herpes zoster)
	Stroke (cerebrovascular accident)
Ear	Ear infection
Eye	Amblyopia
	Cataracts
	Conjunctivitis
	Eyestrain
	Glaucoma
	Vision and focus disorders
Gallbladder	Gallstones
Glands	Adrenal exhaustion
	Cystic fibrosis
	Goiter
	Prostatitis
	Swollen glands

Body Member	Ailment	Body Member	Ailment
Hair/Scalp	Baldness		Impetigo
	Hair problems		Psoriasis
Head	Headache		Scurvy
Heart	Angina pectoris		Shingles (herpes zoster)
	Arteriosclerosis	Stomach	Gastritis
	Hypertension		Gastroenteritis
Intestine	Celiac disease		Stomach ulcer (peptic)
	Constipation	Teeth/Gums	Pyorrhea
	Hemorrhoids		Tooth and gum disorders
Joints	Arthritis	General	Alcoholism
	Bursitis		Arthritis
	Gout		Backache
Kidney	Kidney stones (renal calculi)		Beriberi
	Nephritis		Cancer
Leg	Leg cramp		Chicken pox
	Phlebitis		Fever
	Varicose veins		Infection
Liver	Cirrhosis of liver		Influenza
	Hepatitis		Kwashiorkor
	Jaundice		Overweight and obesity
Lungs/Respiratory system	Allergies		Pregnancy
	Bronchitis		Rheumatic fever
	Common cold		Stress
	Croup		Stroke (cerebrovascular accident)
	Emphysema		
	Hay fever (allergic rhinitis)		
	Influenza		
	Pneumonia		
	Tuberculosis		
Mouth	Canker sore		
	Halitosis		
Muscles	Muscular dystrophy		
	Rheumatism		
Reproductive system	Prostatitis		
Skin	Abscess		
	Acne		
	Athlete's foot		
	Bedsores		
	Boil (furuncle)		
	Bruises		
	Burns		
	Carbuncle		
	Eczema		

VITAMIN D

Description

Vitamin D is a fat-soluble vitamin, and it can be acquired either by ingestion or by exposure to sunlight. It is known as the "sunshine" vitamin because the action of the sun's ultraviolet rays activates a form of cholesterol, which is present in the skin, converting it to vitamin D.

The provitamins D are found in both plant and animal tissue. Vitamin D_2 is known as calciferol, a synthetic; vitamin D_3 is the natural form as it occurs in fish-liver oils. D_3 can be made synthetically by ultraviolet irradiation of 7-dehydrocholesterol, a derivative of cholesterol.

Vitamin D aids in the absorption of calcium from the intestinal tract and the breakdown and assimilation of phosphorus, which is required for bone formation.[85] It

[85] Hoover (ed.), *Remington's Pharmaceutical Sciences* (Emmaus: Mack Pub. Co., 1970), p. 1017.

helps synthesize those enzymes in the mucous membranes which are involved in the active transport of available calcium. Vitamin D is necessary for normal growth in children, for without it bones and teeth do not calcify properly.

Adults also benefit from vitamin D. It is valuable in maintaining a stable nervous system, normal heart action, and normal blood clotting because all these functions are related to the body's supply and utilization of calcium and phosphorus. Vitamin D is best utilized when taken with vitamin A. Fish-liver oils are the best natural source of vitamins A and D.

Absorption and Storage

Ingested vitamin D is absorbed with the fats through the intestinal walls with the aid of bile. Vitamin D from dehydrocholesterol by sun radiation is formed in the skin and absorbed into the circulatory system. Pigmentation is a factor in the absorption of ultraviolet rays. The more pigment there is in the skin, the less vitamin D is produced in the body by irradiation.

After absorption from the intestine or formation in the skin, vitamin D is transported to the liver for storage; other deposits are found in the skin, brain, spleen, and bones. The body can store sizable reserves of vitamin D. Mineral oil can destroy the vitamin D already stored in the intestinal tract.

Dosage and Toxicity

Most of the body's needs for vitamin D can be met by sufficient exposure to sunlight and from the ingestion of small amounts of food, but the sun's action on the skin can be inhibited by such factors as air pollution, clouds, window glass, or clothing. The National Research Council sets the dietary allowance of vitamin D at 400 IU per day to meet the requirements of practically all healthy individuals who have little or no exposure to ultraviolet light. This same dosage is recommended for infants, provided the calcium consumption at the same time is adequate. During pregnancy and lactation women need to include extra vitamin D in their diets. According to the National Research Council, there are no vitamin D recommendations for adults over twenty-two years of age since there is no data available upon which to base such a recommendation.

The adult rate of calcium and phosphorus loss from the skeletal system is thought to be less rapid than that of the growing organism.

It must be emphasized that good will result from the provision of adequate vitamin D *only* when the calcium and phosphorus requirements are met. No extra benefit is obtained from taking more than 400 IU daily except for therapeutic reasons; then dosages may range from 1,500 to 2,800 IU daily for several months. Increased heart activity requires increased calcium, which is not supplied unless there is enough vitamin D in the system.

It is known that "hypervitaminosis D" can occur and can cause pathological changes in the body. Excessive amounts may cause high levels of calcium and phosphorus in the blood and excessive excretion of calcium in the urine; this leads to calcification of soft tissues and of the walls of the blood vessels and kidney tubules, which is hypercalcemia.[86] Adelle Davis stated, "a toxic dose of vitamin D for adults appears to be 300,000 to 800,000 IU daily for many months. 30,000 IU daily or more over a period of time can easily produce toxic symptoms in babies and 50,000 IU are dangerous for children."[87]

Symptoms of acute overdosage are increased frequency of urination, loss of appetite, nausea, vomiting, diarrhea, muscular weakness, dizziness, weariness, and calcification of the soft tissues of the heart, blood vessels, and lungs. These symptoms will disappear within a few days when the overdosage is terminated.

Deficiency Effects and Symptoms

A deficiency of vitamin D leads to inadequate absorption of calcium from the intestinal tract and retention of phosphorus in the kidney, leading to faulty mineralization of bone structures. The inability of the soft bones to withstand the stress of weight results in skeletal malformations. Rickets, a bone disorder in children, is a direct result of vitamin D deficiency. Signs of rickets are softening of the skull; softening of the fragile bones with bowing of the legs and spinal curvature; enlargement of the wrist, knee, and ankle joints; poorly developed muscles; and nervous irritability.[88] "Adult rickets" called osteomalacia may also occur.

It is believed that vitamin D and parathyroid hormones work together to regulate the transport of calcium. A deficiency may cause tetany, a condition characterized by muscular numbness, tingling, and spasm.

[86]Chaney and Ross, *Nutrition*, pp. 223-224.
[87]Rodale and Staff, *The Complete Book of Vitamins*, p. 340.
[88]Hoover (ed.), *Remington's Pharmaceutical Sciences*, p. 1017.

Thyroid glands need vitamin D to manufacture their hormones, so a vitamin D deficiency may cause flabbiness, poor metabolism, and diabetic distress.

Dr. Arthur A. Knapp, an ophthamologist, reported tests indicating that a vitamin D deficiency may cause myopia, or nearsightedness. An imbalance in calcium is the root of this disorder (see Animal and Human Tests). A vitamin D deficiency may also lead to faulty development of tooth structure.

Beneficial Effect on Ailments

Vitamin D helps prevent and cure rickets, a disease resulting from insufficient calcium, phosphorus, or vitamin D. It also aids in repairing osteomalacia in adults.

Vitamin D plays an important role in dentition. Besides being necessary for proper tooth eruption and linear growth, it continually strengthens the teeth. According to Adelle Davis, vitamin D helps in preventing tooth decay and pyorrhea, an inflammation of the sockets of the teeth.

Vitamins D and A have been beneficial in reducing incidences of colds. The two vitamins taken along with vitamin C act as a preventive measure. Researchers have reported that the acidity of gastric juices is affected by the amount of vitamin D in the diet. These juices are named as a cause of stomach ulcers. Therefore an ulcer patient should be checked to see whether his diet has a sufficient supply of vitamin D.

Human Tests

1. Vitamin D and Myopia. 50,000 USP units of vitamin D in capsule and 1 gram of calcium, in the form of milk or dicalcium phosphate tables, were given daily to selected patients.

Results. In one group, 18 of 52 vitamin-fed patients showed a reduction in myopia, and 8 remained unchanged. (Rodale, ed., *Prevention*, May 1973, p. 95.)

2. Vitamin D and Conjunctivitis. 41 patients suffering from allergic conjunctivitis were given 50,000 units of vitamin D daily for seven weeks.

Results. 29 patients experienced complete relief with vitamin D therapy, 11 showed marked improvement, and 1 remained unchanged. (Dr. Arthur A. Knapp, Columbia College of Physicians and Surgeons, as re-ported in Rodale, ed., *Prevention*, September 1969, pp. 80-82.)

3. Vitamins D and A and Colds. 54 patients suffering from frequent colds, accompanied by high fever, were put into three groups. Group 1 received only vitamin A; Group 2 received only vitamin D; Group 3 received both vitamins D and A. Children under twelve were given half the adult dosage.

Results. None of the patients who received either vitamin D or A alone benefited by the treatment. In the group that received both vitamins, 80 percent showed a significant reduction in both the number and severity of common colds.

Animal Tests

1. Vitamin D and Myopia. Animals fed diets deficient in vitamin D and calcium developed axial myopia, keratoconus (a conical protrusion of the cornea), cataracts, and even arteriosclerosis comparable to the senile type observed clinically in human beings. (Dr. Arthur A. Knapp, Columbia College of Physicians and Surgeons, as reported in Rodale, ed., *Prevention*, September 1969, pp. 80-82.)

2. Vitamin D and Bone Growth. Experiments in which the calcium intake varied in rats showed that vitamin D was responsible for suppressing growth when dietary calcium was high and for stimulating growth when dietary calcium intake was low. (H. Steenback and D.C. Herting, *Nutrition Reviews,* vol. 14, p. 191, 1956.)

VITAMIN D MAY BE BENEFICIAL FOR THE FOLLOWING AILMENTS:

Body Member	Ailment
Bladder	Cystitis
Blood/Circulatory system	Cholesterol level, high
	Diabetes
Bones	Fracture
	Osteomalacia
	Osteoporosis
	Rickets
Brain/Nervous system	Epilepsy
	Meningitis
Eye	Bitot spots
	Cataracts

Body Member	Ailment
	Eyestrain
	Glaucoma
	Vision and focus disorders
Glands	Cystic fibrosis
Gallbladder	Gallstones
Head	Fever
Intestine	Celiac disease
	Constipation
	Worms
Joints	Arthritis
Leg	Leg cramp
	Sciatica
Liver	Cirrhosis of liver
	Jaundice
Lungs/Respiratory system	Allergies
	Bronchitis
	Common cold
	Emphysema
	Tuberculosis
Mouth	Canker sores
Muscles	Tetany
Reproductive system	Vaginitis
Skin	Acne
	Bedsores
	Burns
	Carbuncles
	Eczema
	Psoriasis
	Shingles (herpes zoster)
Teeth/Gums	Pyorrhea
General	Aging
	Alcoholism
	Backache
	Cancer
	Fatigue
	Insomnia
	Kwashiorkor
	Pregnancy
	Rheumatic fever
	Stress

VITAMIN E (TOCOPHEROL)

Description

Vitamin E, a fat-soluble vitamin, is composed of a group of compounds called tocopherols. Seven forms of tocopherol exist in nature: alpha, beta, delta, epsilon, eta, gamma, and zeta. Of these, alpha tocopherol is the most potent form of vitamin E and has the greatest nutritional and biological value. Tocopherols occur in highest concentrations in cold-pressed vegetable oils, all whole raw seeds and nuts, and soybeans. Wheat-germ oil is the source from which vitamin E was first obtained.

Vitamin E is an antioxidant, which means it opposes oxidation of substances in the body. It prevents saturated fatty acids and vitamin A from breaking down and combining with other substances that may become harmful to the body. The vitamin B complex and ascorbic acid are also protected against oxidation when vitamin E is present in the digestive tract.[89] Fats and oils containing vitamin E are less susceptible to rancidity than those devoid of vitamin E. Vitamin E has the ability to unite with oxygen and prevent it from being converted into toxic peroxides; this leaves the red blood cells more fully supplied with the pure oxygen that the blood carries to the heart and other organs.

Vitamin E plays an essential role in cellular respiration of all muscles, especially cardiac and skeletal. Vitamin E makes it possible for these muscles and their nerves to function with less oxygen, thereby increasing their endurance and stamina. It also causes dilation of the blood vessels, permitting a fuller flow of blood to the heart. Vitamin E is a highly effective antithrombin in the bloodstream, inhibiting coagulation of blood by preventing clots from forming. It also aids in bringing nourishment to the cells, strengthening the capillary walls, and protecting the red blood cells from destruction by poisons, such as hydrogen peroxide, in the blood.

Vitamin E prevents both the pituitary and adrenal hormones from being oxidized and promotes proper functioning of linoleic acid, an unsaturated fatty acid. Because aging in the cells is due primarily to oxidation, vitamin E is useful in retarding this process. It is also necessary for proper focusing of the eyes in middle-aged persons.

[89] Guthrie, *Introductory Nutrition*, pp. 210-211.

Vitamin E is effective in the prevention of elevated scar formation on the body surface and within the body. In ointment form it is used on burns to promote healing and lessen the formation of scars. It stimulates urine excretion, which helps heart patients whose body tissues contain an excessive amount of tissue fluid (edema). As a diuretic, vitamin E helps lower elevated blood pressure. It protects against the damaging effects of many environmental poisons in the air, water, and food.[90] It protects the lungs and other tissues from damage by polluted air. Vitamin E has a dramatic effect on the reproductive organs; it helps prevent miscarriages, increases male and female fertility, and helps restore male potency.

Absorption and Storage

Vitamin E, as other fat-soluble vitamins, is absorbed in the presence of bile salts and fat. From the intestines, it is absorbed into the lymph and is transported in the bloodstream as tocopherol to the liver, where high concentrations of it are stored. It is also stored in the fatty tissues, heart, muscles, testes, uterus, blood, and adrenal and pituitary glands. Vitamin E in ointment form can be absorbed through the skin and mucous membranes. Excessive amounts of vitamin E are excreted in the urine, and all effects of vitamin E disappear within three days.

There are several substances that interfere with, or even cause a depletion of, vitamin E in the body. For example, when iron, especially the inorganic form, and vitamin E are administered together, the absorption of both substances is impaired. Dr. Wilfred Shute, in *Vitamin E for Ailing and Healthy Hearts*, suggests that vitamin E should be taken in one dose and all iron taken 8 to 12 hours later for proper absorption. The best time to take vitamin E is before mealtime or bedtime. Chlorine in drinking water, ferric chloride, rancid oil or fat, and inorganic iron compounds destroy vitamin E in the body. Mineral oil used as a laxative depletes vitamin E. Vegetable oils dissolve alpha tocopherol and readily release it in the body, whereas mineral oil dissolves it but does not readily release it.

Large amounts of polyunsaturated fats or oils in the diet increase the rate of oxidation of vitamin E; the more unsaturated fats or oils consumed, the more vita-

min E is necessary.[91] The female hormone estrogen is a vitamin E antagonist. Intake of this hormone makes it very difficult to estimate the amount of alpha tocopherol the individual is lacking.

Improper absorption may be partly responsible for muscular problems, such as muscular dystrophy and poor performance in athletes, and digestive problems, such as peptic ulcers and cancer of the colon.[92] Poor absorption can impair the survival of red blood cells.

Dosage and Toxicity

The daily intake of vitamin E recommended by the National Research Council is based upon the metabolic body size and the level of polyunsaturated fatty acids in the diet rather than upon weight or calorie intake. The requirements increase with gains in polyunsaturated fatty acids in the diet. Air pollution also increases the need for vitamin E. The RDA for infants is 4 to 5 IU daily; for children and adolescents the range is 7 to 12 IU; for adult males, 15 IU; for adult females, 12 IU; in pregnancy and lactation, needs increase to 15 IU daily. Many nutritionists consider these daily allowances exceedingly low. Adelle Davis recommends 30 IU daily for infants and children and 100 IU for adolescents and adults.[93] In cases of illness, doctors recommend 300 to 600 IU daily, although 2,000 IU have been used therapeutically with excellent results.[94]

Vitamin E has a tendency to raise blood pressure when it is given in large doses to someone whose body is not accustomed to it; therefore initial intake should be small, and as tolerance rises, the dosage should be gradually increased. It has been suggested that men start with 100 IU and gradually increase to 600 IU when used for preventive purposes. Women should begin with 100 IU and gradually increase to 400 IU.[95] The best way to determine the correct dosage is with the help of a doctor who is learned in vitamin E therapy.

Vitamin E is considered nontoxic except in two conditions: in high blood pressure patients, it elevates the

---

[90] Airola, *How to Get Well*, p. 206.

[91] Clark, *Know Your Nutrition*, p. 49.
[92] Ruth Winter, *Vitamin E the Miracle Worker* (New York: Arco Publ. Co., 1972), p. 84.
[93] Davis, *Let's Get Well*, p. 398.
[94] Davis, *Let's Get Well*, p. 398.
[95] Carlson Wade, *The Rejuvenated Vitamin* (New York: Award Books, 1970), p. 21.

pressure; starting a chronic rheumatic heart disease patient on high doses can lead to rapid deterioration or death. It is best to begin with small doses, gradually increasing the amount. When using vitamin E externally, Shute states that it is a good idea to take it orally while simultaneously applying it to the body. These methods complement each other.[96]

Deficiency Effects and Symptoms

The first clinical sign of a vitamin E deficiency is the rupture of red blood cells which results from their increased fragility. A deficiency could result in a reduction of membrane stability and a shrinkage in collagen, connective tissue. A vitamin E deficiency may result in a tendency toward muscular wasting or abnormal fat deposits in the muscles and an increased demand for oxygen. Without sufficient amounts of vitamin E in the body, the essential fatty acids are altered so that blood cells break down and hemoglobin formation is impaired. In addition, several amino acids cannot be utilized, and pituitary and adrenal glands reduce their level of functioning. Iron absorption and hemoglobin formation also are impaired. A severe deficiency can cause damage to the kidneys and liver.

Perhaps the widest incidence of vitamin E deficiency among adults in the United States is in gastrointestinal disease, where prolonged deficiency can cause faulty absorption of fat and of fat-soluble vitamins, possibly resulting in cystic fibrosis, blockage of the bile ducts, and chronic inflammation of the pancreas.[97] Poor utilization of the vitamin or an increased vitamin E demand peculiar to the individual can cause anemia and edema in premature and malnourished infants. Serious deficiencies of vitamin E in men may lead to degeneration of tissues in the testes. No amount of vitamin E therapy can repair the permanent damage, and such men may become sterile.[98] Women who are severely deficient in vitamin E cannot carry a pregnancy term successfully and often have miscarriages. Premature births frequently result from insufficient intake of vitamin E during pregnancy, leaving the infants more susceptible to anemia.[99]

Hemorrhaging can occur in newborn infants who lack vitamin E. The blood cells of vitamin E–deficient babies are prone to weakness (hemolysis).

Vitamin E deficiencies can result in nephritis. This occurs when kidney tubules plug up with dead cells so that urine is unable to pass; dropsy and progressive degeneration then occur. Vitamin E deficiency appears to make red blood cells more susceptible to damage from medication and from environmental stresses.

A deficiency of vitamin E can produce heart disease.[100] Approximately 25,000 children are born with heart defects every year in the United States, where 50 percent of all deaths result from heart-related ailments. Evidence is accumulating to indicate that a lack of sufficient vitamin E may be a contributing factor in atherosclerosis and cancer.

According to Dr. Wilfred Shute, the lack of vitamin E in the American diet is partially due to the milling process which eliminates the highly perishable wheat germ, a significant source of vitamin E. About 90 percent of the vitamin E is lost in the milling process.

Beneficial Effect on Ailments

Vitamin E works to treat and prevent heart diseases such as coronary thrombosis, a heart attack in which the vessels are blocked by blood clots and part of the heart is deprived of its blood supply. Vitamin E causes arterial blood clots to disintegrate. Angina pectoris, a chest pain resulting from an insufficient supply of blood to the heart tissues, is successfully treated with alpha tocopherol.

According to Shute, rheumatic heart disease is responsible for 90 percent of defective hearts among children. Vitamin E aids rheumatic heart disease and early stages of cardiac complications by returning abnormal capillaries to normal and reducing fluid accumulation within and between cells. This promotes normal gas interchange across the cell membranes, which seems to arrest the disease.[101] Congenital heart disease results in structural defects of the heart. Vitamin E cannot alter the defective structure, but its oxygen-saving effects and its antithrombin activity are vital for patients who are not treated surgically. Many congenital heart disease patients have cyanosis, insufficient supply of oxygen in the

[96]Wilfred E. Shute and Harold J. Taub, *Vitamin E for Ailing and Healthy Hearts* (New York: Pyramid House, 1969), pp. 75-77.

[97]Martin Ebon, *The Truth about Vitamin E* (New York: Bantam Books, 1972), p. 7.

[98]Ebon, *The Truth about Vitamin E*, p. 30.

[99]Davis, *Let's Get Well*, p. 281.

[100]J.I. Rodale, *Complete Book of Minerals for Health* (Emmaus, Pa.: Rodale Books, 1972), p. 439.

[101]Shute and Taub, *Vitamin E for Ailing and Healthy Hearts*, pp. 61-64.

blood, and with adequate dosage of vitamin E the cyanosis has disappeared.

Vitamin E is able to bring relief to intermittent claudication, a severe pain in calf muscles which results from inadequate blood supply caused by arterial spasm, atherosclerosis, or arteriosclerosis. Vitamin E is beneficial to persons with atherosclerosis if vitamin E therapy is used before irrepairable damage has occurred. It relieves pain in the extremities, speeds up blood flow, and reduces clotting tendencies.[102]

Vitamin E can aid in the healing of burned tissue, skin ulcers, and abrasions. It prevents or dissolves scar tissues. Vitamin E helps remove old acne scars, particularly if x-ray treatments have been given.[103] It is needed also to help dissolve scars in the arterial walls caused by toxic substances.

Vitamin E is helpful in counteracting premature aging of the skin.[104] It is useful to apply vitamin E to the skin in ointment form while taking it orally, because it affects the cell formation by replacing the cells on the outer layer of the skin. Vitamin E also helps counter the gradual decline in metabolic processes during aging. Dry, itchy skin is often part of the aging process; vitamin E ointment is able to relieve the itching.

Under normal conditions vitamin E reduces the formation of thrombin, a clotting agent; this tends to reduce the likelihood of thrombosis, the formation of a blood clot. The intake of estrogen, found in contraceptive pills, may neutralize the effect of vitamin E. Intake of estrogen causes the collection of fibrin, an insoluble protein that promotes blood clotting by forming a fibrous network, to become greater. The greater amount of fibrin increases the chances of thromboembolism, the blocking of blood vessels.[105]

Vitamin E has been successful in regulating excessive or scanty flows during menstruation.[106] When vitamin E is added to the diet, it can correct menstrual rhythm. Vitamin E is recognized as a treatment for hot flashes and headaches during menopause. It has helped relieve itching and inflammation of the vagina when applied in ointment form and simultaneously ingested.

Bursitis, wry-neck, gout, and arthritis have improved with vitamin E therapy. Ingestion of large amounts has improved conditions of nearsightedness and crossed eyes. Vitamin E has also been used to prevent calcification of the kidneys caused by excessive vitamin D or other toxic substances.

Vitamin E has been used to help treat varicose veins, as an alternative to surgery. It also can relieve the pain of varicose veins by decreasing the amount of oxygen needed by the tissues involved.

Vitamin E has been successful in treating thrombosis and phlebitis, which are clots in the veins. In large doses it prevents clots from spreading, dissolves existing clots, and provides indirect circulation around obstructed veins. It should be used to prevent initial attacks of clotting after operations or childbirth.[107]

Individuals suffering from muscular dystrophy have benefited from massive doses of vitamin E.[108] Vitamin E may be able to clear up or control many forms of kidney disease, including nephritis. It also aids in restoring the functions of damaged livers.[109]

Vitamin E helps promote body defenses against virus infections and in some cases may be utilized as a flu vaccine.[110] High doses may build both the serum and the cellular levels of the body to high levels of immunity against flu.

Vitamin E therapy has been able to help diabetics. After administration of the vitamin, some patients found that their blood sugar levels became normal or near normal, and the amount of insulin required was reduced. Vitamin E has also been used to prevent and treat gangrene in diabetics.

Vitamins A and E may be beneficial in lowering blood cholesterol by preventing fat deposits. The vitamins help offset the high cholesterol accumulations deposited on the arterial walls.

Vitamin E is used for easing headaches because it preserves the oxygen in the blood for an extended period. This results in more efficiency as the blood is pumped through the blood vessels of the head. Vitamin E has also relieved migraine attacks. Vitamins C and E work together to keep blood vessels flexible, healthy, and less subject to painful disturbances.[111]

[102]Shute and Taub, *Vitamin E for Ailing and Healthy Hearts*, pp. 70-73.
[103]Davis, *Let's Get Well*, pp. 375-376.
[104]Ebon, *The Truth about Vitamin E*, p. 75.
[105]Ebon, *The Truth about Vitamin E*, p. 77.
[106]Ebon, *The Truth about Vitamin E*, p. 80.
[107]Ebon, *The Truth about Vitamin E*, p. 80.
[108]Herbert Bailey, *Vitamin E, Your Key to a Healthy Heart* (New York: Arc Books 1971), pp. 97-98.
[109]Bailey, *Vitamin E, Your Key to a Healthy Heart*, p. 99.
[110]Wade, *The Rejuvenation Vitamin*, p. 85.
[111]Wade, *The Rejuvenation Vitamin*, p. 155.

Human Tests

1. Vitamin E and Menopause. A woman had undergone a complete hysterectomy due to cancer of an ovary. The patient suffered from hot flashes. She was given 75 IU of alpha tocopherol daily.

Results. Administration of the vitamin proved valuable in diminishing or entirely removing the hot flashes. (*Journal of the American Medical Association*, vol. 167, p. 1806, 1958, as reported in Rodale, *The Encyclopedia for Healthful Living*, p. 980.)

2. Vitamin E and Varicose Veins. 51 patients with varicose veins were given 300 to 500 milligrams of vitamin E daily. They were kept on this treatment from two months to three years, depending upon the severity of the ailment.

Results. 9 of the patients showed improvement within 30 days; 7 were completely healed; and the other 35 all showed some relief of congestion, pain, and edema. No side effects were noted. (*La Riforma Medical*, Vol. 69, pp. 853-856, 1955, as reported in Rodale, *The Encyclopedia for Healthful Living*, p. 978.)

3. Vitamin E and Menstrual Pain. 100 women between eighteen and twenty-one years of age were suffering from pain and discomfort during their menstrual periods. They were divided into two groups. Each woman in the first group was given 50 milligrams of vitamin E daily for ten days before menstruation and for the next four days. Each woman in the second group was given a placebo. Treatment lasted three months.

Results. 76 percent of the women in the first group noted improvement; only 29 percent of the women in the second group noted any improvement in three months. The patients experienced a recurrence of their pain two to six months after treatment ceased. (*The Lancet*, vol. I, pp. 844-847, 1955, as reported in Rodale, *The Encyclopedia for Healthful Living*, p. 988.)

4. Vitamin E and Coronary Occlusion (Blood Clot in the Coronary Artery). A forty-year-old male suffering from a coronary occlusion was treated with 60 IU of alpha tocopherol daily.

Results. The symptoms of angina (sense of suffocation) disappeared completely in four weeks. (Shute, *Vitamin E for Ailing and Healthy Hearts*, p. 39.)

5. Vitamin E and Athletic Performance. In a controlled study athletes were given large doses of alpha tocopherol.

Results. Their muscle performance, endurance, and speed of recovery improved. The effect was transient but persisted as long as the treatment was maintained. ("Resolving the Vitamin E Controversy," *Percival*, Summary 3.55, 1951.)

Animal Test

1. Vitamin E and Muscular Stamina in Racehorses. Dr. Evan Shute and William Gutterson devised an experiment with vitamin E and its effect on racehorses.

Results. The percentage of wins for each horse given vitamin E was 2.7, compared to 2.3 the year before, when a smaller dose of vitamin E was given. Two years before, when no vitamin E was given, the percentage of wins per horse had been 1.8. Although there was an improvement in the first year, the horses hit their peak the following year, when the dosages were doubled or tripled. (*The Summary*, December 1956, published by the Shute Foundation for Medical Research, London, Canada, as reported in Rodale, *The Encyclopedia for Healthful Living*, p. 777.)

VITAMIN E MAY BE BENEFICIAL FOR THE FOLLOWING AILMENTS:

Body Member	Ailment
Bladder	Cystitis
Blood/Circulatory system	Anemia
	Angina pectoris
	Arteriosclerosis
	Atherosclerosis
	Bruising
	Coronary thrombosis
	Diabetes
	Hypertension
	Pernicious anemia
	Phlebitis
	Stroke (cerebrovascular accident)
	Thrombophlebitis
	Varicose veins

Body Member	Ailment
Bones	Osteoporosis
Bowel	Colitis
Brain/Nervous system	Epilepsy
	Mental illness
	Multiple sclerosis
	Parkinson's disease
	Stroke (cerebrovascular accident)
Ear	Ménière's syndrome
Eye	Amblyopia
	Cataracts
	Eyestrain
Gallbladder	Gallstones
Glands	Cystic fibrosis
	Hyperthyroidism
	Prostatitis
Hair/Scalp	Baldness
	Dandruff
Head	Headache
	Sinusitis
Heart	Angina pectoris
	Arteriosclerosis
	Atherosclerosis
	Congestive heart failure
	Coronary thrombosis
	Hypertension
	Myocardial infarction
Intestine	Celiac disease
	Constipation
	Hemorrhoids
Joints	Arthritis
	Bursitis
	Gout
Kidney	Kidney stones (renal calculi)
	Nephritis
Leg	Leg cramp
	Phlebitis
	Sciatica
	Varicose veins
Lungs/Respiratory system	Allergies
	Bronchitis
	Common cold
	Emphysema
	Hay fever (allergic rhinitis)

Body Member	Ailment
Muscles	Muscular dystrophy
	Rheumatism
Reproductive system	Miscarriage
	Prostatitis
	Vaginitis
Skin	Abscess
	Acne
	Athlete's foot
	Bedsores
	Boil (furuncle)
	Bruises
	Burns
	Carbuncle
	Impetigo
	Ulcers
	Warts
Stomach	Gastritis
	Stomach ulcer (peptic)
General	Backache
	Cancer
	Measles
	Overweight and obesity
	Pregnancy
	Sunburn
	Thrombophlebitis

VITAMIN F (UNSATURATED FATTY ACIDS)

Description

Vitamin F is a fat-soluble vitamin consisting of the unsaturated fatty acids. Unsaturated fatty acids usually come in the form of liquid vegetable oils, while saturated fatty acids are usually found in solid animal fat. The saturated fatty acids are more slowly metabolized by the body than are the unsaturated fatty acids.

The body cannot manufacture the essential unsaturated fatty acids, linoleic, linolenic, and arachidonic, and they must be obtained from foods. Wheat germ; seeds; natural golden vegetable oils, such as safflower, soy, and corn; and cod-liver oil contain lecithin and are the best sources of the unsaturated fatty acids.

Unsaturated fatty acids are important for respiration

of vital organs and make it easier for oxygen to be transported by the bloodstream to all cells, tissues, and organs. They also help maintain resilience and lubrication of all cells and combine with protein and cholesterol to form living membranes that hold the body cells together.[112]

Vitamin F helps to regulate the rate of blood coagulation and performs a vital function in breaking up cholestrol deposited on arterial walls. It is essential for normal glandular activity, especially of the adrenal glands and the thyroid gland.[113] Vitamin F nourishes the skin cells and is essential for healthy mucous membranes and nerves.

The unsaturated fatty acids function in the body by cooperating with vitamin D in making calcium available to the tissues, assisting in the assimilation of phosphorus, and stimulating the conversion of carotene into vitamin A. Fatty acids are related to normal functioning of the reproductive system.

Absorption and Storage

The stomach, small intestine, and pancreas normally produce liberal amounts of fat-splitting digestive enzymes necessary for conversion of fats into fatty acids and glycerols (broken-down fatty acids). These are absorbed through the walls of the intestinal tract and are then transported through the portal vein to the liver, where they are usually metabolized as a source of energy. These changes must take place before the nutrients can enter the blood without causing food allergies.[114]

The digested fat is taken from the gastrointestinal tract as fatty acids and gylcerol. These then enter fat-collecting ducts that finally carry the fat to the lymphatic system, which is primarily concerned with collecting body fluids and returning them to the general circulatory system.[115] The fatty acids are stored in the adipose (containing massive amounts of fat cells) tissues.

Absorption of fat is decreased when there is increased movement in the gastrointestinal tract and when there is an absence of bile to break down the fat. X-ray treatments and radiation destroy the essential fatty acids within the body, although destruction can be prevented

if large doses of vitamin E are taken. Vitamin F is easily destroyed when exposed to air and may become rancid.

Dosage and Toxicity

The National Research Council states that the fat intake should include essential unsaturated fatty acids to the extent of at least 1 percent of the total calories.[116] The level of essential fatty acids needed by infants has been set at 3 percent of the total calories.[117] The need for essential fatty acids is usually met when 2 percent of the calories are produced by linoleic acid, which is found in food sources such as the vegetable oils of soy, corn, sunflower, and wheat germ.

Men usually need five times more saturated fatty acids than women do. A balance of twice as much unsaturated fatty acids as saturated fatty acids in the daily diet is beneficial for heart and arterial health. About four or five tablespoons of vegetable oils per day are needed to maintain this balance.

The need for linoleic acid increases in proportion to the amount of solids eaten. If the intake of saturated fats is high, a deficiency of linoleic acid can occur even though oils are included in the diet, and increased consumption of such foods as butter, cream, and saturated fat increases the need for vitamin F. Eating a great deal of carbohydrates also increases the need for unsaturated fatty acids. When there is sufficient linoleic acid in the diet, the other two essential fatty acids can be synthesized from it.

In order to get the full benefit of vitamin F, one should take vitamin E with it at mealtimes. This ensures the best absorption. In addition, it is important that as the amount of oils and fats is increased, the dosage of vitamin E is increased.

There are no known toxic effects of vitamin F; however, excessive amounts of saturated fats may cause metabolic disturbances and abnormal weight gain.

Deficiency Effects and Symptoms

A vitamin F deficiency causes changes to occur in the structure and enzyme function within the nucleus of the cells, resulting in a number of disorders. A deficiency may be responsible for brittle and lusterless hair, nail problems, dandruff, and allergic conditions.[118] In addi-

---

[112] Arthur W. Snyder, *Vitamins and Minerals* (Los Angeles: Hansens, 1969), p. 10.

[113] Airola, *How to Get Well*, p. 272.

[114] Davis, *Let's Get Well*, p. 171.

[115] Guthrie, *Introductory Nutrition*, p. 40.

[116] Rodale, *The Complete Book of Vitamins*, p, 410.

[117] Guthrie, *Introductory Nutrition*, p. 44.

[118] Rodale, *The Complete Book of Vitamins*, p. 411.

tion, diarrhea, varicose veins, underweight, and gall-stones may be a result of vitamin F deficiency. Skin disorders such as eczema, acne, and dry skin[119] have been linked with vitamin F deficiency; also ailments, such as diseases of the heart, circulatory system, and kidneys, associated with faulty fat metabolism. Without vitamin F, growth is retarded, teeth do not form properly, and prostaglandins, a group of fatty acids found in tissues of the prostrate gland, brain, kidney, and seminal and menstrual fluid, cannot be made by the cells.

Beneficial Effects on Ailments

Unsaturated fatty acids have been used to treat external ulcers, especially leg ulcers, with good results. The unsaturated fat preparation causes rapid granulation and regeneration of the skin.[120] It can also be used orally and externally for treating infantile eczema and the nonallergenic eczema that occurs in adolescents and adults. Psoriasis can benefit from treatment with unsaturated fatty acids. Arachidonic acid is effective in curing dermatitis.

Linoleic acid is effective in restoring growth. Hay fever has been successfully treated with vitamin F. It is also essential for the prevention and treatment of bronchial asthma and rheumatoid arthritis.

Vitamin F has been used in preventing heart disease. Vitamin F keeps cholesterol soft and prevents it from forming any hard deposits in the lumen of the blood vessels or under the skin.[121] This is especially important for the atherosclerosis patient. Because vitamin F lowers blood cholesterol, it helps prevent high blood pressure and hardening of the arteries.

Unsaturated fatty acids have helped prevent diarrhea and underweight. They have been useful in preventing prostate trouble and arthritis.[122] Any person who has gallbladder problems or has had one removed needs to take extra bile in the form of a food supplement so as to ensure proper breakdown of fats.

Human Tests

1. Unsaturated Fatty Acids and Prostate Glands. 19 cases of prostate gland disorders were treated with unsaturated fatty acids.

[119] Airola, *How to Get Well*, p. 272.
[120] Rodale, *The Health Seeker*, p. 732.
[121] Rodale, *Best Health Articles from* Prevention *Magazine*, p. 821.
[122] Rodale, *Best Health Articles from* Prevention *Magazine*, p. 205.

Results. All 19 cases had a lessening of residual urine, that is, the urine that cannot be released from the bladder due to pressure from the enlarged prostate gland. In 12 cases there was no residual urine at the end of treatment. There was also a decrease in leg pains, fatigue, kidney disorders, and excessive urination at night. (James P. Hart and William de Grande Cooper, *Lee Report*, No. 1, as reported in Rodale, *The Health Builder*, p. 352.)

2. Fatty Acids and Asthma. Two doctors observed the effects of a diet supplement plus fatty acids in patients suffering from asthma.

Results. 40 percent of the patients were either entirely relieved of asthmatic symptoms or noticed some improvement. The other 60 percent did not respond to treatment. (*The Journal of Applied Nutrition*, Spring 1955, as reported in Rodale, *The Health Builder*, p. 357.)

3. Unsaturated Fatty Acids and Eczema. 87 chronic eczema patients were treated daily with corn oil (rich in unsaturated fatty acids) for a period of over four and one-half years.

Results. Standard treatments had been used but not with the same success that corn oil had on the patients. All patients responded and showed improvement with the corn oil treatment. (Lee Foundation Report, February 1942, as reported in Rodale, *The Encyclopedia for Healthful Living*, p. 777.)

VITAMIN F MAY BE BENEFICIAL FOR THE FOLLOWING AILMENTS:

Body Member	Ailment
Blood/Circulatory system	Cholesterol level, high
	Diabetes
Bowel	Colitis
	Diarrhea
Brain/Nervous system	Mental illness
	Multiple sclerosis
Ear	Ménière's syndrome
Glands	Prostatitis
Heart	Coronary thrombosis
Intestine	Constipation
Joints	Arthritis

Body Member	Ailment
Legs	Leg cramp
Lungs/Respiratory system	Asthma
	Bronchitis
Skin	Acne
	Dermatitis
	Eczema
	Psoriasis
Teeth/Gums	Tooth and gum disorders
General	Allergies
	Common cold
	Overweight and obesity
	Underweight

VITAMIN K

Description

There are three main K vitamins: K_1 and K_2 are fat-soluble and can be manufactured in the intestinal tract in the presence of certain intestinal flora (bacteria); K_3 is produced synthetically for the treatment of patients who are unable to utilize naturally occurring vitamin K because they lack bile, an enzyme necessary for the absorption of all fat-soluble vitamins.

If yogurt, kefir (a preparation of curdled milk), or acidophilus milk (fermented milk used to change intestinal bacteria) is included in the diet, the body may be able to manufacture sufficient amounts of vitamin K. In addition, unsaturated fatty acids and a low-carbohydrate diet increase the amounts of vitamin K produced by intestinal flora.[123]

Vitamin K is necessary for the formation of prothrombin, a chemical required in blood clotting. Vitamin K is involved in a body process, phosphorylation, in which phosphate, when combined with glucose, is passed through the cell membranes and converted into glycogen, a form in which carbohydrates are stored in the body.[124] It is also vital for normal liver functioning and is an important vitality and longevity factor.

Some natural sources of vitamin K are kelp, alfalfa, green plants, and leafy green vegetables. Cow's milk, yogurt, egg yolks, blackstrap molasses, safflower oil, fish-liver oils, and other polyunsaturated oils are other good sources. The most dependable supply is the intestinal bacteria.

[123]Clark, *Know Your Nutrition*, p. 62.
[124]Guthrie, *Introductory Nutrition*, p. 216.

Vitamin K can be safely used as a preservative to control fermentation in foods. It has no bleaching effect, no unpleasant odor, and when added to naturally colored fruits, helps maintain a stable and effective condition of the food.

Absorption and Storage

Vitamin K is absorbed in the upper intestinal tract with the aid of bile or bile salts and is transported to the liver, where it is essential for synthesis of prothrombin and several related proteins involved in the clotting of blood. Vitamin K is stored in very small amounts, and considerable quantities are excreted after administration of therapeutic doses.

Factors interfering with absorption of vitamin K include any obstruction of the bile duct limiting the secretion of fat-emulsifying bile salts; failure of the liver to secrete bile;[125] and dicumarol, an anticoagulant that reduces the activity of prothrombin in the blood plasma.

Frozen foods, rancid fats, radiation, x-rays, aspirin, and industrial air pollution all destroy vitamin K. Excessive use of antibiotics can destroy the intestinal flora.[126] Ingestion of mineral oil will cause rapid excretion of vitamin K.

Dosage and Toxicity

The National Research Council states that the abundance of vitamin K in most diets, along with synthesis by the intestinal bacteria, provides adequate intake of vitamin K.[127] The newborn infant needs a daily intake of 1 to 5 milligrams to prevent hemorrhagic disease, which is abnormal bleeding.[128] It is estimated that the average daily intake is between 300 and 500 micrograms, which is considered an adequate supply of vitamin K.[129]

Therapeutic dosages of vitamin K are often given before and after operations to reduce blood losses. Vitamin K injections are sometimes given to women prior to labor to protect against hemorrhaging.

Excessive doses of synthetic vitamin K can cause toxic reactions because the supplements will build up in the blood. Toxicity brings about a form of anemia

[125]Guthrie, *Introductory Nutrition*, p. 216.
[126]Clark, *Know Your Nutrition*, p. 61.
[127]Krause and Hunscher, *Food, Nutrition and Diet Therapy*, p. 129.
[128]Guthrie, *Introductory Nutrition*, p. 216.
[129]Goodhart and Shils, *Modern Nutrition in Health and Disease*, p. 172.

that results in an increased breakdown in the red blood cells. In infants, kernicterus, a condition in which yellow pigment infiltrates the spinal cord and brain areas, can result, usually developing during the second to eighth days of life. Heinz bodies, or granules in the red blood cells resulting from damage to the hemoglobin molecules, are seen in infants suffering from an overdose. Toxicity has occurred when large dosages of synthetic vitamin K were injected into pregnant women. Flushing, sweating, and chest constrictions are symptoms of synthetic vitamin K toxicity. Natural vitamin K is stored in the body and produces no toxicity signs.

Deficiency Effects and Symptoms

Deficiencies of vitamin K usually result from inadequate absorption or the body's inability to utilize vitamin K in the liver.[130] Vitamin K deficiency is common in diseases such as celiac disease (intestinal malabsorption), sprue (malabsorption in adulthood), and colitis, which affect the absorbing mucosa of the small intestine and cause a rapid loss of intestinal contents. In such cases, intravenous administration of vitamin K may be needed.

In a deficiency, a condition of hypoprothrombinemia can occur, causing blood-clotting time to be greatly or even indefinitely prolonged. A deficiency can cause hemorrhages in any part of the body, including brain, spinal cord, and intestinal tract. A vitamin K deficiency can cause miscarriages and nosebleeds and can also be a factor in cellular disease and diarrhea.

Beneficial Effect on Ailments

Vitamin K is necessary to promote blood clotting, especially when jaundice is present. It is administered to heart patients who are using anticoagulant drugs to thin the consistency of their blood. Carefully measured doses of vitamin K are given to these patients to raise the prothrombin level slightly while not allowing it to completely counteract the effect of the anticoagulant.[131]

Vitamin K has proved beneficial in reducing the blood flow during prolonged menstruation, clots either diminish or disappear. It has often lessened or relieved menstrual cramps.

Vitamin K is frequently used with vitamin C in the prevention and improvement of hemorrhages in various

parts of the eye.[132] Vitamin K is also used to prevent hemorrhaging following gallbladder operations and to prevent cerebral palsy.[133]

VITAMIN K MAY BE BENEFICIAL FOR THE FOLLOWING AILMENTS:

Body Member	Ailment
Blood/Circulatory system	Bruising
	Hemorrhage
Gallbladder	Gallstones
Glands	Cystic fibrosis
Intestine	Celiac disease
	Worms
Liver	Cirrhosis of liver
	Jaundice
Skin	Ulcers
General	Aging
	Alcoholism
	Cancer
	Hepatitis
	Kwashiorkor

BIOFLAVONOIDS (VITAMIN P)

Description

Bioflavonoids, known as vitamin P, are water-soluble and are composed of a group of brightly colored substances that often appear in fruits and vegetables as companions to vitamin C. The components of the bioflavonoids are citrin, hesperidin, rutin, flavones, and flavonals.

Bioflavonoids were first discovered as a substance in the white segments, not in the juices, of citrus fruits. There is ten times the concentration of bioflavonoids in the edible part of the fruit that there is in the strained juice. Sources of bioflavonoids include lemons, grapes, plums, black currants, grapefruit, apricots, buckwheat, cherries, blackberries, and rose hips.

Bioflavonoids are essential for the proper absorption and use of vitamin C. They assist vitamin C in keeping collagen, the intercellular cement, in healthy condition. They are vital in their ability to increase the strength of the capillaries and to regulate their permeability.[134] These actions help prevent hemorrhages and ruptures in

[130] Krause and Hunscher, *Food, Nutrition and Diet Therapy*, p. 129.
[131] Rodale, *The Complete Book of Vitamins*, p. 439.
[132] Rodale, *The Health Builder*, p. 341.
[133] Clark, *Know Your Nutrition*, p. 61.
[134] Rodale, *The Health Builder*, p. 982.

the capillaries and connective tissues and build a protective barrier against infections.[135]

Absorption and Storage

The absorption and storage properties of bioflavonoids are very similar to those of vitamin C. The bioflavonoids are readily absorbed from the gastrointestinal tract into the bloodstream. Excessive amounts are excreted through urination and perspiration.

Dosage and Toxicity

There is no Recommended Dietary Allowance for this vitamin. Since bioflavonoids occur with vitamin C in natural food sources, synthetic vitamin C does not contain the bioflavonoids. When ingested together, bioflavonoids and C are more helpful than vitamin C taken alone.[136] Rutin, which comes from buckwheat leaves, is a good food source of bioflavonoids. Bioflavonoids are completely nontoxic.

Deficiency Effects and Symptoms

Symptoms of a bioflavonoid deficiency are closely related to those of a vitamin C deficiency. Especially noted is the increased tendency to bleed or hemorrhage and bruise easily. A deficiency of vitamins C and P may contribute to rheumatism and rheumatic fever.[137]

Beneficial Effect on Ailments

The body's utilization of vitamin C is increased when bioflavonoids are present. They are helpful in strengthening the capillaries and may help prevent colds and influenza. Bioflavonoids have proved to be beneficial in treating various degrees of capillary injury and have been found to minimize bruising that occurs in contact sports.[138]

Rutin is especially helpful in the prevention of recurrent bleeding arising from weakened blood vessels. It is sometimes used in the treatment of hemorrhoids and helps prevent the walls of the blood vessels from becoming fragile.

Bioflavonoids have been used successfully to treat ulcer patients and those suffering from dizziness caused by labyrinthitis, a disease of the inner ear. Weakness of the capillaries was found to be a major causative factor in both of these ailments.[139] Asthma has been successfully treated by the administration of bioflavonoids. Bioflavonoids have also been used as a protective agent against the harmful effects of x-rays.[140]

Bioflavonoids and vitamin C when taken together may help prevent habitual miscarriages. They are helpful in the treatment of disorders such as bleeding gums, eczema, and susceptibility to hemorrhaging. Rheumatism and rheumatic fever seem to be helped by vitamins C and P. The blood-vessel disorder of the eye which affects diabetics seems to respond to bioflavonoid–vitamin C treatment.[141] Administered together, these vitamins have also been beneficial in the treatment of muscular dystrophy because they help lower blood pressure moderately.

Human Tests

1. Bioflavonoids and Rheumatoid Arthritis. A fifty-two-year-old woman with rheumatoid arthritis in both hands, wrists, and elbows and in the right shoulder, knees, and ankles was given 3,000 milligrams of bioflavonoid complex.

Results. In seven days she "felt better." Two weeks later the pain had practically disappeared, her digestion was improved, and bowel action was normal. Her blood pressure dropped from 190 to 176, and by the end of five weeks she had more action in her joints and a great deal more endurance. (Dr. James R. West, Morrell Memorial Hospital, Lakeland, Florida, as reported in Rodale, *The Encyclopedia for Healthful Living*, p. 30.)

2. Bioflavonoids and Duodenal Ulcers. 36 cases of bleeding duodenal ulcers were treated with bioflavonoids and a diet consisting of an orange juice-milk-gelatin mixture given in doses of 4 to 6 ounces every two hours with bioflavonoid capsules, until bleeding was arrested. The bioflavonoid capsules were administered orally at the rate of three to nine capsules daily.

[135] Dr. Paavo Airola, *Are You Confused?* (Phoenix, Ariz.: Health Plus Pub., 1971), p. 164.
[136] Rodale, *The Health Builder*, p. 980.
[137] Rodale, *The Health Seeker*, p. 76.
[138] Rodale, *The Health Seeker*, p. 77.

[139] Rodale, *The Encyclopedia for Healthful Living*, p. 70.
[140] Airola, *Are You Confused?*, p. 161.
[141] Rodale, *The Health Seeker*, p. 76.

Results. All bleeding ceased on the fourth day. Then the patients were put on a bland diet. Vitamin supplements and bioflavonoid rations were added to the diet. All 36 patients responded with a return of mucous membrane and duodenal contour to a normal state. Total treatment took from 12 to 22 days. No recurrence of bleeding in two years or more occurred in 23 of the 36 cases. Twelve cases remained ulcer-free for one year or more, and the remaining cases were successfully treated and ulcer-free for four months. (Drs. Samuel Weiss, Jerome Weiss, and Bernard Weiss, *American Journal of Gastroenterology*, July 1958, as reported in Rodale, *The Encyclopedia for Healthful Living*, pp. 70-71.)

3. Bioflavonoids and Labyrinthitis (Disease of the Inner Ear). Nine cases were treated with four to six capsules of bioflavonoids daily with decreased salt intake.

Results. Positive results occurred in three to six days. The symptoms of dizziness, loss of balance, and nausea were successfully treated with no recurrence. (Dr. Theodore R. Miller, *Eye, Ear, Nose and Throat Monthly*, September 1958, as reported in Rodale, *The Encyclopedia for Healthful Living*, pp. 72-73.)

BIOFLAVONOIDS MAY BE BENEFICIAL FOR THE FOLLOWING AILMENTS:

Body Member	Ailment
Blood/Circulatory system	Arteriosclerosis
	Atherosclerosis
	Bruising
	Cholesterol level, high
	Hemophilia
	Hypertension
	Leukemia
	Stroke (cerebrovascular accident)
	Varicose veins
Heart	Arteriosclerosis
	Atherosclerosis
	Hypertension
	Hypoxia
Intestine	Hemorrhoids
Joints	Arthritis
	Rheumatic fever
	Rheumatism
Lungs/Respiratory system	Pneumonia
Skin	Ulcers
Teeth/Gums	Pyorrhea
	Scurvy
General	Common cold

VITAMIN T

Description

Vitamin T is often referred to as the "sesame seed factor." It reestablishes blood coagulation and is useful in correcting nutritional anemia. Vitamin T promotes the formation of blood platelets (round disks in the blood) and combats anemia and hemophilia, a hereditary blood disease characterized by prolonged coagulation time. It can also be useful in improving a fading memory.[142] Some natural sources of vitamin T are sesame seeds, raw sesame butter, and egg yolks.

VITAMIN U

Description

Vitamin U is a vitaminlike factor found in some vegetables. It promotes healing activity in peptic ulcers[143] and is particularly vital in healing duodenal ulcers. Important natural sources of vitamin U are raw cabbage juice, fresh cabbage, and homemade sauerkraut.[144]

MINERALS

ALUMINUM

Description

Aluminum is a trace mineral, but it can be dangerous, even fatal, if consumed in excessive amounts. There is no established function of aluminum in human nutri-

[142] Airola, *How to Get Well*, p. 273.
[143] Airola, *How to Get Well*, p. 273.
[144] Airola, *How to Get Well*, p. 273.

tion. It is found in many plant and animal foods. It is also an ingredient in the bases of false teeth, children's aspirin tablets, some baking powders, and some white flour.

Aluminum weakens the living tissue of the alimentary canal, the digestive tube from the mouth to the anus. Many of aluminum's harmful effects result from its destruction of vitamins. It binds with many other substances and is never found alone in nature.

Absorption and Storage

Aluminum is easily absorbed by the body and is accumulated in the arteries. Foods cooked in aluminum utensils may absorb minute quantities of the mineral.

Dosage and Toxicity

The total aluminum content of the adult body is from 50 to 150 milligrams. The daily amount ingested in the average diet ranges from 10 milligrams to more than 100 milligrams.

Excessive amounts of aluminum can result in symptoms of poisoning. These symptoms include constipation, colic, loss of appetite, nausea, skin ailments, twitching of leg muscles, excessive perspiration, and loss of energy. Patients with aluminum poisoning should discontinue the use of aluminum cookware. Doctors often recommend that the drinking of tap water be discontinued.

Small quantities of soluble salts of aluminum present in the blood cause a slow form of poisoning characterized by motor paralysis and areas of local numbness, with fatty degeneration of the kidney and liver.[145] There are also anatomical changes in the nerve centers and symptoms of gastrointestinal inflammation. These symptoms result from the body's effort to eliminate the poison.

Deficiency Effects and Symptoms

No available information.

Beneficial Effect on Ailments

No available information.

[145] Rodale, *Complete Book of Minerals for Health*, p. 387.

BERYLLIUM

Description

Beryllium is a mineral that has definite adverse effects on the human body. This mineral can deplete the body's store of magnesium, allowing disease to result. When beryllium is absorbed into the bloodstream, it often lodges in vital organs and keeps them from performing their functions. It interferes with a number of the body's enzyme systems.[146] It does not allow the enzyme system to carry on its function in the body.

Beryllium is used in neon signs, electronic devices, some alloys including steel, bicycle wheels, fishing rods, and many common household products.[147]

Beryllium is a dangerous substance in industrial toxicology. Beryllium dust makes breathing difficult. This condition may lead to injury of the lungs, causing scarring or fibrosis. Some victims of beryllium poisoning become completely disabled by serious lung destruction.

CADMIUM

Description

Cadmium is a toxic trace mineral that has many structural similarities to zinc. There is no biological function for this element in humans. Its toxic effects are kept under control in the body by the presence of zinc.

Refining processes disturb the important cadmium-zinc balance. In whole wheat, cadmium is present in proportion to zinc in a ratio of 1 to 120.

Cadmium is found primarily in refined foods such as flour, rice, and white sugar. It is present in the air as an industrial contaminant. In addition, soft water usually contains higher levels of cadmium than does hard water. Coffee and tea also contain high levels of cadmium; drinking about five cups of either per day doubles the average daily intake of cadmium.

Absorption and Storage

The liver and kidneys are storage areas for both cadmium and zinc. The total body concentration of cadmium increases with age and varies in different areas of the world.

[146] Rodale, *Complete Book of Minerals for Health*, p. 405.
[147] Rodale, *Complete Book of Minerals for Health*, p. 408.

When a deficit of zinc occurs in the diet, the body may make it up by storing cadmium instead. If the daily intake of zinc is high, zinc will be stored and cadmium will be excreted.

Dosage and Toxicity

Daily intakes of cadmium have been estimated at 0.2 to 0.5 milligram, with considerable variation according to sources and types of food.[148] Cadmium's toxic effects may stem from its being stored for use in the body in place of zinc when the proportion between the two metals is unfavorably out of balance.[149] Zinc is a natural antagonist to cadmium.

Dr. Henry A. Shroeder, a trace mineral researcher, has developed a theory about cadmium being a major causative factor in hypertension and related heart ailments.[150] Testing his theories on rats because of their biological similarity to humans, Dr. Schroeder found that regular high doses of cadmium caused increased tension. When he stopped administering the cadmium to the rats, they returned to normotension.

In humans, the urine of hypertensive patients contains up to 40 percent more cadmium than does the urine of normotensive persons. These findings may lend credibility to the theory that excessive cadmium can directly lead to hypertension.[151]

Deficiency Effects and Symptoms

No available information.

Beneficial Effect on Ailments

No available information.

CALCIUM

Description

Calcium is the most abundant mineral in the body. About 99 percent of the calcium in the body is deposited in the bones and teeth, and the remainder is in the soft tissues. The ratio of calcium to phosphorus in the bones is 2.5 to 1. To function properly, calcium must be accompanied by magnesium, phosphorus, and vitamins A, C, and D.

The major function of calcium is to act in cooperation with phosphorus to build and maintain bones and teeth. It is essential for healthy blood, eases insomnia, and helps regulate the heartbeat. An important calcium partner in cardiovascular health is magnesium.

In addition, calcium assists in the process of blood clotting and helps prevent the accumulation of too much acid or too much alkali in the blood. It also plays a part in muscle growth, muscle contraction, and nerve transmission. Calcium aids in the body's utilization of iron, helps activate several enzymes (catalysts important for metabolism), and helps regulate the passage of nutrients in and out of the cell walls.

Calcium is present in significant amounts in a very limited number of foods. Milk and dairy products are dependable sources. The most common supplemental source is bone meal; it is well absorbed and utilized by most people. Those who are unable to use bone meal may use calcium gluconate or calcium lactate, natural derivatives of calcium which are even easier to absorb than is bone meal.

Absorption and Storage

Calcium absorption is very inefficient, and usually only 20 to 30 percent of ingested calcium is absorbed. Unabsorbed calcium is excreted in the feces. Absorption takes place in the duodenum and ceases in the lower part of the intestinal tract when the food content becomes alkaline. The amount absorbed depends largely on the diet, for unless calcium is in a water-soluble form in the intestine, it will not be absorbed properly.

Many other factors influence the actual amount of calcium absorbed. When in need, the body absorbs calcium more effectively; therefore the greater the need and the smaller the dietary supply, the more efficient the absorption. Absorption is also increased during periods of rapid growth.[152]

Calcium needs acid for proper assimilation. If acid in some form is not present in the body, calcium is not dissolved and therefore cannot be used as needed by the body. Instead it can build up in tissues or joints as calcium deposits, leading to a variety of disturbances.

[148] National Academy of Sciences, *Toxicants Occurring Naturally in Foods*, p. 64.
[149] Rodale, *Complete Book of Minerals for Health*, p. 410.
[150] Rodale, *Complete Book of Minerals for Health*, p. 413.
[151] Rodale, *Complete Book of Minerals for Health*, p. 277.

[152] Krause and Hunscher, *Food, Nutrition and Diet Therapy*, p. 102.

Calcium absorption also depends upon the presence of adequate amounts of vitamin D, which works with the parathyroid hormone to regulate the amount of calcium in the blood. Phosphorus is needed in at least the same amount as calcium. Vitamins A and C are necessary for calcium absorption. Fat content in moderate amounts, moving slowly through the digestive tract, helps facilitate absorption. A high intake of protein also aids in the absorption of calcium.

Certain substances interfere with the absorption of calcium. When excessive amounts of fat combine with calcium, an insoluble compound is formed which cannot be absorbed. Oxalic acid, found in chocolate, spinach, and rhubarb, when combined with calcium makes another insoluble compound and may form into stones in the kidney or gallbladder. Large amounts of phytic acid, present in cereals and grains, may inhibit the absorption of calcium by the body. Other interfering factors include lack of exercise, excessive stress, and too rapid a flow of food through the intestinal tract.

Dosage and Toxicity

The National Research Council recommends 800 milligrams as a daily calcium intake; since only 20 to 30 percent is absorbed, 800 milligrams would maintain the necessary balance.[153] During pregnancy and lactation, this amount increases to 1,200 milligrams. With age, it seems the requirement also increases because the rate of absorption is reduced. If the calcium intake is high, the magnesium levels also need to be high.

A high intake of calcium and vitamin D is a potential source of hypercalcemia. This condition may result in excessive calcification of the bones and some tissues, such as the kidney's.

Deficiency Effects and Symptoms

One of the first signs of a calcium deficiency is a nervous affliction, tetany, characterized by muscle cramps and numbness and tingling in the arms and legs. A calcium deficiency can result in bone malformation, causing rickets in children and osteomalacia in adults. Another calcium deficiency ailment is osteoporosis, in which the bones become porous and fragile because calcium is withdrawn from the bones and other body areas faster than it is deposited in them.

Moderate cases of calcium deficiency may lead to cramps, joint pains, heart palpitation, slow pulse rates, tooth decay, insomnia, impaired growth, and excessive irritability of nerves and muscles. In extreme cases of deficiency, brittle or porous bone and tooth formation, slow blood clotting, or hemorrhaging may result.

Beneficial Effect on Ailments

Calcium has been successfully used in the treatment of osteoporosis. The hormones involved are stimulated by the concentration of calcium ions in the blood. Calcium is a natural tranquilizer and tends to calm the nerves.

Calcium has been beneficial in the treatment of cardiovascular disorders. In addition, calcium is a recognized aid for cramps in the feet or legs. It also helps patients suffering from "growing pains."

Calcium has been used in the treatment and prevention of sunburn. In addition to giving protection against effects of sun damage such as redness and subsequent peeling, it also protects against sun-caused skin cancers.[154] Calcium helps the skin to remain healthy. Vitamin A and calcium are a good combination for protection of the skin. This combination can also be used as a neutralizing agent against the poison of a black widow spider or a bee sting.

Arthritis, structural rigidity often caused by depletion of bone calcium, can be helped with regular supplements of bone meal. Early consumption of bone meal may help prevent arthritis. Rheumatism can also be treated successfully with calcium therapy.

Problems of menopause, such as nervousness, irritability, insomnia, and headaches, have been overcome with administration of calcium, magnesium, and vitamin D.[155] When there is not enough calcium in the body to be absorbed, the output of estrogen decreases. Calcium can help prevent premenstrual tension and menstrual cramps.

High intakes of calcium may relieve the symptoms commonly associated with aging. Some of the disorders include bone pain, backaches, insomnia, brittle teeth with cavities, and tremors of the fingers.[156]

The parathyroid glands located in the neck help adjust the body's storage of calcium. If these glands are not functioning properly, calcium accumulation may occur. The remedy for this situation is to renew the

[153] Krause and Hunscher, *Food, Nutrition and Diet Therapy*, p. 102.

[154] Rodale, *Complete Book of Minerals for Health*, p. 37.
[155] Rodale, *Complete Book of Minerals for Health*, p. 37.
[156] Davis, *Let's Get Well*, p. 309.

proper function of the parathyroid glands rather than to cut down on calcium intake.[157]

Calcium treatments have been used successfully in treating rickets in children and osteomalacia in adults. In addition, nephritis has been cleared up with administration of calcium and other nutrients. Tooth and gum disorders are also relieved by higher intakes of calcium in the diet. A high dietary intake of calcium may protect against the harmful effects of radioactive strontium 90.

CALCIUM MAY BE BENEFICIAL FOR THE FOLLOWING AILMENTS:

Body Member	Ailment
Blood/Circulatory system	Anemia
	Diabetes
	Hemophilia
	Pernicious anemia
Bones	Fracture
	Osteomalacia
	Osteoporosis
	Rickets
Bowel	Colitis
	Diarrhea
Brain/Nervous system	Dizziness
	Epilepsy
	Insomnia
	Mental illness
	Parkinson's disease
Ear	Ménière's syndrome
Eye	Cataracts
Head	Fever
Heart	Arteriosclerosis
	Atherosclerosis
	Hypertension
Intestine	Celiac disease
	Constipation
	Hemorrhoids
	Worms
Joints	Arthritis
Kidney	Nephritis
Leg	Leg cramp
Lungs/Respiratory system	Allergies
	Common cold
	Tuberculosis

Body Member	Ailment
Muscles	General muscle cramps
	Tetany
Nails	Nail problems
Skin	Acne
Stomach	Stomach ulcer (peptic)
Teeth/Gums	Pyorrhea
	Tooth and gum disorders
General	Aging
	Fever
	Overweight and Obesity
	Sunburn

CHLORINE

Description

Chlorine is an essential mineral, occurring in the body mainly in compound form with sodium or potassium. It is widely distributed throughout the body in the form of chloride in amounts less than 15 percent of the total body weight.[158] Chlorine compounds such as sodium chloride, or salt, are found primarily within the cells.

Chlorine helps regulate the correct balance of acid and alkali in the blood and maintains pressure that causes fluids to pass in and out of cell membranes until the concentration of dissolved particles is equalized on both sides. It stimulates production of hydrochloric acid, an enzymatic juice needed in the stomach for digestion of tough, fibrous foods.

Chlorine stimulates the liver to function as a filter for wastes and helps clean toxic waste products out of the system.[159] It aids in keeping joints and tendons in youthful shape, and it helps to distribute hormones. Chlorine is sometimes added to water for purification purposes because it destroys waterborne diseases such as typhoid and hepatitis.

Chlorine in the diet is provided almost exclusively by sodium chloride, or table salt. It is also found in kelp, dulse, rye flour, ripe olives, and sea greens.

Absorption and Storage

Chlorine is absorbed in the intestine and excreted through urination and perspiration. The highest body

[157]Rodale, *Best Health Articles from* Prevention *Magazine,* p. 598.

[158]Guthrie, *Introductory Nutrition,* p. 132.

[159]Carlson Wade, *Magic Minerals: Key to Better Health* (West Nyack, N.Y.: Parker, 1967), p. 26.

concentrations are stored in the cerebrospinal fluid and in the secretions of the gastrointestinal tract. Muscle and nerve tissues are relatively low in chloride.[160] Excess chlorine is excreted; additional loss may be caused by conditions such as vomiting, diarrhea, or sweating.

There has been much controversy over the relative merits of adding chlorine to drinking water supplies because it is a highly reactive chemical and may join with inorganic minerals and other chemicals to form possibly harmful substances. It is known that chlorine in the drinking water destroys vitamin E. It also destroys many of the intestinal flora that help in the digestion of food.

Dosage and Toxicity

There is no Recommended Dietary Allowance for chlorine because the average person's salt intake is high and usually provides between 3 and 9 grams daily. Diets sufficient in sodium and potassium provide adequate chlorine. Daily intake of 14 to 28 grams of salt is considered excessive.[161]

Deficiency Effects and Symptoms

A deficiency of chlorine can cause hair and tooth loss, poor muscular contraction, and impaired digestion.[162]

Beneficial Effect on Ailments

Chlorine is beneficial in treating diarrhea and vomiting.

CHLORINE MAY BE BENEFICIAL FOR THE FOLLOWING AILMENTS:

Body Member	Ailment
Bowel	Diarrhea
Stomach	Vomiting

CHROMIUM

Description

Chromium is an essential mineral found in concentrations of 20 parts of chromium per 1 billion parts of blood.[163] It has functions in both animal and human nutrition.

Chromium stimulates the activity of enzymes involved in the metabolism of glucose for energy and the synthesis of fatty acids and cholesterol. Chromium also appears to increase the effectiveness of insulin, thereby facilitating the transport of glucose into the cell. In the blood it competes with iron in the transport of protein. Chromium may also be involved in the synthesis of protein through its binding action with RNA molecules.

Sources of chromium include corn oil, clams, whole-grain cereals, and meats. Fruits and vegetables contain trace amounts. Brewer's yeast provides a dependable supply without the problems of high carbohydrate intake and high cholesterol levels.

Absorption and Storage

Chromium is difficult to absorb. Only about three percent of dietary chromium is retained in the body.[164] The mineral is stored primarily in the spleen, kidneys, and testes; small amounts are also stored in the heart, pancreas, lungs, and brain. Chromium has been found in some enzymes and in RNA.[165] Excretion occurs mainly through urination, with minor amounts lost in the feces. The amount of chromium stored in the body decreases with age.

Dosage and Toxicity

There is no Recommended Dietary Allowance for chromium. The daily chromium intake of humans is estimated to range from 80 to 100 micrograms.[166]

Deficiency Effects and Symptoms

Even a very slight chromium deficiency will have serious effects on the body.[167] Tests indicate systematic deficiency of chromium to be common in the United States, although it rarely occurs in other countries. Americans tend to be deficient because their soil does not contain an adequate supply and thus chromium cannot be absorbed by the crops or reach the water supply. The refining of natural carbohydrates is another probable cause of chromium loss.

---

[160] Guthrie, *Introductory Nutrition*, p. 132.
[161] National Academy of Sciences, *Toxicants Occurring Naturally in Foods*, p. 30.
[162] Wade, *Magic Minerals: Key to Better Health*, p. 26.

[163] Rodale, *Complete Book of Minerals for Health*, p. 171.
[164] Guthrie, *Introductory Nutrition*, p. 166.
[165] Chaney and Ross, *Nutrition*, p. 172.
[166] Krause and Hunscher, *Food, Nutrition and Diet Therapy*, p. 118.
[167] Rodale, *Complete Book of Minerals for Health*, p. 171.

A chromium deficiency may be a factor that will upset the function of insulin and result in depressed growth rates and severe glucose intolerance in diabetics. It is also believed that the interaction of chromium and insulin is not limited to glucose metabolism but also applies to amino acid metabolism.[168] Chromium may inhibit the formation of aortic plaques, and a deficiency may contribute to atherosclerosis.

Beneficial Effect on Ailments

Chromium helps to regulate sugar levels in the blood. Infants suffering from kwashiorkor have benefited from oral administration of chromium.

CHROMIUM MAY BE BENEFICIAL FOR THE FOLLOWING AILMENTS:

Body Member	Ailment
Blood/Circulatory system	Diabetes
General	Kwashiorkor

COBALT

Description

Cobalt is considered an essential mineral and is an integral part of vitamin B_{12}, or cobalamin. Vitamin B_{12} and cobalt are so closely connected that the two terms can be used interchangeably.

Cobalt activates a number of enzymes in the body. It is necessary for normal functioning and maintenance of red blood cells as well as all other body cells.

The body does not have the ability to synthesize cobalt and must depend on animal sources for an adequate supply of this nutrient.[169] For this reason, strict vegetarians are more susceptible to cobalt deficiency than are meat eaters. The best food sources are meats, especially liver and kidney, oysters, clams, and milk. Cobalt is present in ocean and sea vegetation but is lacking in almost all land green foods, although cobalt-enriched soil can yield minute amounts.

Absorption and Storage

Cobalt is not easily assimilated, and most of it passes through the intestinal tract unabsorbed. Most of what is absorbed is excreted in the urine after being used by the body. Cobalt is stored in the red blood cells and plasma; some storage occurs also in the liver, kidneys, pancreas, and spleen.[170]

Dosage and Toxicity

There is no Recommended Dietary Allowance for cobalt because the dietary need for it is low and can be supplied in protein foods. The average daily intake of cobalt is 5 to 8 micrograms.

There is evidence that high intakes of cobalt may result in an enlarged thyroid gland. Reduction in the cobalt intake should allow an enlarged thyroid to return to normal size.

Deficiency Effects and Symptoms

A deficiency of cobalt may be responsible for the symptoms of pernicious anemia and a slow rate of growth. If cobalt deficiency is not treated, permanent nervous disorders may result.[171]

Beneficial Effect on Ailments

Therapeutic doses of cobalt have been beneficial in the treatment of pernicious anemia. This action is attributed to cobalt's importance as a builder of red blood cells.

COBALT MAY BE BENEFICIAL FOR THE FOLLOWING AILMENTS:

Body Member	Ailment
Blood/Circulatory system	Pernicious anemia

COPPER

Description

Copper is a trace mineral found in all body tissues. Copper assists in the formation of hemoglobin and red blood cells by facilitating iron absorption.

---

[168] Chaney and Ross, *Nutrition*, p. 173.
[169] Guthrie, *Introductory Nutrition*, p. 166.

[170] Chaney and Ross, *Nutrition*, p. 188.
[171] Rodale, *Complete Book of Minerals For Health*, p. 187.

Copper is present in many enzymes that break down or build up body tissue. It aids in the conversion of the amino acid tyrosine into a dark pigment that colors the hair and skin. It is also involved in protein metabolism and in healing processes. Copper is required for the synthesis of phospholipids, substances essential in the formation of the protective myelin sheaths surrounding nerve fibers. Copper helps the body to oxidize vitamin C and works with this vitamin in the formation of elastin, a chief component of the elastic muscle fibers throughout the body. Copper is necessary for proper bone formation and maintenance. It is also necessary for the production of RNA.

Among the best food sources of copper are liver, whole-grain products, almonds, green leafy vegetables, and dried legumes. The amounts vary in plant sources, according to the mineral content in the soil in which they were grown. Most seafoods are also good sources of copper.

Absorption and Storage

Approximately 30 percent of ingested copper is used by the body; absorption takes place in the stomach and upper intestine. The copper moves from the intestine into the bloodstream 15 minutes after ingestion. Most of the dietary copper is excreted in the feces and bile, with very little lost in the urine.

Copper is stored in the tissues; highest concentrations of copper are in the liver, kidneys, heart, and brain. Bones and muscles have lower concentrations of copper, but because of their mass, they contain over 50 percent of the total copper in the body.[172]

Dosage and Toxicity

The National Research Council recommends a daily dietary intake of 2 milligrams of copper for adults. The average person ingests 2.5 to 5.0 milligrams per day. Toxicity is rare, since only a small amount of copper is absorbed and stored while the greatest part is excreted. However, the possibility of copper toxicity occurs with Wilson's disease, a rare genetic disorder that results from abnormal copper metabolism, bringing about excess copper retention in the liver, brain, kidney, and corneas of the eyes.[173]

[172]Krause and Hunscher, *Food, Nutrition and Diet Therapy*, p. 114.
[173]Guthrie, *Introductory Nutrition*, p. 165.

Deficiency Effects and Symptoms

Although copper deficiencies are relatively unknown, low blood levels of copper have been noted in children with iron-deficiency anemia, edema, and kwashiorkor. Symptoms of deficiency include general weakness, impaired respiration, and skin sores.[174]

Beneficial Effect on Ailments

Copper works with iron to form hemoglobin, thereby helping in the treatment of anemia. Copper is beneficial in the prevention and treatment of edema and kwashiorkor in children.

COPPER MAY BE BENEFICIAL FOR THE FOLLOWING AILMENTS:

Body Member	Ailment
Blood/Circulatory system	Anemia
	Leukemia
Bones	Osteoporosis
Hair	Baldness
Skin	Bedsores
General	Edema

FLUORINE (FLUORIDES)

Description

Fluorine is an essential trace mineral that is present in minute amounts in nearly every human tissue but is found primarily in the skeleton and teeth. Fluorine occurs in the body in compounds called fluorides. There are two types of fluorides: sodium fluoride is added to drinking water and is not the same as calcium fluoride, which is found in nature.

Recent research indicates that fluorine increases the deposition of calcium, thereby strengthening the bones. Fluorine also helps to reduce the formation of acid in the mouth caused by carbohydrates, thereby reducing the likelihood of decayed tooth enamel.[175] Although traces of fluorine are beneficial to the body, excessive amounts are definitely harmful. Fluorine can destroy the enzyme phosphotase, which is vital to many body processes including the metabolism of vitamins. Fluorine inhibits the activities of other important enzymes and

[174]Wade, *Magic Minerals: Key to Health*, p. 24.
[175]Guthrie, *Introductory Nutrition*, p. 170.

appears to be especially antagonistic towards brain tissues.

Fluoridated water supplies are by far the most common source of this mineral, although this form (sodium fluoride) may be toxic. Toxic levels occur when the content of fluorine in drinking water exceeds 2 parts per million. Calcium is an antidote for fluoride poisoning. Other rich sources of fluorine include seafoods and gelatin. The fluorine content in plant foods varies according to environmental conditions such as type of soil, intensity of prevailing winds, and use of fertilizers and sprays that contain fluorine.

Absorption and Storage

Fluorine is absorbed primarily in the intestine, although some may be taken up by the stomach. About 90 percent of ingested fluorine appears in the bloodstream.[176] Half of this is excreted in the urine, and the other half is readily absorbed by the teeth and bones.

Substances interfering with absorption include aluminum salts of fluorine and insoluble calcium.

Dosage and Toxicity

An average diet will provide 0.25 to 0.35 milligram of fluorine daily. In addition, the average adult may ingest 1.0 to 1.5 milligrams from drinking and cooking water containing 1 part per million (ppm) of fluorine. Dental fluorosis may occur at fluoride concentrations of 2 to 8 ppm; osteosclerosis, at 8 to 20 ppm.[177] Higher levels can depress growth, cause calcification of the ligaments and tendons, and bring about degenerative changes in the kidneys, liver, adrenal glands, heart, central nervous system, and finally the reproductive organs. Fatal poisoning can occur at 50 ppm, or 2,500 times the recommended level.[178] There are some areas in the United States where fluorine levels in the water are high and tooth mottling (enamel discoloration) is epidemic, and there are other areas where fluorine is not added to the water and dental decay is high.

Dr. Ionel Rapaport, a University of Wisconsin researcher, suggests that there is a direct relationship between the incidence of mongolism and fluoridated drinking water.[179] Higher than average incidences of

mongolism have been noted in areas where mottled teeth indicate an excess concentration of fluorides in the water.[180]

Deficiency Effects and Symptoms

A diet deficient in fluorine may lead to poor tooth development and subsequent dental caries. Fluorine deficiencies are unusual in the American diet.

Beneficial Effect on Ailments

Fluorides have been used in the treatment and prevention of osteoporosis and dental caries.

FLUORINE MAY BE BENEFICIAL FOR THE FOLLOWING AILMENTS:

Body Member	Ailment
Bones	Osteoporosis
Teeth/Gums	Tooth decay
	Tooth and gum disorders

IODINE (IODIDE)

Description

Iodine is a trace mineral most of which is converted into iodide in the body. Iodine aids in the development and functioning of the thyroid gland and is an integral part of thyroxine, a principal hormone produced by the thyroid gland. It is estimated that the body contains 25 milligrams of iodine, about 0.0004 percent of the total weight.[181]

Iodine plays an important role in regulating the body's production of energy, promotes growth and development, and stimulates the rate of metabolism, helping the body burn excess fat. Mentality; speech; and the condition of hair, nails, skin, and teeth are dependent upon a well-functioning thyroid gland.[182] The conversion of carotene to vitamin A, the synthesis of protein by ribosomes, and the absorption of carbohydrates from the intestine all work more efficiently when thyroxine production is normal.[183] The synthesis of cholesterol is stimulated by thyroxine levels.

[176] Guthrie, *Introductory Nutrition*, p. 170.
[177] Krause and Hunscher, *Food, Nutrition and Diet Therapy*, p. 115.
[178] Guthrie, *Introductory Nutrition*, p. 171.
[179] Rodale, *Complete Book of Minerals for Health*, pp. 367–370.
[180] Rodale, *Complete Book of Minerals for Health*, pp. 367-370.
[181] Chaney and Ross, *Nutrition*, p. 158.
[182] Rodale, *Complete Book of Minerals for Health*, p. 204.
[183] Gunthrie, *Introductory Nutrition*, p. 151.

Both types of sea life, plant and animal, absorb iodine from seawater and are excellent sources of this mineral. Mushrooms and Irish moss are good sources, too, but only if they are grown in soil rich in iodine.

Absorption and Storage

Iodine is readily absorbed from the gastrointestinal tract and is transported via the bloodstream to the thyroid gland, where it is oxidized and converted into thyroxine.[184] About 30 percent of the iodide in the blood is absorbed by the thyroid gland; the rest is absorbed by the kidneys and excreted in the urine.

Dosage and Toxicity

The National Research Council has suggested that an intake of 1 microgram of iodine per kilogram of body weight is adequate for most adults.[185] They recommend a daily intake of 130 micrograms for men and 100 micrograms for women, 125 micrograms during pregnancy, and 150 micrograms during lactation.

There have been no reported cases of toxicity resulting from too much iodine as it naturally occurs in food or water. However, iodine prepared as a drug or medicine must be carefully prescribed, because an overdose can be serious.[186] Sudden large doses of iodine administered to humans with a normal thyroid may impair the synthesis of thyroid hormones. For individuals on low-salt therapeutic diets, iodine supplements may be desirable.

Deficiency Effects and Symptoms

An iodine deficiency results in simple goiter characterized by thyroid enlargement and hypothyroidism (an abnormally low rate of secretion of thyroid hormones, including thyroxine).

Iodine deficiency may lead to hardening of the arteries, obesity, sluggish metabolism, slowed mental reactions, dry hair, rapid pulse, heart palpitation, tremor, nervousness, restlessness, and irritability. An iodine deficiency may also result in cretinism, which is a congenital disease characterized by physical and mental retardation in children born to mothers who have had a limited iodine intake during adolescence and pregnancy. Polio has also been associated with iodine deficiency. The higher rate of occurrence of polio cases in the summer may be caused in part by higher losses of iodine through perspiration.[187]

An iodine deficiency may be caused by certain compounds present in some raw foods, such as cabbage and nuts, which may interfere with the utilization of iodine in thyroid-hormone production. This will not occur unless excessive amounts of these raw foods are eaten and the intake of iodine is low to begin with.

Beneficial Effect on Ailments

Iodine therapy has been used successfully in the treatment and prevention of simple goiter.

Hardening of the arteries occurs when a disturbance in normal fat metabolism allows cholesterol to collect in the arteries instead of being used or expelled. Iodine is needed to prevent this metabolic malfunction. Sufficient dietary iodine will also reduce the danger of radioactive iodine collecting in the thyroid gland.

Iodine is beneficial to children suffering from cretinism, if treatment is started soon after birth. Many of the symptoms are reversible, but if conditions persist beyond childbirth, the mental and physical retardation will be permanent.

IODINE MAY BE BENEFICIAL FOR THE FOLLOWING AILMENTS:

Body Member	Ailment
Blood/Circulatory system	Angina pectoris
Hair	Hair problems
Heart	Arteriosclerosis
	Atherosclerosis
Joints	Arthritis
Thyroid	Goiter
	Hyperthyroidism
	Hypothyroidism
General	Cretinism
	Loss of physical and mental vigor

---

[184] Krause and Hunscher, *Food, Nutrition and Diet Therapy*, p. 116.
[185] Guthrie, *Introductory Nutrition*, p. 152.
[186] Rodale, *Complete Book of Minerals for Health*, p. 215.
[187] Rodale, *Complete Book of Minerals for Health*, p. 207.

IRON

Description

Iron is a mineral concentrate in the blood which is present in every living cell. All iron exists in the body combined with protein.

The major function of iron is to combine with protein and copper in making hemoglobin, the coloring matter of red blood cells. Hemoglobin transports oxygen in the blood from the lungs to the tissues, which need oxygen to maintain the basic life functions. Thus iron builds up the quality of the blood and increases resistance to stress and disease. Iron is also necessary for the formation of myoglobin, which is found only in muscle tissue. Myoglobin is also a transporter of oxygen; it supplies oxygen to the muscle cells for use in the chemical reaction that results in muscle contraction.

Iron is present in enzymes that promote protein metabolism, and it works with other nutrients to improve respiratory action. Calcium and copper must be present for iron to function properly.

The best source of dietary iron is liver, with oysters, heart, lean meat, and tongue as second choices. Leafy green vegetables are the best plant sources.

Absorption and Storage

The body can utilize either ferric or ferrous iron, but evidence indicates that naturally occurring ferrous iron is used more efficiently and that most iron is reduced to ferrous iron before being absorbed.[188] It is absorbed from food in regulated amounts into the blood and bone marrow. Absorption occurs in the upper part of the small intestines. Iron is usually absorbed within four hours after ingestion; from 2 to 4 percent of the iron found in the food is used by the body. It is primarily stored in the liver, spleen, bone marrow, and blood.

The iron in the body is normally used efficiently. It is neither used up nor destroyed, but it is conserved to be used repeatedly. Only very small amounts are normally excreted from the body. Virtually no iron is excreted in the urine, but unabsorbed iron is detected in the feces.

There are many factors that influence the absorption of iron. Ascorbic acid enhances absorption by helping reduce ferric to ferrous iron. Vitamin E also aids in the assimilation of iron. The iron found in animal protein is more readily absorbed than the iron in vegetables. The degree of gastric acidity regulates the solubility and availability of the iron in food.[189]

The balance of calcium, phosphorus, and iron is very important. Excess phosphorus hinders iron absorption, although if calcium is present in sufficient amounts, it will combine with the phosphates and free the iron for use. In addition, the lack of hydrochloric acid; the administration of alkalis; a high intake of cellulose, coffee, and tea; the presence of insoluble iron complexes (phytates, oxalates, and phosphates); and increased intestinal mobility all interfere with iron absorption.[190]

Dosage and Toxicity

The National Research Council suggests a daily iron intake of 18 milligrams for women and 10 milligrams for men. The need for iron increases during menstruation, hemorrhage, periods of rapid growth, or whenever there is a loss of blood. Additional iron is required during pregnancy, when the developing fetus builds up his own reserve supply of iron in the liver.

A toxic level of iron may occur in an individual due to a genetic error of metabolism, due to blood transfusion, or due to a prolonged oral intake of iron. Excessive deposits of iron in the liver and spleen, in certain individuals, may result from such conditions as cirrhosis of the liver, diabetes, and pancreas insufficiency.[191]

Deficiency Effects and Symptoms

The most common deficiency of iron is iron-deficiency anemia (hypochromic anemia), in which the amount of hemoglobin in the red blood cells is reduced and the cells consequently become smaller. As in other forms of anemia, iron-deficiency anemia reduces the oxygen-carrying capacity of the blood, resulting in pale skin and abnormal fatigue. Symptoms of anemia may include constipation, lusterless, brittle nails, and difficult breathing.

---

[188] Guthrie, *Introductory Nutrition*, p. 140.

[189] Krause and Hunscher, *Food, Nutrition and Diet Therapy*, p. 106.
[190] Krause and Hunscher, *Food, Nutrition and Diet Therapy*, p. 106.
[191] Goodhart and Shils, *Modern Nutrition in Health and Disease*, pp. 320-321.

Hemorrhagic anemia, marked by internal hemorrhaging, may not be detected for some time, especially when associated with the bleeding that may occur in peptic ulcers.[192] Excessive donation of blood may cause this type of anemia.

Infections and peptic ulcers may also lead to anemia.

Beneficial Effect on Ailments

When iron-deficiency anemia, with its symptoms of pallor, easy fatigue and decreased resistance to disease, is diagnosed, a diet high in iron-rich foods with a concurrent intake of vitamin C will speed up the restoration of hemoglobin levels to normal. Pernicious anemia is successfully treated with therapeutic doses of organic and inorganic iron salts.

Iron is the most important mineral for the prevention of anemia during menstruation. Iron may also be beneficial in the treatment of leukemia and colitis.

IRON MAY BE BENEFICIAL FOR THE FOLLOWING AILMENTS:

Body Member	Ailment
Blood/Circulatory system	Anemia
	Diabetes
	Leukemia
	Menstruation
	Pernicious anemia
Bowel	Colitis
	Diarrhea
Brain/Nervous system	Alcoholism
Intestine	Celiac disease
	Colitis
	Worms
Joint	Gout
Kidney	Nephritis
Lungs/Respiratory system	Tuberculosis
Nails	Nail problems
Reproductive system	Menstruation
	Pregnancy
Skin	Scurvy
	Ulcers
Stomach	Gastritis
	Stomach ulcer (peptic)
Teeth/Gums	Tooth and gum disorders

Body Member	Ailment
General	Aging
	Alcoholism
	Bruises
	Cancer
	Pregnancy

LEAD

Description

Lead is a highly toxic trace mineral. In recent years human exposure to lead poisoning has changed in origin and probably has increased in magnitude.[193]

The human body can tolerate only 1 to 2 milligrams (about 0.00003 of an ounce) of lead without suffering toxic effects.[194] Two pounds of food contaminated by only one part per million of lead contain almost a milligram of lead, so there is not a very wide margin of safety.

The single most effective way to prevent lead poisoning is to include a small amount of algin in the daily diet. Algin is a nonnutritive substance found in Pacific kelp, which is sometimes used as a thickening agent in the preparation of various foods. It attaches itself to any lead that is present and carries it harmlessly out of the system.[195]

Absorption and Storage

Lead contained in food is poorly absorbed and is excreted mainly in the feces. Lead may enter the body via the skin and the gastrointestinal tract. The lead that is absorbed enters the blood and is stored in the bones and the soft tissues, including the liver. Up to certain levels of consumption, lead excretion keeps pace with ingestion so that retention is negligible.

Dosage and Toxicity

Critical levels of intake, above which significant lead retention occurs, cannot be quoted with any accuracy.[196] Toxic intake can come from consumption of

[192]Chaney and Ross, *Nutrition*, p. 149.

[193]National Academy of Sciences, *Toxicants Occurring Naturally in Foods*, p. 61.
[194]Rodale, *Complete Book of Minerals for Health*, p. 446.
[195]"Problem Children, Lead and What to Do about It," *Prevention*, October 1973, p. 87.
[196]National Academy of Sciences, *Toxicants Occurring Naturally in Foods*, pp. 61-62.

moonshine whiskey and fruit juices stored in lead-glazed earthenware pottery. Sources of poisoning include drinking water, food from lead-lined containers, lead-based paint, lead in water pipes, cosmetics, cigarette smoking, and motor vehicle exhausts. The accumulation of lead in the body from motor vehicle exhausts is caused directly by inhalation and indirectly through deposition in the soil and plants along highways and in urban areas.

Acute lead toxicity is manifested in abdominal colic, encephalopathy (dysfunction of the brain), myelopathy (any pathological condition of the spinal cord), and anemia. The anemia is hypochromic and is rarely severe. Acute lead poisoning attacks the central nervous system and is a possible cause of hyperactivity in children.[197]

There is considerable difference of opinion as to the treatment for lead poisoning. The usual treatment during acute stages consists of a diet high in calcium plus injections of a calcium chloride solution and administration of vitamin D.[198] The additional calcium and vitamin D help prevent lead from being leeched out of the bones into the circulatory system. Calcium and vitamin D also appear to facilitate the return of lead from the blood to the bones.

Deficiency Effects and Symptoms

No available information.

Beneficial Effect on Ailments

No available information.

MAGNESIUM

Description

Magnesium is an essential mineral that accounts for about 0.05 percent of the body's total weight. Nearly 70 percent of the body's supply is located in the bones together with calcium and phosphorus, while 30 percent is found in the soft tissues and body fluids.

Magnesium is involved in many essential metabolic processes. Most magnesium is found inside the cell, where it activates enzymes necessary for the metabolism of carbohydrates and amino acids. By countering the stimulative effect of calcium, magnesium plays an important role in neuromuscular contractions.[199] It also helps regulate the acid-alkaline balance in the body.

Magnesium helps promote absorption and metabolism of other minerals, such as calcium, phosphorus, sodium, and potassium. It also helps utilize the B complex and vitamins C and E in the body. It aids during bone growth and is necessary for proper functioning of the nerves and muscles, including those of the heart. Evidence suggests that magnesium is associated with the regulation of body temperature. Sufficient amounts of magnesium are needed in the conversion of blood sugar into energy.

Magnesium appears to be widely distributed in foods, being found chiefly in fresh green vegetables, where it is an essential element of chlorophyll. Other excellent sources include raw, unmilled wheat germ, soybeans, figs, corn, apples, and oil-rich seeds and nuts, especially almonds. Dolomite, a natural dietary supplement, is also rich in magnesium and is a good source of calcium and essential trace minerals as well.

Absorption and Storage

Nearly 50 percent of the average daily intake of magnesium is absorbed in the small intestine. The rate of absorption is influenced by the parathyroid hormones, the rate of water absorption, and the amounts of calcium, phosphate, and lactose (milk sugar) in the body.[200] When the intake of magnesium is low, the rate of absorption may be as high as 75 percent; when the intake is high, the rate of absorption may be as low as 25 percent.[201]

The adrenal gland secretes a hormone called aldosterone, which helps to regulate the rate of magnesium excretion through the kidneys. Losses tend to increase with the use of diuretics and with the consumption of alcohol.

Dosage and Toxicity

The National Research Council recommends a daily magnesium intake of 350 milligrams for the adult male and 300 milligrams for the adult female. The amount increases to 450 milligrams during pregnancy and lactation.[202] It is estimated that the typical American diet

[197]"Problem Children, Lead and What to Do about It," pp. 81-88.
[198]Krause and Hunscher, *Food, Nutrition and Diet Therapy*, p. 519.
[199]Guthrie, *Introductory Nutrition*, p. 133.
[200]Ruth L. Pike and Myrtle L. Brown, *Nutrition: An Integrated Approach* (New York: Wiley, 1971), p. 444.
[201]Guthrie, *Introductory Nutrition*, p. 133.
[202]Krause and Hunscher, *Food, Nutrition and Diet Therapy*, p. 109.

provides 120 milligrams per 1000 kilocalories, a level that will barely provide the recommended daily intake.

Evidence suggests that the balance between calcium and magnesium is especially important. If calcium consumption is high, magnesium intake needs to be high also. The amounts of protein, phosphorus, and vitamin D in the diet also influence the magnesium requirement. The need for magnesium is increased when blood cholesterol levels are high and when consumption of protein is high. Magnesium oxide is preferred over dolomite, but if dolomite is taken, additional supplementation of hydrochloric acid is needed to ensure that the dolomite is dissolved properly. Because magnesium acts as an alkali, it should not be taken after meals.

Large amounts of magnesium can be toxic, especially if the calcium intake is low and the phosphorus intake is high. Excessive magnesium is usually excreted adequately, but in the event of a kidney failure, there is greater danger of toxicity because the rate of excretion will be much lower.

Deficiency Effects and Symptoms

Magnesium deficiency can occur in patients with diabetes, pancreatitis, chronic alcoholism, kwashiorkor, kidney malfunction, a high-carbohydrate diet, or severe malabsorption as caused by chronic diarrhea or vomiting. Some hormones when used as drugs can upset metabolism and cause local deficiencies.[203]

Magnesium deficiency is thought to be closely related to coronary heart disease.[204] An inadequate supply of this mineral may result in the formation of clots in the heart and brain and may contribute to calcium deposits in the kidneys, blood vessels, and heart.

Symptoms of magnesium deficiency may include apprehensiveness, muscle twitch, tremors, confusion, and disorientation. The first step in treating the symptoms of a magnesium deficiency, especially among children, is to eliminate milk from the diet.[205] Calciferol (synthetic vitamin D), like fluorine, tends to bind with magnesium and carry it out of the body; since milk contains high amounts of this substance, it contributes to the deficiency. Herein lies another good reason to supplement the diet with natural fish-liver oil instead of synthetic vitamin D, which is ten times more active as a magnesium-binding agent.

Beneficial Effect on Ailments

Magnesium is vital in helping prevent heart attacks and severe coronary thrombosis. Magnesium seems to be important in controlling the manner in which electrical charges are utilized by the body to induce the passage of nutrients in and out of cells. It has been successfully used to treat prostate troubles, polio, and depression. It has also proved beneficial in the treatment of neuromuscular disorders, nervousness, tantrums, sensitivity to noise, and hand tremor.[206]

In alcoholics, the magnesium levels in the blood and muscles are low. Magnesium treatment helps the body retain magnesium and often helps control delirium tremens.

Magnesium helps to protect the accumulation of calcium deposits in the urinary tract. It makes the calcium and phosphorus soluble in the urine and prevents them from turning into hard stones. Adequate amounts of magnesium can help reduce blood cholesterol and help keep the arteries healthy.

Magnesium, not calcium, helps form the kind of hard tooth enamel that resists decay.[207] No matter how much calcium is ingested, only a soft enamel will be formed unless magnesium is present. The magnesium supplement dolomite is beneficial in fighting tooth decay.

Magnesium therapy has been effective in treating diarrhea, vomiting, nervousness, and kwashiorkor. Since magnesium works to preserve the health of the nervous system, it has been successfully used in controlling convulsions in pregnant women and epileptic patients. Because magnesium is very alkaline, it acts as an antacid and can be used in place of over-the-counter antacid compounds.

Human Tests

1. Magnesium and Kidney Stones. A thirty three-year-old pregnant woman had passed at least 8 to 12 stones during previous pregnancies. She was given 500 to 1,500 milligrams of magnesium daily over a period of 6 weeks.

Results. The pregnancy during which she was given the oral dose of magnesium was the first one during which she did not pass a single kidney stone. (F. Peter Kohler and Charles A. W. Uhle, *Journal of Urology*, November

---

[203] Rodale, *Complete Book of Minerals for Health*, p. 82.
[204] Williams, *Nutrition against Disease*, p. 80.
[205] Rodale, *Complete Book of Minerals for Health*, p. 99.

[206] Linda Clark, *Get Well Naturally* (New York: Pyramid Communications, 1968), p. 122.
[207] Rodale, *Complete Book of Minerals for Health*, p. 105.

1966, as reported in Rodale, *Complete Book of Minerals for Health,* p. 78.)

MAGNESIUM MAY BE BENEFICIAL FOR THE FOLLOWING AILMENTS:

Body Member	Ailment
Blood/Circulatory system	Arteriosclerosis
	Atherosclerosis
	Cholesterol level, high
	Diabetes
	Hypertension
Bones	Fracture
	Osteoporosis
	Rickets
Bowel	Colitis
	Diarrhea
Brain/Nervous system	Alcoholism
	Epilepsy
	Mental illness
	Multiple sclerosis
	Nervousness
	Neuritis
	Parkinson's disease
Heart	Arteriosclerosis
	Atherosclerosis
	Hypertension
Intestine	Celiac disease
Joint	Arthritis
Kidney	Kidney stones (renal calculi)
	Nephritis
Leg	Leg cramp
Muscles	Muscular excitability
Skin	Psoriasis
Stomach	Vomiting
General	Alcoholism
	Backache
	Kwashiorkor
	Overweight and obesity

MANGANESE

Description

Manganese is a trace mineral and plays a role in activating numerous enzymes. Manganese aids in the utilization of choline and is an activator of enzymes that are necessary for utilization of biotin, thiamine, and ascorbic acid.[208] Manganese is a catalyst in the synthesis of fatty acids and cholesterol. It also plays a part in protein, carbohydrate, and fat production; is necessary for normal skeletal development; and may be important for the formation of blood.[209] Manganese is important for the production of milk and the formation of urea, a part of the urine. It helps maintain sex-hormone production. Manganese also helps nourish the nerves and brain.

Whole-grain cereals, egg yolks, and green vegetables are among the better sources of manganese, but the content will vary depending upon the amount present in the soil.

Absorption and Storage

Manganese is very poorly absorbed while in the intestinal tract. Large intakes of calcium and phosphorus in the diet will depress the rate of absorption. Excretion of manganese occurs via the feces, much of it in the form of choline complex in the bile.[210]

The adult body contains only 10 to 20 milligrams of manganese. The highest concentrations of it are in the bones, liver, pancreas, and pituitary gland.

Dosage and Toxicity

The National Research Council sets no Recommended Dietary Allowance for manganese. The average daily diet contains approximately four milligrams, which is within the amount (3 to 9 milligrams) estimated to be required for an adult.[211]

A high calcium and phosphorus intake will increase the need for manganese. Very high dosages of manganese result in reduced storage and utilization of iron.

Industrial workers frequently exposed to manganese dust may absorb enough of the metal in the respiratory tract to develop toxic symptoms.[212] Weakness and psychological and motor difficulties can result from high tissue levels of manganese.

[208] Rodale, *Complete Book of Minerals for Health*, pp. 228-229.
[209] Linnea Anderson, Marjorie V. Dibble, Helen S. Mitchell, and Hendrika J. Rynbergen, *Cooper's Nutrition in Health and Disease* (Philadelphia: J.B. Lippincott Co., 1968), p. 73.
[210] Chaney and Ross, *Nutrition*, p. 182.
[211] Krause and Hunscher, *Food, Nutrition and Diet Therapy*, p. 116.
[212] Rodale, *Complete Book of Minerals for Health*, p. 223.

Deficiency Effects and Symptoms

A deficiency of manganese can affect glucose tolerance, resulting in the inability to remove excess sugar from the blood by oxidation and/or storage.[213] Ataxia, the failure of muscular coordination, has been linked with the inadequate intake of manganese. Deficiencies may also lead to paralysis, convulsion, blindness, and deafness in infants. Dizziness, ear noises, and loss of hearing may occur in adults.

Beneficial Effect on Ailments

Manganese has been beneficial in the treatment of diabetes. When combined with the B vitamins, manganese has helped children and adults who are suffering from devastating weakness by stimulating the transmission of impulses between nerve and muscle. Manganese also helps treat myasthenia gravis (failure of muscular coordination and loss of muscle strength).[214] Research suggests that manganese may play a role in the treatment of multiple sclerosis.[215]

MANGANESE MAY BE BENEFICIAL FOR THE FOLLOWING AILMENTS:

Body Member	Ailment
Blood/Circulatory system	Diabetes
Brain/Nervous system	Epilepsy
	Multiple sclerosis
Lungs/Respiratory system	Allergies
	Asthma
General	Fatigue

MERCURY

Description

Mercury occurs widely in the biosphere and is a toxic element presenting occupational hazards associated with both ingestion and inhalation. Mercury has no essential function in the human body.

Dr. Henry A. Shroeder, a prominent trace mineral researcher, has stated that the only fish that need to be avoided for fear of mercury poisoning are fish from inland waters known to be polluted by toxic-mercury dumping. People eating well-balanced meals, not exclusively fish, have not reported any mercury poisoning.

Mercury's danger to the body lies in exposure to specific compounds, rather than inorganic forms, of this trace mineral. Methyl mercury and ethyl mercury are two highly toxic forms.[216] Methyl mercury can be found throughout agriculture and industry in pesticides, in fungicides, in the chemical by-product of chlorine, and in a form of mercury vapor from smokestacks. All of these chemicals can threaten the environment and the human body because they are retained in the tissues for long periods and adversely effect the central nervous system.

Symptoms of subacute mercury poisoning may be salivation, stomatitis, and diarrhea; or they may be neurological, such as Parkinsonian tremors, vertigo, irritability, moodiness, and depression.[217] Methyl mercury attacks the central nervous system and can cause brain damage. It usually takes the body 70 days to flush out half of the amount that originally was ingested. Symptoms of methyl mercury poisoning include loss of coordination, intellectual ability, vision, and hearing.

The average intake of mercury from food is estimated to be only 0.5 milligram daily. Oral ingestion of as little as 100 milligrams of mercury chloride produces toxic symptoms, and 500 milligrams is usually always fatal unless immediate treatment is given.

MOLYBDENUM

Description

Molybdenum is a trace mineral found in practically all plant and animal tissues. It is an essential part of two enzymes: xanthine oxidase, which aids in the mobilization of iron from the liver reserves; and aldehyde oxidase, which is necessary for the oxidation of fats.

Food sources of molybdenum include legumes, cereal grains, and some of the dark-green leafy vegetables. The food's mineral content is completely dependent upon the soil content.

Absorption and Storage

Molybdenum is found in minute amounts in the body, being readily absorbed from the gastrointestinal tract

[213] Rodale, *Complete Book of Minerals for Health*, p. 224.
[214] Clark, *Know Your Nutrition*, pp. 166-167.
[215] Clark, *Know Your Nutrition*, pp. 166-167.
[216] Rodale, *Complete Book of Minerals for Health*, p. 419.
[217] National Academy of Sciences, *Toxicants Occurring Naturally in Foods*, p. 67.

and excreted in the urine. Molybdenum is stored in the liver, kidneys, and bones.[218]

Dosage and Toxicity

There is no Recommended Dietary Allowance for molybdenum because it is so widely distributed in commonly used foods. Toxicity symptoms include diarrhea, anemia, and depressed growth rate.[219] High intake may also result in a copper deficiency.[220]

Deficiency Effects and Symptoms

There are no known molybdenum deficiency effects.

Beneficial Effect on Ailments

Molybdenum may play a part in the prevention of anemia.

MOLYBDENUM MAY BE BENEFICIAL FOR THE FOLLOWING AILMENTS:

Body Member	Ailment
Liver	Anemia

NICKEL

Description

Nickel is a trace mineral found in large amounts in the body. Nickel catalysts are involved in the hydrogenation of edible vegetable oils such as corn, peanut, and cottonseed oil. This is one reason for large amounts of nickel being present in the human body tissue. Nickel is an essential mineral, but its application in human nutrition is unknown.[221]

PHOSPHORUS

Description

Phosphorus is the second most abundant mineral in the body and is found in every cell. It often functions along with calcium, and the healthy body maintains a specific calcium-phosphorus balance in the bones of 2.5 parts calcium to 1 part phosphorus, although phosphorus is in higher ratio in the soft tissues. This balance of calcium and phosphorus is needed for these minerals to be effectively used by the body.

Phosphorus plays a part in almost every chemical reaction within the body because it is present in every cell. It is important in the utilization of carbohydrates, fats, and protein for the growth, maintenance, and repair of cells and for the production of energy. It stimulates muscle contractions, including the regular contractions of the heart muscle. Niacin and riboflavin cannot be digested unless phosphorus is present. Phosphorus is an essential part of nucleoproteins, which are responsible for cell division and reproduction and the transference of hereditary traits from parents to offspring. It is also necessary for proper skeletal growth, tooth development, kidney functioning, and transference of nerve impulses.

Phospholipids, such as lecithin, help break up and transport fats and fatty acids. They help prevent the accumulation of too much acid or too much alkali in the blood, assist in the passage of substances through the cell walls, and promote the secretion of glandular hormones. They are also needed for healthy nerves and efficient mental activity.

Foods rich in protein are also rich in phosphorus. Meat, fish, poultry, eggs, whole grains, seeds, and nuts are primary sources of phosphorus.

Absorption and Storage

Unlike calcium, which is poorly absorbed, most dietary phosphorus is absorbed from the intestine into the bloodstream. About 70 percent of the phosphorus ingested in foods is absorbed. About 88 percent of the absorbed phosphorus is stored in the bones and teeth, along with calcium, although antacids can deplete the storage. There is relatively little control over the rate of absorption, so the body content is regulated by urinary excretion.

Phosphorus absorption depends on the presence of vitamin D and calcium. Absorption can be interfered with by excessive amounts of iron, aluminum, and magnesium, which tend to form insoluble phosphates.[222] The calcium-phosphorus balance is disturbed in the presence of white sugar. High fat diets or digestive conditions that prevent the absorption of fat increase

[218]Guthrie, *Introductory Nutrition*, p. 165.
[219]Chaney and Ross, *Nutrition*, p. 183.
[220]Chaney and Ross, *Nutrition*, p. 183.
[221]National Academy of Sciences, *Recommended Dietary Allowances*, Washington, p. 102.
[222]Guthrie, *Introductory Nutrition* p. 126.

the absorption of phosphorus in the intestine, but such conditions are not healthful because they also decrease the amount of calcium absorbed and upset the calcium-phosphorus balance.[223]

Dosage and Toxicity

The National Research Council recommends a daily dietary intake of 800 milligrams of phosphorus for men and women. During pregnancy and lactation the amount increases to 1,200 milligrams. This is equal to the daily requirement for calcium. If the phosphorus content of the body is high, additional calcium should be taken to maintain a proper balance. There is no known toxicity of phosphorus.

Deficiency Effects and Symptoms

An insufficient supply of phosphorus, calcium, or vitamin D may result in stunted growth, poor quality of bones and teeth, or other bone disorders. A deficiency in the calcium-phosphorus balance may result in diseases such as arthritis, pyorrhea, rickets, and tooth decay.[224]

A phosphorus deficiency can cause lack of appetite and weight loss or, conversely, overweight. Irregular breathing, mental and physical fatigue, and nervous disorders may occur.

Beneficial Effect on Ailments

Dietary phosphate has speeded up the healing process in bone fractures and has reduced the expected loss of calcium in such patients. It has been used successfully in the treatment of osteomalacia and osteoporosis. It also helps to prevent or cure rickets and to prevent stunted growth in children.

Mental stress can cause an upset in the body chemistry and bring on strong arthritic symptoms such as aching joints. The calcium-phosphorus balance can help treat the stressful condition and can also help alleviate the arthritis.

Recent research has shown that phosphorus may be important in cancer prevention. Investigators have discovered that phosphorus is more easily lost from cancerous cells than from normal cells.[225] Phosphorus is essential in treating disorders of the teeth and gums.

[223]Rodale, *Complete Book of Minerals for Health*, p. 65.
[224]Rodale, *Complete Book of Minerals for Health*, p. 65.
[225]Rodale, *The Health Builder*, p. 664.

PHOSPHORUS MAY BE BENEFICIAL FOR THE FOLLOWING AILMENTS:

Body Member	Ailment
Bones	Fracture
	Osteomalacia
	Osteoporosis
	Rickets
	Stunted growth
Bowel	Colitis
Brain/Nervous system	Mental illness
Heart	Arteriosclerosis
	Atherosclerosis
Joints	Arthritis
Leg	Leg cramp
Teeth/Gums	Tooth and gum disorders
General	Backache
	Cancer
	Pregnancy
	Stress

POTASSIUM

Description

Potassium is an essential mineral found mainly in the intracellular fluid; a small amount occurs in the extracellular fluid. Potassium constitutes 5 percent of the total mineral content of the body.[226] Potassium and sodium help regulate water balance within the body; that is, they help regulate the distribution of fluids on either side of the cell walls.

Potassium is necessary for normal growth, to stimulate nerve impulses for muscle contraction, and to preserve proper alkalinity of the body fluids. It aids in keeping the skin healthy. Potassium assists in the conversion of glucose to glycogen, the form in which glucose can be stored in the liver. It functions in cell metabolism, enzyme reactions, and the synthesis of muscle protein from amino acids in the blood. It stimulates the kidneys to eliminate poisonous body wastes.

Potassium works with sodium to help normalize the heartbeat and nourish the muscular system.[227] It unites

[226]Krause and Hunscher, *Food, Nutrition and Diet Therapy*, p. 110.
[227]Wade, *Magic Minerals: Key to Health*, p. 22.

with phosphorus to send oxygen to the brain and also functions with calcium in the regulation of neuromuscular activity.[228]

Food sources of potassium include all vegetables, especially green leafy vegetables, oranges, whole grains, sunflower seeds, and mint leaves. Large amounts of potassium are found in potatoes, especially in the peelings, and in bananas.

Absorption and Storage

Potassium is rapidly absorbed from the small intestine. It is excreted mainly through urination and perspiration, with very little lost in the feces. The kidneys are able to maintain normal serum levels through their ability to filter, secrete, and excrete potassium. Aldosterone, an adrenal hormone, stimulates potassium excretion.

Excessive potassium buildup may result from kidney failure or from severe lack of fluid.

Because sodium and potassium must be in balance, the excessive use of salt depletes the body's conservation of its often scarce potassium supplies. In addition, potassium can be depleted by prolonged diarrhea, excessive sweating, vomiting, and the use of diuretics.

Alcohol and coffee increase the urinary excretion of potassium. Alcohol is a double antagonist since it also depletes the magnesium reserve.[229] Excessive intake of sugar is also antagonistic towards potassium.

A low blood sugar level is a stressful condition that strains the adrenal glands, causing additional potassium to be lost in the urine while water and salt are held in the tissues. An adequate supply of magnesium is needed to retain the storage of potassium in the cells.

Dosage and Toxicity

A Recommended Dietary Allowance for potassium has not been established, but many authorities suggest that between 2,000 and 2,500 milligrams be included in the diet daily. The amount of potassium in the average American's daily diet has been estimated at 2,000 to 6,000 milligrams per day, since it is distributed in many different foods.[230]

Deficiency Effects and Symptoms

Excessive urinary losses induced by high salt intake have caused potassium deficiencies to be commonplace. A potassium deficiency can result from an excessive intake of sodium chloride or from an inadequate intake of fruits and vegetables. Refined sugar can cause the urine to become alkaline so that minerals cannot be held in solution. Deficiency can be caused by prolonged intravenous administration of saline, which induces potassium excretion.[231] Vomiting, severe malnutrition, and stress, both mental and physical, may also lead to potassium deficiency.

A potassium deficiency may cause nervous disorders, insomnia, constipation, slow and irregular heartbeat, and muscle damage. When a deficiency of potassium impairs glucose metabolism, energy is no longer available to the muscles and they become more or less paralyzed.

When the body is lacking potassium, the sodium content of the heart and muscles increases. Infants suffering from diarrhea may have a potassium deficiency because the passage of the intestinal contents is so rapid that there is decreased absorption of potassium.[232] Diabetic patients are often deficient in potassium.[233] Persons suffering from diseases of the digestive tract are frequently found to be potassium-deficient. A person loses potassium when taking hormone products such as cortisone and aldosterone. Sodium is retained and potassium is excreted when these drugs are administered.

Early symptoms of potassium deficiency include general weakness and impairment of neuromuscular function, poor reflexes, and soft, sagging muscles. In adolescents, acne can result; in older persons, dry skin may occur.

Beneficial Effect on Ailments

Potassium has been used to treat cases of high blood pressure which were directly caused by excessive salt intake. Colic in infants has disappeared after injections of potassium chloride. Potassium chloride has also proven effective in treating allergies.

Giving potassium to patients with mild diabetes can reduce blood pressure and blood sugar levels.[234] Since

[228]Krause and Hunscher, *Food, Nutrition and Diet Therapy*, p. 110.
[229]Lisa Cosman, "Potassium: The Neglected Mineral," *Bestways*, October 1973, p. 19.
[230]Guthrie, *Introductory Nutrition*, p. 128.

[231]Williams, *Nutrition against Disease*, pp. 156-157.
[232]Guthrie, *Introductory Nutrition*, p. 128.
[233]Davis, *Let's Get Well*, p. 115.
[234]Rodale, *The Health Builder*, p. 695.

potassium is essential for the transmission of nerve impulses to the brain, it has been effective in the treatment of headache-causing allergies.[235]

Potassium has also been used in the treatment of diarrhea in infants and adults. Therapeutic doses of potassium are sometimes used to slow the heartbeat in cases of severe injury, such as burns.

POTASSIUM MAY BE BENEFICIAL FOR THE FOLLOWING AILMENTS:

Body Member	Ailment
Blood/Circulatory system	Angina pectoris
	Diabetes
	Hypertension
	Mononucleosis
	Stroke (cerebrovascular accident)
Bones	Fracture
Bowel	Colitis
	Diarrhea
Brain/Nervous system	Alcoholism
	Hypertension
	Insomnia
	Polio
Glands	Mononucleosis
Head	Fever
	Headache
Intestine	Constipation
	Worms
Heart	Angina pectoris
	Congestive heart failure
	Hypertension
	Myocardial infarction
Joints	Arthritis
	Gout
Lungs/Respiratory system	Allergies
Muscles	Impaired muscle activity
	Muscular dystrophy
	Rheumatism
Skin	Acne
	Burns
	Dermatitis
Stomach	Gastroenteritis
Teeth/Gums	Tooth and gum disorders
General	Alcoholism
	Cancer
	Fever
	Stress

[235]Rodale, *The Best Health Articles from* Prevention *Magazine*, p. 578.

SELENIUM

Description

Selenium is an essential mineral found in minute amounts in the body. It works closely with vitamin E in some of its metabolic actions and in the promotion of normal body growth and fertility. Selenium is a natural antioxidant and appears to preserve elasticity of tissue by delaying oxidation of polyunsaturated fatty acids that can cause solidification of tissue proteins.[236]

The selenium content of food is dependent upon the extent of its presence in the soil, whether directly as in plant foods or indirectly as in animal products whose selenium levels are derived from feed. Selenium is found in the bran and germ of cereals; in vegetables such as broccoli, onions, and tomatoes; and in tuna.

Archives of Environmental Health, September/October, 1976, reports that in a study of the relationship between cancer incidence and soil distribution of selenium in the United States, areas with high selenium levels showed significantly lower overall male cancer death rates. Also in these areas, in both men and women, fewer cancers were noted in those organ systems involved with the assimilation, metabolism, and excretion of selenium.

Absorption and Storage

The liver and kidneys contain four to five times as much selenium as do the muscles and other tissues. Selenium is normally excreted in the urine; its presence in the feces is an indication of improper absorption.[237]

Dosage and Toxicity

The Recommended Dietary Allowance of selenium for adults is extremely minute; 5 to 10 parts per million is considered toxic. This is due to the tendency of selenium to replace sulfur in biological compounds and inhibit the action of some enzymes.[238] Selenium can be toxic in its pure form, so supplements should be taken with care. Reported instances of toxicity have occurred in areas where the selenium content of the soil was high.

[236]Rodale, *Complete Book of Minerals for Health*, p. 235.
[237]Guthrie, *Introductory Nutrition*, p. 162.
[238]Guthrie, *Introductory Nutrition*, p. 162.

Deficiency Effects and Symptoms

A deficiency of selenium may lead to premature aging. This is because selenium preserves tissue elasticity.

Beneficial Effect on Ailments

Selenium when combined with protein is beneficial in treating kwashiorkor, a protein-deficiency disease.

Dr. Julian E. Spallholz of the Veterans Administration Hospital in Long Beach, California, has demonstrated through experiments with mice that selenium may increase resistance to disease by increasing the number of antibodies that neutralize toxins. Selenium supplements enabled mice to produce significantly more antibodies than those that were not given the trace element.

SELENIUM MAY BE BENEFICIAL FOR THE FOLLOWING AILMENT:

Body Member	Ailment
General	Kwashiorkor

SODIUM

Description

Sodium is an essential mineral found predominantly in the extracellular fluids; the vascular fluids within the blood vessels, arteries, veins, and capillaries; and the intestinal fluids surrounding the cells.[239] About 50 percent of the body's sodium is found in these fluids and the remaining amount is found within the bones.[240]

Sodium functions with potassium to equalize the acid-alkali factor in the blood. Along with potassium, it helps regulate water balance within the body; that is, it helps regulate the distribution of fluids on either side of the cell walls. Sodium and potassium are also involved in muscle contraction and expansion and in nerve stimulation.

Another important function of sodium is keeping the other blood minerals soluble, so that they will not build up as deposits in the bloodstream.[241] It acts with chlorine to improve blood and lymph health, helps purge carbon dioxide from the body and aids digestion.[242] Sodium is also necessary for hydrochloric acid production in the stomach.

Sodium is found in virtually all foods, especially sodium chloride, or salt. High concentrations are contained in seafoods, carrots, beets, poultry, and meat. Kelp is an excellent supplemental source of sodium.

Absorption and Storage

Sodium is readily absorbed in the small intestine and the stomach and is carried by the blood to the kidneys, where it is filtered out and returned to the blood in amounts needed to maintain blood levels required by the body.[243] The absorption of sodium requires energy. Any excess, which usually amounts to 90 to 95 percent of ingested sodium, is excreted in the urine.[244]

The adrenal hormone aldosterone is an important regulator of sodium metabolism. Excessive salt in food interferes with absorption and utilization, especially in the case of protein foods.[245] Vomiting, diarrhea, or excessive perspiration may result in a depletion of sodium. Sodium supplements to prevent sodium deficiency may be needed in such cases. The levels of sodium in the urine reflect the dietary intake; therefore when there is a high intake of sodium the rate of excretion is high, and if the intake is low the excretion rate is low.

Dosage and Toxicity

There is no established dietary requirement for sodium, but it is generally observed that the usual intake far exceeds the need. The average American ingests 3 to 7 grams of sodium and 6 to 18 grams of sodium chloride each day.[246] The National Research Council recommends a daily sodium chloride intake of 1 gram per kilogram of water consumed.[247]

An excess of sodium in the diet may cause potassium to be lost in the urine. Abnormal fluid retention accompanied by dizziness and swelling of such areas as legs and face can also occur. An intake of 14 to 28 grams of salt (sodium chloride) daily is considered excessive.[248]

Diets containing excessive amounts of sodium contribute to the increasing incidences of high blood pressure. The simplest way to reduce sodium intake is to eliminate the use of table salt.

[239]Guthrie, *Introductory Nutrition*, p. 129.
[240]Guthrie, *Introductory Nutrition*, p. 129.
[241]Wade, *Magic Minerals: Key to Health*, p. 21.
[242]Rodale, *Complete Book of Minerals for Health*, p. 133.
[243]Guthrie, *Introductory Nutrition*, p. 129.
[244]Krause and Hunscher, *Food, Nutrition and Diet Therapy*, p. 110.
[245]Rodale, *The Health Builder*, pp. 841-842.
[246]Krause and Hunscher, *Food, Nutrition and Diet Therapy*, p. 110.
[247]Krause and Hunscher, *Food, Nutrition and Diet Therapy*, p. 110.
[248]National Academy of Sciences, *Toxicants Occurring Naturally in Foods*, p. 270.

Deficiency Effects and Symptoms

Deficiencies are very uncommon because nearly all foods contain some sodium, with meats containing especially high amounts. A sodium deficiency can cause intestinal gas, weight loss, vomiting, and muscle shrinkage. The conversion of carbohydrates into fat for digestion is impaired when sodium is absent. Arthritis, rheumatism, and neuralgia, a sharp pain along a nerve, may be caused by acids that accumulate in the absence of sodium.

Beneficial Effect on Ailments

An individual suffering from high blood pressure is advised to maintain a low-sodium diet, since sodium may aggravate this ailment. Resistance to heat cramps and heat strokes may be increased by moderate sodium intake. Sodium helps keep calcium in a solution that is necessary for nerve strength.[249] Clinical studies indicate that low-sodium diets are effective in preventing or relieving the symptoms of toxemia (bacterial poisoning), edema (swelling), proteinuria (albumin in the urine), and blurred vision.

SODIUM MAY BE BENEFICIAL FOR THE FOLLOWING AILMENTS:

Body Member	Ailment
Bowel	Diarrhea
Glands	Adrenal exhaustion
	Cystic Fibrosis
Leg	Leg cramp
Teeth/Gums	Tooth and gum disorders
General	Dehydration
	Fever
	Polio

SULFUR

Description

Sulfur is a nonmetallic element that occurs widely in nature, being present in every cell of animals and plants. Sulfur makes up 0.25 percent of the human body weight. It is called nature's "beauty mineral" because it keeps the hair glossy and smooth and keeps the complexion clear and youthful.

Sulfur has an important relationship with protein. It is contained in the amino acids methionine, cystine, and cysteine, and it appears to be necessary for collagen synthesis.[250] Sulfur is prevalent in keratin, a tough protein substance necessary for health and maintenance of the skin, nails, and hair.[251] It is found in insulin, the hormone that regulates carbohydrate metabolism.[252] It also occurs in carbohydrates such as heparin, an anti-coagulant found in the liver and other tissues.

Sulfur works with thiamine, pantothenic acid, biotin, and lipoic acid, which are needed for metabolism and strong nerve health. In addition, sulfur plays a part in tissue respiration, the process whereby oxygen and other substances are used to build cells and release energy. It works with the liver to secrete bile. Sulfur also helps to maintain overall body balance.

Sulfur is found in protein-containing foods such as meat, fish, legumes, and nuts. Other natural sources include eggs, cabbage, dried beans, and brussels sprouts.

Absorption and Storage

Sulfur is stored in every cell of the body. The highest concentrations are found in the hair, skin, and nails. Excess sulfur is excreted in the urine and the feces.

Dosage and Toxicity

There is no Recommended Dietary Allowance for sulfur because it is assumed that a person's sulfur requirement is met when the protein intake is adequate.[253] Sulfur can be used in various forms such as ointments, creams, lotions, and dusting powders. Excessive intake of inorganic sulfur may result in toxicity.

Deficiency Effects and Symptoms

There are no known deficiency effects or symptoms.

Beneficial Effect on Ailments

Sulfur is important in the treatment of arthritis. The level of cystine, a sulfur-containing amino acid, in arthritic patients is usually much lower than normal.

When used topically in the form of an ointment, sulfur is helpful in treating skin disorders, such as

---

[249]Wade, *Magic Minerals: Key to Health*, p. 22.

[250]Guthrie, *Introductory Nutrition*, pp. 128–129.
[251]Wade, *Magic Minerals: Key to Health*, p. 24.
[252]Krause and Hunscher, *Food, Nutrition and Diet Therapy*, p. 108.
[253]Chaney and Ross, *Nutrition*, p. 187.

psoriasis, eczema, and dermatitis. It also may be beneficial in treating ringworm.

SULFUR MAY BE BENEFICIAL FOR THE FOLLOWING AILMENTS:

Body Member	Ailment
Intestine	Worms
Joints	Arthritis
Skin	Dermatitis
	Eczema
	Psoriasis

VANADIUM

Description

Vanadium is a trace mineral found in varying quantities in vegetables. Marine life is the most reliable source.

Vanadium is part of the natural circulatory regulating system. The presence of it in the brain inhibits cholesterol formation in the blood vessels. In addition, the formation of cholesterol in the human central nervous system can be reduced by administering vanadium orally.[254]

It is difficult to measure vanadium levels in humans, although 90 percent of ingested vanadium is eliminated in the urine. An overdose of vanadium, even in synthetic form, is easily induced. Vanadium should be taken in the natural form, and fish is an excellent source.

ZINC

Description

Zinc is an essential trace mineral occurring in the body in larger amounts than any other trace element except iron. The human body contains approximately 1.8 grams of zinc compared to nearly 5 grams of iron.

Zinc has a variety of functions. It is related to the normal absorption and action of vitamins, especially the B complex. It is a constituent of at least 25 enzymes involved in digestion and metabolism, including carbonic anhydrase, which is necessary for tissue respiration. Zinc is a component of insulin, and it is part of the enzyme that is needed to break down alcohol. It also plays a part in carbohydrate digestion and phosphorus

metabolism. In addition, it is essential in the synthesis of nucleic acid, which controls the formation of different proteins in the cell. Zinc is essential for general growth and proper development of the reproductive organs and for normal functioning of the prostate gland.

Recent medical findings indicate that zinc is important in healing wounds and burns. It may also be required in the synthesis of DNA, which is the master substance of life, carrying all inherited traits and directing the activity of each cell.[255]

The best sources of all trace elements in proper balance are natural unprocessed foods, preferably those grown in organically enriched soil. Diets high in protein, whole-grain products, brewer's yeast, wheat bran, wheat germ, and pumpkin seeds are usually high in zinc. The zinc content of most municipal drinking water is negligible.[256]

Absorption and Storage

Zinc is readily absorbed in the upper small intestine. The major route of excretion is through the gastrointestinal tract; little is lost in the urine. The largest storage of zinc occurs in the liver, pancreas, kidney, bones, and voluntary muscles. Zinc is also stored in parts of the eyes, prostate gland and spermatozoa, skin, hair, fingernails, and toenails as well as being present in the white blood cells.[257]

A high intake of calcium and phytic acid, found in certain grains, may prevent absorption of zinc. If the intake of calcium and phytic acid is higher, zinc consumption should be increased.

Dosage and Toxicity

The National Research Council recommends a daily dietary intake of 15 milligrams of zinc for adults. An additional 15 milligrams is recommended during pregnancy, and an additional 25 milligrams is recommended during lactation. The average zinc content of a mixed diet is between 10 and 15 milligrams.[258]

Zinc is relatively nontoxic, although poisoning may result from eating foods that have been stored in

[254]Rodale, *Complete Book of Minerals for Health,* p. 251.
[255]Rodale, *Complete Book of Minerals for Health,* p. 259.
[256]National Academy of Sciences, *Recommended Dietary Allowances,* p. 101.
[257]Krause and Hunscher, *Food, Nutrition and Diet Therapy,* p. 117.
[258]National Academy of Sciences, *Recommended Dietary Allowances,* p. 100.

galvanized containers. High intakes of zinc interfere with copper utilization, causing incomplete iron metabolism. Excessive intake of zinc may result in a loss of iron and copper from the liver. When zinc is added to the diet, vitamin A is also needed in larger amounts.

Deficiency Effects and Symptoms

The most common cause of zinc deficiency is an unbalanced diet, although other factors may also be responsible. For example, the consumption of alcohol may precipitate a deficiency by flushing stored zinc out of the liver and into the urine.[259] Zinc deficiency is also a factor in increased fatigue, susceptibility to infection, injury, and decreased alertness.[260]

Zinc deficiency can cause retarded growth, delayed sexual maturity, and prolonged healing of wounds. A deficiency of zinc, copper, and vanadium may result in atherosclerosis. Stretch marks in the skin and white spots in the fingernails may be signs of a zinc deficiency.

Cadmium, a toxic mineral, also plays an important role in zinc deficiencies. High intakes of cadmium will accentuate the signs of a zinc deficiency, and the cadmium will be stored in the body in the absence of zinc. This creates a detrimental situation that can be reversed by increasing the consumption of zinc.

Recent studies demonstrate conclusively that zinc deficiency causes sterility and dwarfism in humans. The deficiency leads to unhealthy changes in the size and structure of the prostate gland, which contains more zinc than any other part of the human anatomy. In prostate problems, particularly prostate cancer, the levels of zinc in the prostate gland decline.

James A. Halstead and J. Cecil Smith, Jr., of the Trace Element Research Laboratory, Washington, D.C., have made interesting studies on zinc. They found low zinc levels in the blood plasma of people suffering from alcoholic cirrhosis, other types of liver disease, ulcers, heart attacks, mongolism, and cystic fibrosis. Pregnant women and women taking oral contraceptives also had low levels of zinc in their blood plasma.

Excessive zinc excretion occurs in leukemia and Hodgkin's disease, but the causes of this are unknown. A zinc deficiency is characterized by abnormal fatigue and may cause a loss of normal taste sensitivity, poor appetite, and suboptimal growth.

[259]Rodale, *Complete Book of Minerals for Health*, p. 226.
[260]Clark, *Know Your Nutrition*, p. 168.

Beneficial Effect on Ailments

Zinc helps eliminate cholesterol deposits and has been successfully used in the treatment of atherosclerosis. Zinc may contribute to the rapid healing of internal wounds or any injury to the arteries. Zinc supplements given in therapeutic doses will speed up the rate at which the body heals certain external wounds and injuries.

Zinc is beneficial in the prevention and treatment of infertility. It also helps in the proper growth and maturity of the sex organs.

The administration of zinc may benefit patients suffering from Hodgkin's disease and leukemia. It also is used in treatment of cirrhosis of the liver and alcoholism.

Zinc is beneficial to the diabetic because of its regulatory affect on insulin in the blood. It has been found that the addition of zinc to insulin prolongs its effect on blood sugar.[261] A diabetic pancreas contains only about half as much zinc as does a healthy one.

ZINC MAY BE BENEFICIAL FOR THE FOLLOWING AILMENTS:

Body Member	Ailment
Blood/Circulatory system	Arteriosclerosis
	Atherosclerosis
	Cholesterol level, high
	Diabetes
	Hodgkin's disease
Brain/Nervous system	Alcoholism
Eye	Night blindness
Glands	Prostatitis
Heart	Arteriosclerosis
	Atherosclerosis
Joints	Rheumatoid arthritis
Reproductive system	Prostatitis
	Retarded sexual activity
Skin	Acne
	Burns
	Dermatitis
	Eczema
	Wounds
General	Alcoholism
	Retarded growth
	Ulcers

[261]Rodale, *The Encyclopedia of Common Disease*, p. 273.

BORON, LITHIUM, SILICON, STRONTIUM, TIN, AND TRITIUM

These are essential trace minerals, but their role in human nutrition is unknown.

WATER

Water is not only the most abundant nutrient found in the body (accounting for roughly two-thirds of body weight), it also is by far the most important nutrient. Responsible for and involved in nearly every body process, including digestion, absorption, circulation, and excretion, water is the primary transporter of nutrients throughout the body and is necessary for all building functions in the body. Water helps maintain a normal body temperature and is essential for carrying waste material out of the body.

Nearly all foods contain water that is absorbed by the body during digestion. Fruits and vegetables are especially good sources of chemically pure water, which is 100 percent pure hydrogen and oxygen.

The average adult body contains approximately 45 quarts of water and loses about 3 quarts daily through excretion and perspiration. Rate of water loss depends almost entirely upon level of activity and environmental conditions and may range from less than 1 quart per day for a sedentary person in a temperate climate to more than 10 quarts per day in a desert.[262] If severe deficiencies are not corrected as soon as possible, salt depletion and dehydration will occur, eventually resulting in death.

There are nearly as many types of water as there are uses for it. Most *tap water* comes from streams, rivers, and lakes. This surface water may contain pollutants and agricultural wastes, such as fertilizer and insecticide residue that is carried by rainwater runoff into nearby waterways. Air pollutants, such as lead from automobile and factory exhausts, also end up in our rivers and streams. Chemicals, including chlorine, fluorine, phosphates, alum, sodium aluminates, soda ash, carbon, and lime, are frequently added to drinking water for purification. These substances are needed to kill bacteria, but questions have been raised regarding potential cancer-causing effects of some of these chemicals. Poisonous substances such as arsenic, cadmium, cyanides, asbestos, etc.—common industrial wastes—can combine with other chemicals in water and form carcinogenic substances. Boiling water, whether hot or cold tap water or bottled water, for long periods of time for purification is *not* recommended because, although the bacteria will be destroyed, the purest water will be lost in the form of steam and any heavy metals or nitrates in the water will be more concentrated in the final amount.

Another source of tap water is *well water*. Unlike most surface water, which has relatively uniform mineral content, well water varies so drastically in mineral content from one location to the next that the hardness and total dissolved solids in the water can range from nearly nothing to excessive extremes.

Because drinking water is polluted—even rainwater, which collects atmospheric pollutants as it descends—it may be desirable to purchase a home-purification unit. In November 1975, data identified 253 different specific organic chemicals (such as chloroform and pesticides) in drinking water in the United States. The occurrence of these compounds in drinking water suggests that other organics that are not yet identified may also be present, and that the total number of compounds could be considerably larger.[263] In laboratory tests, the purification process of distilling and reverse osmosis was the most efficient in removing and reducing the widest range of contaminants.

It has been suggested that a person switching to purified water should make an effort to provide an adequate mineral intake by eating mineral-rich foods or supplementing the diet. This diet allows the consumption of minerals in manageable quantities that will fill individual needs. This is the only way to ensure a proper mineral balance without taking the risk of pollutants, chemicals, and bacteria.

---

[262]National Academy of Sciences, *Recommended Dietary Allowances*, p. 22.

[263]*Preliminary Assessment of Suspected Carcinogens in Drinking Water*, Report to Congress (Washington, D.C.: U.S. Environmental Protection Agency, Dec. 1975), p. 3.

SUMMARY CHART OF NUTRIENTS

Nutrients	Importance	Deficiency Symptoms	RDA*	Toxicity Level
Carbohydrate	Provides energy for body functions and muscular exertions. Assists in digestion and assimilation of foods.	Loss of energy. Fatigue. Excessive protein breakdown. Disturbed balance of water, sodium, potassium, and chloride.	See "Nutrient Allowance Chart," p. 235.	Intake should not exceed what is needed to maintain desirable weight.
Fat	Provides energy. Acts as a carrier for fat-soluble vitamins A, D, E, and K. Supplies essential fatty acids needed for growth, health, and smooth skin.	Eczema or skin disorders. Retarded growth.	See "Nutrient Allowance Chart," p. 235.	Intake should not exceed what is needed to maintain desirable weight.
Protein	Is necessary for growth and development. Acts in formation of hormones, enzymes, and antibodies. Maintains acid-alkali balance. Is source of heat and energy.	Fatigue. Loss of appetite. Diarrhea and vomiting. Stunted growth. Edema.	See "Nutrient Allowance Chart," p. 235.	Intake should not exceed what is needed to maintain desirable weight.

VITAMINS

Nutrients	Importance	Deficiency Symptoms	RDA*	Toxicity Level
Vitamin A (Carotene)	Is necessary for growth and repair of body tissues. Is important to health of the eyes. Fights bacteria and infection. Maintains healthy epithelial tissue. Aids in bone and teeth formation.	Night blindness. Rough, dry, scaly skin. Increased susceptibility to infections. Frequent fatigue. Loss of smell and appetite.	5,000 IU.	50,000 or more IU may be toxic if there is no deficiency. 10,000 IU is the maximum single dose that can be bought without a prescription.
Vitamin B Complex	Is necessary for carbohydrate, fat, and protein metabolism. Helps functioning of the nervous system. Helps maintain muscle tone in the gastrointestinal tract.	Dry, rough, cracked skin. Acne. Dull, dry, or gray hair. Fatigue. Poor appetite. Gastrointestinal tract disorders.	See individual B vitamins.	See individual B vitamins; relatively nontoxic.

*Recommended Dietary Allowances.

Nutrients	Importance	Deficiency Symptoms	RDA*	Toxicity Level
	Maintains health of skin, hair, eyes, mouth, and liver.			
Vitamin B$_1$ (Thiamine)	Is necessary for carbohydrate metabolism. Helps maintain healthy nervous system. Stabilizes the appetite. Stimulates growth and good muscle tone.	Gastrointestinal problems. Fatigue. Loss of appetite. Nerve disorders. Heart disorders.	0.5 mg per 1000 calories consumed. 1.4 mg for men, 1.0 mg for women.	No known oral toxicity. Single doses of up to 500 mg are available without prescription.
Vitamin B$_2$ (Riboflavin)	Is necessary for carbohydrate, fat, and protein metabolism. Aids in formation of antibodies and red blood cells. Maintains cell respiration.	Eye problems. Cracks and sores in mouth. Dermatitis. Retarded growth. Digestive disturbances.	0.55 mg per 1000 calories consumed. 1.6 mg for adults.	No known oral toxicity. Single doses of 100 mg are available without prescription.
Vitamin B$_6$ (Pyridoxine)	Is necessary for carbohydrate, fat, and protein metabolism. Aids in formation of antibodies. Helps maintain balance of sodium and phosphorus.	Anemia. Mouth disorders. Nervousness. Muscular weakness. Dermatitis. Sensitivity to insulin.	0.2 mg for each 100 mg of protein. 1.8 mg men, 1.5 mg women.	No known oral toxicity. Single doses up to 100 mg are available without prescription.
Vitamin B$_{12}$ (Cyanocobalamin)	Is essential for normal formation of blood cells. Is necessary for carbohydrate, fat, and protein metabolism. Maintains healthy nervous system.	Pernicious anemia. Brain damage. Nervousness. Neuritis.	3 mcg for adults.	No known oral toxicity even with intake as high as 600-1,200 mcg.
Vitamin B$_{13}$ (Orotic acid)	Is needed for metabolism of some B vitamins.	Degenerative disorders.	No RDA.	No known toxicity.
Biotin	Necessary for carbohydrate, fat, and protein metabolism. Aids in utilization of other B vitamins.	Dermatitis. Grayish skin color. Depression. Muscle pain. Impairment of fat metabolism. Poor appetite.	150-300 mcg usually meets daily needs. No RDA.	No known oral toxicity. Single doses up to 50 mcg are available without prescription.

*Recommended Dietary Allowances.

Nutrients	Importance	Deficiency Symptoms	RDA*	Toxicity Level
Choline	Is important in normal nerve transmission. Aids metabolism and transport of fats. Helps regulate liver and gallbladder.	Fatty liver. Hemorrhaging kidneys. High blood pressure.	No RDA, but the average diet yields 500-900 mg per day.	No known oral toxicity, even with intake as high as 50,000 mg daily for one week.
Folic acid (Folacin)	Is important in red blood cell formation. Aids metabolism of proteins. Is necessary for growth and division of body cells.	Poor growth. Gastrointestinal disorders. Anemia. B_{12} deficiency.	400 mcg for adults.	No toxic effects. Single doses up to 400 mcg are available without prescription.
Inositol	Is necessary for formation of lecithin. May be indirectly connected with metabolism of fats, including cholesterol. Is vital for hair growth.	Constipation. Eczema. Hair loss. High blood cholesterol.	No RDA.	No known toxicity. Single doses up to 500 mg are available without prescription.
Laetrile	Has been linked to cancer prevention.	Diminished resistance to malignancies.	No RDA.	More than 1.0 g taken at one time may prove toxic. 0.25-1.0 g at a mealtime is usual dosage.
Niacin (Nicotinic acid, Niacinamide)	Is necessary for carbohydrate, fat, and protein metabolism. Helps maintain health of skin, tongue, and digestive system.	Dermatitis. Nervous disorders.	6.6 mg per 1000 calories. 1.8 mg men, 13 mg women.	100-300 mg nicotinic acid orally or 30 mg intraveneously may produce side effects for some individuals. No effects with niacinamide.
PABA	Aids bacteria in producing folic acid. Acts as a coenzyme in the breakdown and utilization of proteins. Aids in formation of red blood cells. Acts as a sunscreen.	Fatigue. Irritability. Depression. Nervousness. Constipation. Headache. Digestive disorders. Graying hair.	No RDA.	Single doses of 100 mg are available without prescription. Continued high ingestion may be toxic.
Pangamic acid	Helps eliminate hypoxia. Helps promote protein metabolism. Stimulates nervous and glandular system.	Diminished oxygenation of cells.	No RDA.	500 mg tolerated daily with no toxic effect.

*Recommended Dietary Allowances.

Nutrients	Importance	Deficiency Symptoms	RDA*	Toxicity Level
Pantothenic acid	Aids in formation of some fats. Participates in the release of energy from carbohydrates, fats, and protein. Aids in the utilization of some vitamins. Improves body's resistance to stress.	Vomiting. Restlessness. Stomach stress. Increased susceptibility to infection. Sensitivity to insulin.	0.5-10.0 mg for both adults and children is considered adequate.	10,000-20,000 mg as a calcium salt may have side effects in some persons.
Vitamin C	Maintains collagen. Helps heal wounds, scar tissue, and fractures. Gives strength to blood vessels. May provide resistance to infections. Aids in absorption of iron.	Bleeding gums. Swollen or painful joints. Slow-healing wounds and fractures. Bruising. Nosebleeds. Impaired digestion.	45 mg for adults.	Essentially nontoxic. 5,000-15,000 mg daily over a prolonged period may have side effects in some persons.
Vitamin D	Improves absorption and utilization of calcium and phosphorus required for bone formation. Maintains stable nervous system and normal heart action.	Poor bone and tooth formation. Softening of bones and teeth. Inadequate absorption of calcium. Retention of phosphorus in kidney.	400 IU for adults.	25,000 IU may be toxic in some individuals over extended period of time. 400 IU is the maximum single dose that can be purchased without a prescription.
Vitamin E	Protects fat-soluble vitamins. Protects red blood cells. Is essential in cellular respiration. Inhibits coagulation of blood by preventing blood clots.	Rupture of red blood cells. Muscular wasting. Abnormal fat deposits in muscles.	15 IU men, 12 IU women.	Essentially nontoxic. 4.0-12.0 g (4,000-30,000 IU) of tocopherol for prolonged periods produces side effects in some persons.
Vitamin F	Is important for respiration of vital organs. Helps maintain resilience and lubrication of cells. Helps regulate blood coagulation. Is essential for normal glandular activity.	Brittle, lusterless hair. Brittle nails. Dandruff. Diarrhea. Varicose veins.	No RDA, 10% of total calories. Men need five times more than women.	Intake should not exceed what is needed to maintain desirable weight.

*Recommended Dietary Allowances.

Nutrients	Importance	Deficiency Symptoms	RDA*	Toxicity Level
Vitamin K	Is necessary for formation of prothrombin; is needed for blood coagulation.	Lack of prothrombin, increasing the tendency to hemorrhage.	No RDA; 300-500 mcg daily is considered adequate.	The menadione (synthetic vitamin K) may have side effects in newborn infants. Available in alfalfa tablet form.
Bioflavonoids	Help increase strength of capillaries.	Tendency to bleed and bruise easily.	No RDA.	No known toxicity.
MINERALS				
Calcium	Sustains development and maintenance of strong bones and teeth. Assists normal blood clotting, muscle action, nerve function, and heart function.	Tetany. Softening bones. Back and leg pains. Brittle bones.	800-1,400 mg, depending upon age.	Excessive intakes of calcium may have side effects in certain persons. No known oral toxicity.
Chlorine	Regulates acid-base balance. Maintains osmotic pressure. Stimulates production of hydrochloric acid. Helps maintain joints and tendons.	Loss of hair and teeth. Poor muscular contractibility. Impaired digestion.	No RDA.	Daily intake of 14-28 g of salt (sodium chloride) is considered excessive. Excess intake of chlorine may have adverse effects.
Chromium	Stimulates enzymes in metabolism of energy and synthesis of fatty acids, cholesterol, and protein. Increases effectiveness of insulin.	Depressed growth rate. Glucose intolerance in diabetics. Atherosclerosis.	No RDA; average daily intake is 80-100 mcg for adults.	No known toxicity.
Cobalt	Functions as part of vitamin B_{12}. Maintains red blood cells. Activates a number of enzymes in the body.	Pernicious anemia. Slow rate of growth.	No RDA; average daily intake is 5.0-8.0 mcg.	Excessive intakes of cobalt may have side effects in certain persons. Available by prescription only.
Copper	Aids in formation of red blood cells. Is part of many enzymes. Works with vitamin C to form elastin.	General weakness. Impaired respiration. Skin sores.	0.08 mg per kilogram of body weight. 2 mg for adults.	20 times RDA over prolonged period may cause toxicity.

*Recommended Dietary Allowances.

Nutrients	Importance	Deficiency Symptoms	RDA*	Toxicity Level
Fluorine	May reduce tooth decay by discouraging the growth of acid-forming bacteria.	Tooth decay.	No RDA.	Excessive intake of fluorine may have side effects in some persons.
Iodine	Is essential part of the hormone thyroxine. Is necessary for the prevention of goiter. Regulates production of energy and rate of metabolism. Promotes growth.	Enlarged thyroid gland. Dry skin and hair. Loss of physical and mental vigor. Cretinism in children born to iodine-deficient mothers.	100 mcg women, 130 mcg men.	Up to 1,000 mcg daily produced no toxic effects in persons with a normal thyroid.[†]
Iron	Is necessary for hemoglobin and myoglobin formation. Helps in protein metabolism. Promotes growth.	Weakness. Paleness of skin. Constipation. Anemia.	10 mg men, 18 mg women.	100 mg daily over prolonged period of time may be toxic in some individuals.
Magnesium	Acts as a catalyst in the utilization of carbohydrates, fats, protein, calcium, phosphorus, and possibly potassium.	Nervousness. Muscular excitability. Tremors.	350 mg men, 300 mg women.	30,000 mg daily may be toxic in certain individuals with kidney malfunctions.
Manganese	Is enzyme activator. Plays a part in carbohydrate and fat production. Is necessary for normal skeletal development. Maintains sex-hormone production.	Paralysis. Convulsions. Dizziness. Ataxia. Blindness and deafness in infants.	No RDA. Average diet supplies 3.0-9.0 mg.	Excessive intake may have side effects in certain persons. Single doses of up to 60 mg are available without prescription.
Molybdenum	Acts in oxidation of fats and aldehydes. Aids in mobilization of iron from liver reserves.	Premature aging.	No RDA. Minute amounts found in body.	5.0-10 ppm is considered toxic.
Phosphorus	Works with calcium to build bones and teeth. Utilizes carbohydrates, fats, and proteins.	Loss of weight and appetite. Irregular breathing. Pyorrhea.	800 mg for adults.	No known toxicity.

*Recommended Dietary Allowances.
[†]Goodhart and Shils, *Modern Nutrition in Health and Disease*, p. 365.

Nutrients	Importance	Deficiency Symptoms	RDA*	Toxicity Level
	Stimulates muscular contraction.			
Potassium	Works to control activity of heart muscles, nervous system, and kidneys.	Poor reflexes. Respiratory failure. Cardiac arrest.	No RDA. Average daily intake is 2,000-2,500 mg.	No known toxicity.
Selenium	Works with vitamin E. Preserves tissue elasticity.	Premature aging.	No RDA.	5.0-10 ppm is considered toxic.
Sodium	Maintains normal fluid levels in cells. Maintains health of the nervous, muscular, blood, and lymph systems.	Muscle weakness. Muscle shrinkage. Nausea. Loss of appetite. Intestinal gas.	3.0-7.0 g sodium. 6.0-18 g sodium chloride.	Excessive sodium intake may have adverse effects. Intake of 14-28 g of sodium chloride (salt) is considered excessive.
Sulfur	Is part of amino acids. Is essential for formation of body tissues. Is part of the B vitamins. Plays a part in tissue respiration. Is necessary for collagen synthesis.	—	The RDA of protein supplies sufficient amounts of sulfur.	Not available for over-the-counter sales.
Vanadium	Inhibits cholesterol formation.	—	No RDA.	No known toxicity.
Zinc	Is component of insulin and male reproductive fluid. Aids in digestion and metabolism of phosphorus. Aids in healing process.	Retarded growth. Delayed sexual maturity. Prolonged healing of wounds.	15 mg for adults.	Relatively nontoxic. 50 mg available without prescription.
Water	Part of blood, lymph, and body secretions. Aids in digestion. Regulates body temperature. Transports nutrients and body wastes.	Dehydration.	—	—

*Recommended Dietary Allowances.

NUTRIENTS THAT FUNCTION TOGETHER

When nutrients are taken in supplemental form, they function best when taken together in particular combinations. Some nutrients are so closely interrelated that their effectiveness in the body is markedly improved when they are taken together with other nutrients. Minerals are especially important in aiding the effectiveness of specific vitamins.

For example, if one is suffering from athlete's foot (see p. 114), vitamin A is recommended for treatment. Vitamin A can be utilized more effectively within the body when taken with the B-complex vitamins, choline, and vitamins C, D, E, and F. Calcium, phosphorus, and zinc are also recommended to increase the effectiveness of vitamin A.

The following chart provides a basic guide to nutrients that function best when taken together.

A. VITAMINS

1. VITAMIN A IS MORE EFFECTIVE WHEN TAKEN WITH

Vitamin B complex	Helps preserve stored vitamin A.
Choline	
Vitamin C	Helps protect against toxic effects of vitamin A.
	Helps prevent oxidation.
Vitamin D	1 part vitamin D to 10 parts vitamin A.
Vitamin E	Acts as an antioxidant.
Vitamin F	When vitamin E dosage is increased, increase supply of vitamin A.
Calcium	When vitamin A dosage is increased, increase supply of calcium and phosphorus.
Phosphorus	When vitamin A dosage is increased, increase supply of calcium and phosphorus.
Zinc	Helps in the absorption of vitamin A.

VITAMIN A EFFECTIVENESS IS DIMINISHED BY

Mineral oil

Lack of vitamin D in the body

2. VITAMIN B COMPLEX IS MORE EFFECTIVE WHEN TAKEN WITH

Vitamin C

Vitamin E

Calcium

Phosphorus

3. VITAMIN B_1 (THIAMINE) IS MORE EFFECTIVE WHEN TAKEN WITH

Vitamin B complex	
Vitamin B_2 (riboflavin)	
Folic acid	
Niacin	
Vitamin C	Helps protect against oxidation.
Vitamin E	
Manganese	
Sulfur	

4. VITAMIN B_2 (RIBOFLAVIN) IS MORE EFFECTIVE WHEN TAKEN WITH

Vitamin B complex	
Vitamin B_6	Vitamin B_2 and vitamin B_6 doses should always be the same.
Niacin	
Vitamin C	Helps protect against oxidation.

5. VITAMIN B_6 (PYRIDOXINE) IS MORE EFFECTIVE WHEN TAKEN WITH

Vitamin B complex	
Vitamin B_1 (thiamine)	Vitamin B_1 and vitamin B_6 doses should always be the same.
Vitamin B_2 (riboflavin)	Vitamin B_2 and vitamin B_6 doses should always be the same.
Pantothenic acid	
Vitamin C	
Magnesium	
Potassium	
Linoleic acid	
Sodium	

6. VITAMIN B_{12} (CYANOCOBALAMIN) IS MORE EFFECTIVE WHEN TAKEN WITH
Vitamin B complex
Vitamin B_6 (pyridoxine)　　　Helps increase absorption of vitamin B_{12}.
Choline
Folic acid
Inositol
Vitamin C　　　Helps increase absorption of vitamin B_{12}.
Potassium
Sodium

7. BIOTIN IS MORE EFFECTIVE WHEN TAKEN WITH
Vitamin B complex
Vitamin B_{12} (cyanocobalamin)
Folic acid
Pantothenic acid
Vitamin C
Sulfur

8. CHOLINE IS MORE EFFECTIVE WHEN TAKEN WITH
Vitamin A
Vitamin B complex
Vitamin B_{12}　　　Helps synthesize choline.
Folic acid　　　Helps synthesize choline.
Inositol
Linoleic acid

9. FOLIC ACID IS MORE EFFECTIVE WHEN TAKEN WITH
Vitamin B complex
Vitamin B_{12}
Biotin
Pantothenic acid
Vitamin C　　　Helps protect against oxidation.

10. INOSITOL IS MORE EFFECTIVE WHEN TAKEN WITH
Vitamin B complex
Vitamin B_{12}
Choline
Linoleic acid

11. LAETRILE IS MORE EFFECTIVE WHEN TAKEN WITH
Vitamin A
Vitamin B complex
Pangamic acid
Vitamin C
Vitamin E

12. NIACIN IS MORE EFFECTIVE WHEN TAKEN WITH
Vitamin B complex
Vitamin B_1 (thiamine)
Vitamin B_2 (riboflavin)
Vitamin C　　　Helps protect against oxidation.

13. PARA-AMINOBENZOIC ACID (PABA) IS MORE EFFECTIVE WHEN TAKEN WITH
    Vitamin B complex
    Folic acid
    Vitamin C

14. PANGAMIC ACID IS MORE EFFECTIVE WHEN TAKEN WITH
    Vitamin B complex
    Vitamin C
    Vitamin E

15. PANTOTHENIC ACID IS MORE EFFECTIVE WHEN TAKEN WITH
    Vitamin B complex
    Vitamin B_6 (pyridoxine)
    Vitamin B_{12} (cyanocobalamin)
    Biotin   Aids in the absorption of pantothenic acid.
    Folic acid   Aids in the absorption of pantothenic acid.
    Vitamin C   Helps protect against oxidation.
    Sulfur

16. VITAMIN C IS MORE EFFECTIVE WHEN TAKEN WITH
    All vitamins and minerals
    Bioflavonoids
    Calcium   Helps body utilize vitamin C.
    Magnesium   Helps body utilize vitamin C.

17. VITAMIN D IS MORE EFFECTIVE WHEN TAKEN WITH
    Vitamin A   10 parts vitamin A to 1 part vitamin D.
    Choline   Helps to prevent toxicity.
    Vitamin C   Helps to prevent toxicity.
    Vitamin F
    Calcium
    Phosphorus

18. VITAMIN E IS MORE EFFECTIVE WHEN TAKEN WITH
    Vitamin A
    Vitamin B complex
    Vitamin B_1 (thiamine)
    Inositol   Helps body utilize vitamin E.
    Vitamin C   Helps protect against oxidation.
    Vitamin F
    Manganese   Helps body utilize vitamin E.
    Selenium

19. VITAMIN F IS MORE EFFECTIVE WHEN TAKEN WITH
    Vitamin A
    Vitamin C
    Vitamin D
    Vitamin E   Helps prevent oxidation and depletion.
    Phosphorus

20. VITAMIN K IS MORE EFFECTIVE WHEN TAKEN WITH
    No information is available at this time.

21. BIOFLAVONOIDS (VITAMIN P) ARE MORE EFFECTIVE WHEN TAKEN WITH
    Vitamin C

B. MINERALS

1. CALCIUM IS MORE EFFECTIVE WHEN TAKEN WITH

Vitamin A	Aids in absorption.
Vitamin C	Aids in absorption.
Vitamin D	Helps in the reabsorption of calcium in kidney tubules and in the retention and utilization of calcium.
Vitamin F	Helps make calcium available to tissues.
Iron	Aids in absorption.
Magnesium	2 parts calcium to 1 part magnesium.
Manganese	
Phosphorus	2.5 parts calcium to 1 part phosphorus.
Hydrochloric acid	

    CALCIUM EFFECTIVENESS IS DIMINISHED BY
    Lack of hydrochloric acid
    Lack of vitamin D
    Lack of magnesium

2. CHLORINE IS MORE EFFECTIVE WHEN TAKEN WITH
    No information is available at this time.

3. CHROMIUM IS MORE EFFECTIVE WHEN TAKEN WITH*
    No information is available at this time.

4. COBALT IS MORE EFFECTIVE WHEN TAKEN WITH*
    Copper
    Iron
    Zinc

5. COPPER IS MORE EFFECTIVE WHEN TAKEN WITH
    Cobalt
    Iron
    Zinc

6. FLUORINE IS MORE EFFECTIVE WHEN TAKEN WITH*
    No information is available at this time.

7. IODINE IS MORE EFFECTIVE WHEN TAKEN WITH*
    No information is available at this time.

8. IRON IS MORE EFFECTIVE WHEN TAKEN WITH*

Vitamin B_{12}	Helps iron function in the body.
Folic acid	

*Denotes essential trace mineral.

Vitamin C	Aids in absorption
Calcium	
Cobalt	
Copper	
Phosphorus	
Hydrochloric acid	Needed for assimilation of iron.

9. MAGNESIUM IS MORE EFFECTIVE WHEN TAKEN WITH

Vitamin B_6	
Vitamin C	
Vitamin D	
Calcium	1 part magnesium to 2 parts calcium.
Phosphorus	
Protein	

10. MANGANESE IS MORE EFFECTIVE WHEN TAKEN WITH*

Vitamin B_1 (thiamine)
Vitamin E
Calcium
Phosphorus

11. MOLYBDENUM IS MORE EFFECTIVE WHEN TAKEN WITH†

No information is available at this time.

12. PHOSPHORUS IS MORE EFFECTIVE WHEN TAKEN WITH

Vitamin A	
Vitamin D	
Vitamin F	
Calcium	1 part phosphorus to 2.5 parts calcium.
Iron	
Manganese	
Protein	

13. POTASSIUM IS MORE EFFECTIVE WHEN TAKEN WITH

Vitamin B_6
Sodium

14. SELENIUM IS MORE EFFECTIVE WHEN TAKEN WITH†

Vitamin E

15. SODIUM IS MORE EFFECTIVE WHEN TAKEN WITH

Vitamin D

SODIUM EFFECTIVENESS IS DIMINISHED BY

Lack of chlorine
Lack of potassium

16. SULFUR IS MORE EFFECTIVE WHEN TAKEN WITH

Vitamin B complex

*Denotes essential trace mineral.
†Denotes trace element whose biological importance to man is unknown.

Vitamin B$_1$ (thiamine)

Biotin

Pantothenic acid

SULFUR EFFECTIVENESS IS DIMINISHED BY

Insufficient protein

17. VANADIUM IS MORE EFFECTIVE WHEN TAKEN WITH†

No information is available at this time.

18. ZINC IS MORE EFFECTIVE WHEN TAKEN WITH*

Vitamin A

Calcium

Copper

Phosphorus

ZINC EFFECTIVENESS IS DIMINISHED BY

Lack of phosphorus

*Denotes essential trace element.
†Denotes trace element whose biological importance to man is unknown.

AVAILABLE FORMS OF NUTRIENT SUPPLEMENTS

NATURAL AND SYNTHETIC

Because of individual differences such as sex, age, environment, stress, and state of health, many people do not receive the full benefit of the nutrients provided in their daily diet. For this reason vitamin and mineral supplements are used.

Vitamin supplements come in two forms, natural and synthetic. A natural vitamin exists in its original state in nature. It is not artificial, and its source is either a plant or an animal. A synthetic vitamin, in most instances, has the same chemical structure as the natural vitamin, but it is produced artificially by synthesis of simpler materials. There may be factors such as enzymes, synergists, catalysts, minerals, proteins, or even unidentified vitamins which are found in the natural nutrient but not in its synthetic counterpart. Compounds found in the natural vitamins contain nutrients in their natural ratios and do not contain potentially harmful ingredients such as artificial coloring or flavorings, as may be found in the synthetic product.

Labels do not always tell the full story. A natural vitamin should be a whole food product with nothing removed. Many so-called natural vitamins are not completely natural but rather are a combination of both natural and synthetic nutrients called "co-natural" vitamins. Synthetic nutrients are added to increase the potency or stability and to standardize the amount of nutrients per capsule or per batch.

Synthetic vitamins and minerals often contain a salt form that is used to increase stability of the nutrient. These salt forms are palmatate, sulfate, nitrate, hydrochloride, chloride, succinate, bitartrate, acetate, and gluconate. This information may aid in the determination of whether a nutrient is natural or synthetic. A label may read "Vitamin A Palmitate," thus indicating that it is synthetic rather than natural.

ORGANIC AND INORGANIC

If a vitamin supplement is labeled "organic," it is composed of, or contains, matter of plant or animal origin. "Inorganic" means that the vitamin supplement is composed of something other than organic materials such as those found in water and soil. Foods and supplements derived from organic sources are probably better assimilated by the body than are inorganic supplements.

FORMS OF SUPPLEMENTAL NUTRIENTS

Nearly all the nutrient supplements are available in many forms: tablet, capsule, liquid, powder, drops, or ointment. This variety allows people to choose a supplement form that best suits their needs.

The *tablet* is a compressed block of material available in a variety of potencies, especially higher ones. If kept in a closed bottle, it can be stored indefinitely. However, once opened, all nutrients in this form should be stored in a cool, dark place because exposure to air will reduce potency.

The *capsule* is a small container made of gelatin or other soluble materials. The ingredients inside the container can either be powder or liquid. The advantage of the powder-filled capsule is that it can be opened and sprinkled on food or in beverages, a useful factor for those people who have difficulty swallowing. The liquid-filled capsule, as in vitamin E, has distinct advantages too. For example, a person suffering from a cold sore may pick up a capsule, insert a pin, gently squeeze, and apply the oil directly to the sore. The capsule will then seal itself, become airtight, and be ready for use again. The capsule is available in the same potencies as the tablet, and its storage properties are also the same.

Nutrients in liquid form are easily taken and are especially good for children or elderly persons who find swallowing a tablet or a capsule difficult. Vitamin C is available in liquid and may be the preferred form if one is suffering from a cold and finds swallowing a pill painful. The liquid is usually found in lower potencies and should be stored in the refrigerator. Once opened, a bottle of liquid nutrients rapidly loses potency.

Nutrients in powdered form can be sprinkled on foods and in beverages and are also easy for children or the elderly to consume. They are an excellent way to provide the essential amino acids. Vegetarians may find this form useful. Powder should be kept in a dark place away from high humidity.

In some cases it may be desirable to obtain the nutrients in drops or ointments. For example, vitamin E ointment is recommended for treatment of burns to promote healing and reduce scarring.

To avoid confusion and insure the best possible benefits from nutrient supplements, it is important to schedule their consumption. Schedules will vary with specific needs, ailments, eating habits, environment, etc. Vitamins and minerals should be taken with meals, and it is advantageous to take the most vitamins with the largest meal for best absorption. It is wise to take the fat-soluble vitamins with fat-containing foods to ensure adequate amounts of bile for absorption. The water-soluble vitamins need to be taken throughout the day because they are lost through excretion. It is also necessary to be aware of which nutrients function together and which are antagonists. For example, vitamin E and iron should be taken 8 to 12 hours apart. For further information, see individual nutrients and "Nutrients That Function Together," pp. 93-99.

The following table gives the various supplemental forms in which a nutrient may be found, together with its source. Supplemental forms are subject to change and may vary in different localities.

Nutrient	Form	Source	Explanation
VITAMINS			
Vitamin A	Fish-liver oils	Natural	Excellent natural sources; good source of oil in diet.
	Carrot (oil)	Natural	Cannot be tolerated by persons suffering from gall-bladder problems and other digestive problems. Not absorbed by the body as easily as fish-liver oils.
	Lemon grass	Natural	An herbal grass that is a good source of oil.
	Vitamin A palmatate	Synthetic	Recommended for pregnant women and persons with fish-liver-oil absorption problems.
	Vitamin A acetate	Synthetic	Recommended for pregnant women and persons with fish-liver-oil absorption problems.
Vitamin B complex	Brewer's yeast	Natural	Low-potency form; all B factors, protein, enzymes, and possibly some unidentified nutrients included.
	Nutritional yeast	Natural	Usually higher potency and better flavor than brewer's yeast.
Vitamin B_1 (thiamine)	Yeast or rice bran	Natural	Natural ingredient in capsule or tablet form.
	Thiamine hydrochloride	Synthetic	High-potency.
	Thiamine chloride	Synthetic	High-potency.
	Thiamine mononitrate	Synthetic	High-potency.
Vitamin B_2 (riboflavin)	Yeast or bran	Natural	Natural ingredient in capsule or tablet form.
	Riboflavin	Synthetic	High-potency.
Vitamin B_6 (pyridoxine)	Yeast or bran	Natural	Natural ingredient in capsule or tablet form.
	Pyridoxine hydrochloride	Synthetic	High potency.
Vitamin B_{12} (cobalamin)	Yeast or rice bran	Natural	Natural ingredient in capsule or tablet form.
	Fermentation concentrate	Natural	More easily absorbed than other forms of B_{12}.
	Cobalamin	Natural	High-potency natural fermentation product.
	Cyanocobalamin	Natural	Natural fermentation product.
Vitamin B_{13} (orotic acid)	Orotic acid	Natural	May not be available yet in health stores in U.S.
Biotin	Yeast	Natural	
	D-biotin	Synthetic	High-potency.
Choline	Soybeans	Natural	Other factors may be present which may not be in synthetic form; found in powder, tablet, and capsule forms.
	Yeast	Natural	Other factors may be present which may not be in synthetic form; found in powder, tablet, and capsule forms.
	Choline bitartrate	Synthetic	Obtained in high-potency dosage.
Folic acid	Yeast	Natural	Other factors may be present which may not be in synthetic form.
	Pleroylglutamic	Synthetic	High-potency.
Inositol	Soybeans	Natural	Other factors may be present which may not be in synthetic form; found in powder, tablet, and capsule forms.
	Corn or yeast	Natural	Other factors may be present which may not be in synthetic form; found in powder, tablet, and capsule forms.

Nutrient	Form	Source	Explanation
Laetrile	Apricot kernels	Natural	More inexpensive and more readily available than amygdalin.
	Amygdalin	Natural	More expensive than apricot kernels.
Niacin	Yeast or bran	Natural	Other factors may be present which may not be in synthetic form.
	Niacinamide	Synthetic	Will not cause flushing or tingling sensation (see "Niacin") when dosage is over 100 mg.
	Nicotinic acid	Synthetic	
	Niacin	Synthetic	Will cause flushing or tingling sensation (100 mg or more); more effective than niacinamide for migraine headaches.
Pantothenic acid	Yeast	—	Other factors may be present which may not be in synthetic forms.
	Calcium D-pantothenate	Synthetic	High-potency.
Para-aminobenzoic acid (PABA)	Yeast	—	Other factors may be present which may not be in synthetic forms.
	Para-aminobenzoic acid	Synthetic	High-potency.
Pangamic acid	Apricot kernels	Natural	More inexpensive and more readily absorbed than other forms.
	Pangamic acid	Synthetic	Russian formula for pangamic acid has recently become available in the U.S.; high-potency.
	Calcium pangamate	—	High-potency.
Vitamin C	Rose hips	Natural	Available in all forms, capsule, tablet, etc.
	Acerola cherries	Natural	Available in all forms, capsule, tablet, etc.
	Citrus fruits	Natural	Available in all forms, capsule, tablet, etc.
	Green peppers	Natural	
	Ascorbic acid	Synthetic	Most economical source but without bioflavonoids; added to vitamin C to increase potency and stability.
Vitamin D	Cod-liver oil	Natural	An excellent natural source; cannot be tolerated by persons suffering from gallbladder or other digestive problems.
	Irradiated ergosterol	Synthetic	High-potency.
	Calciferol	Synthetic	High-potency.
Vitamin E	Vegetable oils	Natural	Good way to get essential oils.
	Wheat germ	Natural	Low-potency.
	Mixed tocopheryl	Natural	D-alpha and other tocopheryls that help alpha function better.
	d-alpha tocopheryl	Natural	Most active form of tocopheryl which helps alpha function better.
	d-alpha tocopheryl acetate	Co-natural	A natural derivative with synthetic products added.
	dl-alpha tocopheryl	Synthetic	Considered by some a more stable form.
	dl-alpha tocopheryl acetate	Synthetic	Considered by some a more stable form.
	dl-alpha tocopheryl succinate	Synthetic	Considered by some a more stable form.

Nutrient	Form	Source	Explanation
Vitamin F	Unsaturated fatty acids	Natural	Good way to provide oil for diet.
	Essential fatty acids	Natural	Good way to provide oil for diet.
Vitamin K	Alfalfa	Natural	Contains chlorophyll enzymes, and other factors; high mineral source.
	Menodoine	Synthetic	
Bioflavonoids	Rutin	Natural	Are factors that make vitamin C more effective.
	Hesperiden	Natural	Are factors that make vitamin C more effective.
	Flavons	Natural	Are factors that make vitamin C more effective.
	Bioflavonoids in combination with vitamin C	Natural	Are factors that make vitamin C more effective.
MINERALS			
Calcium	Calcium lactate	Natural	A salt of lactic acid from milk; easily absorbed; low-potency.
	Calcium gluconate	Natural	A salt of gluconic acid from glucose; easily absorbed; one needs to take more to get equivalent potencies.
	Calcium pantothenate	Natural	A salt of pantothenic acid (from B complex).
	Bone meal	Natural	Dried bones of cattle; type of calcium closest to calcium found in human bones and teeth; poorly absorbed; has high potency with other trace minerals.
	Dolomite	Natural	Calcium and magnesium also available with vitamin A and D; not to be used by the elderly or persons with poor hydrochloric acid secretions.
	Di-cal phosphate	Co-natural	Bone meal or bone ash with additional 22% phosphorus.
	Eggshell calcium	Natural	Dried eggshell.
	Oyster-shell calcium	Natural	Natural calcium form with minimal phosphorus interference but with natural trace minerals.
	Liquid calcium	Natural	Good for person who has calcium-absorption problems.
Chloride	—	—	Not available singly but in some complete-multimineral supplements.
Cobalt	—	—	Not available singly but in some complete-multimineral supplements.
Copper	Copper sulfate	Synthetic	Available in other salt forms.
Chromium	—	—	Not available singly but in some complete-multimineral supplements.
Fluorine	—	—	Not available singly but in some complete-multimineral supplements.
Iodine	Sea kelp	Natural	Includes trace minerals and other substances.
	Sea salt	Natural	Includes trace minerals and other substances.
	Seaweed	Natural	Includes trace minerals and other substances.
	Potassium oxide	Synthetic	Table salt.

Nutrient	Form	Source	Explanation
Iron	Desiccated liver	Natural	Dried liver of cattle; low-potency; good for women.
	Yeast	Natural	Low-potency; good for women.
	Molasses	Natural	Low-potency; good for women.
	Ferrous fumerate	Synthetic	High-potency.
	Ferrous gluconate	Synthetic	High-potency; more readily absorbed than ferrous fumerate.
	Ferrous sulfate	Synthetic	High-potency.
Magnesium	Dolomite	Natural	Calcium and magnesium in natural balance (2:1); not recommended for persons with poor hydrochloric acid secretions.
	Magnesium palmatate	Synthetic	Available in other salt forms; high-potency.
	Magnesium sulfate	Synthetic	Epsom salts; calcium-free.
Manganese	Manganese gluconate	Synthetic	Easily absorbed.
Molybdenum	—	—	
Phosphorus	Bone meal	Natural	Contains additional calcium and other nutrients.
	Calcium phosphate	Synthetic	High-potency.
Potassium	Potassium gluconate	Synthetic	Easily absorbed.
	Potassium chloride	Synthetic	
Selenium	—	—	
Sodium	Sodium chloride	Synthetic	Table salt.
Sulfur	—	—	Available in ointment form and in some complete-multimineral supplements.
Zinc	Zinc gluconate	Synthetic	More readily absorbed than zinc sulfate.
	Zinc sulfate	Synthetic	
Protein	Meat or fish	Natural	Available in powder and tablet forms.
	Eggs or milk	Natural	Available in powder and tablet forms.
	Soybeans	Natural	Good source for vegetarians.
	Amino acid compounds	Natural	Available in tablet, liquid, and powder form.

APPROXIMATE NUTRIENT COMPOSITION OF THE BODY

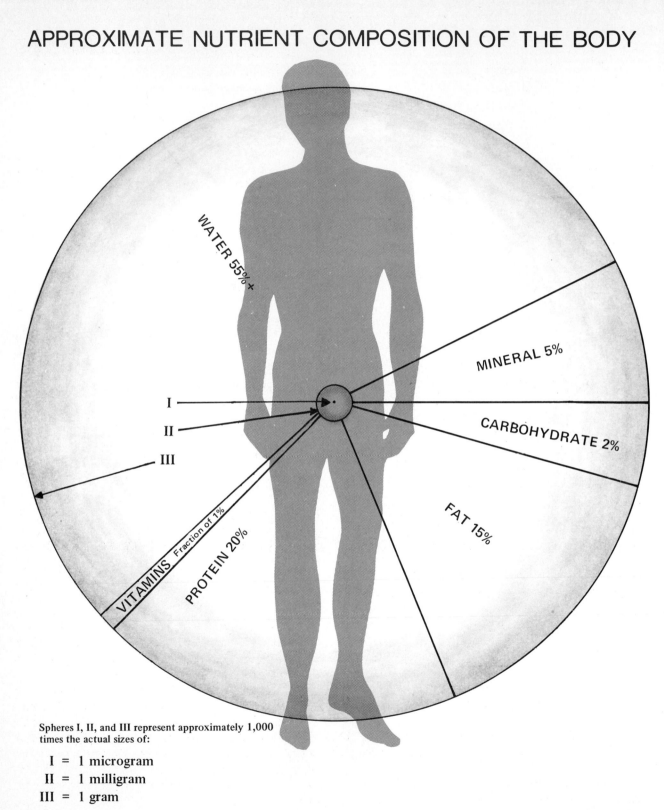

WATER 55%+

MINERAL 5%

CARBOHYDRATE 2%

FAT 15%

VITAMINS Fraction of 1%

PROTEIN 20%

I

II

III

Spheres I, II, and III represent approximately 1,000
times the actual sizes of:

I = 1 microgram
II = 1 milligram
III = 1 gram

Ailments and Other Stressful Conditions

Good health is a product of heredity, environment, and nutrition. Nutritional deficiency, resulting in malnutrition or disease, is one of the major problems in modern society despite adequate food supply, primarily because of ignorance of good nutrition. A well-balanced diet, rich in all essential nutrients, is necessary to maintain a healthy body and mind.

Authorities have found that a number of diseases can appear when there is a deficiency of one or more nutrients. Most diseases caused by such deficiencies can be corrected when all essential nutrients are supplied. However, in some instances of severe deficiency, irreparable damage may be done.

The following pages list common ailments and stressful conditions that many authorities believe are related to nutrition. Common ailments are listed alphabetically by ailment together with explanations, including pertinent nutritional information regarding the nature of most of the ailments. These explanations are designed to give an understanding of the specific ailments.

The body member affected by each ailment is also identified. Nutrient listings for each ailment are given. These include those nutrients found by nutrition researchers to be beneficial in the treatment of the given ailment.

Nutrient quantities are given for some nutrients. They represent amounts of these nutrients which have been found by some researchers to be effective in the treatment of the ailment. All amounts are daily unless otherwise stated. When no quantity is listed, available research did not indicate an amount.

Note: These and the following quantity-of-nutrient listings do not constitute prescriptive amounts. They only represent research findings.

Many of the seemingly high doses result from clinical tests on ailing persons. These amounts would not necessarily be required, or even recommended, for a healthy person. Most dosages used in research are greater than those cited as daily allowances. We repeat:

These amounts are not prescriptive.

Individual tolerances to the nutrients may differ significantly. Each individual must determine, according to his own tolerances, the quantity of each nutrient that will be beneficial in the treatment of disease.

Factors influencing individual tolerances include a person's normal eating habits, previous amounts of vitamins ingested, height, weight, metabolic rate, reaction to stress, and environmental variances. Build up the dosages slowly: it took a long time for your body to become ill, so take your time in trying to heal it. If you wish to take large amounts of a nutrient, it would be wise to consult a physician.

AILMENTS

ABSCESS

An abscess is a localized infection with a collection of pus in any part of the body. An abscess may be located externally or internally and may be initiated by lowered resistance to infection, bacterial contamination, or injury. Symptoms of abscess include tenderness and swelling in the infected area, fever, and chills.

Antibiotics may be used to treat the infection, although in the case of a severe abscess, surgery may be necessary. Because the antibiotics used in treatment may interfere with the absorption of the B vitamins, supplementary B complex may be required. Fever increases the body's need for calories; vitamins A, C, and E; and extra fluids.

NUTRIENTS THAT MAY BE BENEFICIAL IN TREATMENT OF ABSCESS

Body Member	Nutrients	Quantity*
Body/Skin	Vitamin A	100,000 IU for three days
	Vitamin B complex	
	Vitamin C	
	Vitamin E	
	Water	

*See note, p. 169.

ACNE

Acne is a common disorder of the oil glands in the skin characterized by the recurring formation of blackheads, whiteheads, and pimples. Acne occurs primarily on the face and sometimes on the back, shoulders, chest, and arms. The incidence of acne is greatest during puberty and adolescence, when hormones influencing the secretion of the oil glands are at their peak level of activity.

Proper nutrition and skin cleanliness, together with adequate rest, exercise, fresh air, and sunlight, are helpful in the treatment of acne. Many authorities believe overindulgence in carbohydrates and foods with high fat content should be avoided. Candy, sweetened soft drinks, fried foods, and nuts should be avoided. An excess of oxalic acid found in chocolate, cocoa, spinach, and rhubarb may inhibit the body's absorption of calcium. Calcium helps maintain the acid-alkali balance of the blood necessary for a clear complexion.

Vitamin A is especially beneficial for clear, healthy skin. The B-complex vitamins, especially riboflavin, pyridoxine, and pantothenic acid, help reduce facial oiliness and blackhead formation. Vitamin C aids in resisting the spread of acne infection, and vitamin D guards the body's store of calcium from excretion. Vitamin E has been found helpful in the prevention of scarring.[1]

NUTRIENTS THAT MAY BE BENEFICIAL IN TREATMENT OF ACNE

Body Member	Nutrients	Quantity*
Skin	Vitamin A	50,000-100,000 IU daily for one month
	Vitamin B complex	
	Vitamin B$_2$	5-15 mg
	Vitamin B$_6$	
	Niacin	100 mg three times daily
	Pantothenic acid	300 mg
	Vitamin C	1,000 mg
	Vitamin D	200-400 mg
	Vitamin E	
	Vitamin F	
	Calcium	
	Potassium	

*See note, p. 169.

ADRENAL EXHAUSTION

Adrenal exhaustion is the progressive lessening of activity of the adrenal glands, which may eventually lead to complete functional failure. It is characterized by a low energy level in the morning which gradually rises, being highest late at night. The person retires but cannot fall asleep right away, then sleeps soundly but arises exhausted. Adrenal exhaustion is often categorized with insomnia.

The vitamins B$_2$, B$_{12}$, folic acid, and pantothenic acid with potassium and sodium stabilize the activity of the adrenal glands.

NUTRIENTS THAT MAY BE BENEFICIAL IN TREATMENT OF ADRENAL EXHAUSTION

Body Member	Nutrients	Quantity
Glands	Vitamin B complex	
	Vitamin B$_2$	

[1] Adelle Davis, *Let's Get Well* (New York: Harcourt, Brace & World, 1965), p. 161.

Body Member	Nutrients	Quantity
	Vitamin B$_{12}$	
	Folic acid	
	Pantothenic acid	
	Vitamin C	
	Potassium	
	Sodium	

ALCOHOLISM

Alcoholism is a dependence on or addiction to alcohol. The body's outward reaction to alcohol suggests that it acts as a stimulant by producing aggressive social behavior such as loss of inhibitions, increased boldness, and sociability associated with drinking. In fact, alcohol is a depressant that acts to decrease the basic speed of all bodily functions, including muscle contractions, speed of reaction, digestion, and thinking processes.

Prolonged dependence upon this drug may result in severe problems in the pancreas and gastrointestinal tract as well as the emotional and mental problems associated with alcoholism. Severe deficiencies of many nutrients occur because the alcohol itself satisfies the body's caloric needs. (Alcohol contains about 70 calories per ounce.)

As the alcohol enters the bloodstream directly through the walls of the stomach, it begins to act upon the central nervous system by changing the most basic mental functions and by destroying brain cells. Cells are destroyed by the withdrawal of necessary water from the tissues and cells. The liver works to neutralize the effects of alcohol upon the body by breaking down the composition of the alcohol. Under normal circumstances, especially if there is food in the stomach, the liver can effectively perform the function of breaking down the alcohol if not more than one drink per hour is consumed. However, when the liver is overworked, it must compensate by creating an increased tolerance for alcohol. After a time the liver compensates less rapidly, becomes fatty, and is less able to decompose the alcohol. As a result, the alcoholic develops a decreased tolerance for alcohol and less is needed to produce intoxication. As drinking continues over a period of time, the liver cells die and are replaced with scar tissue. This condition is known as cirrhosis of the liver.

Diet and nutrient supplements are very important in the treatment of alcoholism. In some cases, a strict diet adequate in calories and high in protein, which contains all the vitamins and minerals and is especially high in B vitamins, reduced the alcoholic's desire to drink. Protein is necessary for tissue regeneration, particularly when cirrhosis of the liver occurs. Vitamin A is an anti-infective agent for upper respiratory infections such as tuberculosis and pneumonia which are common in alcoholics. The vitamin B complex is essential for the prevention and treatment of alcoholic neuritis, pellagra, and delirium tremens. Vitamin C, which is often deficient in alcoholics, is needed to prevent scurvy. A zinc deficiency may occur, making the alcoholic more prone to cirrhosis of the liver and preventing vitamin K from being absorbed into the body. Iron is needed to correct the anemia that often develops. A magnesium deficiency can contribute to the occurrence of delirium tremens. A deficiency of potassium may also occur in alcoholics, and supplements may be necessary. Choline aids in the decomposition of fat in the liver and helps maintain healthy kidneys jeopardized by heavy drinking.

NUTRIENTS THAT MAY BE BENEFICIAL IN TREATMENT OF ALCOHOLISM

Body Member	Nutrients	Quantity*
Brain/Nervous system	Vitamin A	25,000 IU
	Vitamin B complex	
	Vitamin B$_1$	
	Vitamin B$_2$	
	Vitamin B$_6$	100 mg
	Vitamin B$_{12}$	
	Choline	
	Folic acid	
	Niacin	100 mg in the form of niacinamide
	Pangamic acid	
	Pantothenic acid	
	Vitamin C	Up to 3,000 mg
	Vitamin D	1,000 IU
	Vitamin E	Up to 1,200 IU
	Vitamin K	
	Iron	
	Magnesium	Up to 1,000 mg
	Zinc	

*See note, p. 169.

ALLERGIES

An allergy is a sensitivity to some particular substance known as an allergen. The allergen may be harmless to some people but can cause a reaction in others. Almost any food may be an allergen to some people. The allergic reaction may be hay fever, asthma, hives, high blood pressure, abnormal fatigue, constipation, stomach ulcers, dizziness, headache, mental disorders, hyperactivity, or hypoglycemia. After eating, excessive tiredness, swelled stomach, palpitations, sweating, or mental fuzziness may be experienced.

NUTRIENTS THAT MAY BE BENEFICIAL IN TREATMENT OF ALLERGIES

Body Member	Nutrients	Quantity*
General	Vitamin A	10,000-25,000 IU
	Vitamin B complex	
	Vitamin B_{12}	
	Pantothenic acid	100-200 mg
	Vitamin C	250 mg four times daily; up to 5,000 mg
	Vitamin D	
	Vitamin E	Up to 800 IU
	Vitamin F	
	Calcium	Up to 1,000 mg
	Manganese	5 mg twice weekly for 10 weeks
	Potassium	

*See note, p. 169.

AMBLYOPIA

Amblyopia is an impairment of the ability of the eyes to focus. Vitamin B_1 is used to correct it.

NUTRIENTS THAT MAY BE BENEFICIAL IN TREATMENT OF AMBLYOPIA

Body Member	Nutrient	Quantity*
Eyes	Vitamin A	
	Vitamin B complex	
	Vitamin B_1	20 mg
	Vitamin C	
	Vitamin E	

*See note, p. 169.

ANEMIA

A reduction of the amount of hemoglobin in the bloodstream and/or a reduction in the number of red blood cells themselves reduces the amount of oxygen available to all body cells. Carbon dioxide accumulates in the cells, causing decreased efficiency and lower rate of body processes. When the brain cells are deprived of oxygen, dizziness may result. Additional symptoms of anemia are general weakness, fatigue, paleness, brittle nails, loss of appetite, and abdominal pain.

Anemia often arises from recurrent infections and/or diseases involving the entire body. It may also be caused by inadequate intake or impaired absorption of nutrients or by excessive losses of blood through such conditions as heavy menstruation or peptic ulcer. It has been shown that excess amounts of vitamin K in the diet during pregnancy may cause anemia in newborn infants.[2]

Iron, protein, copper, folic acid, and vitamins B_6, B_{12}, and C are all necessary for the formation of red blood cells. A deficiency in any of these nutrients can cause anemia, although iron-deficiency anemia is the most common form of the condition. Infants, adolescents, and women, particularly during pregnancy, are often deficient in iron and may require iron supplements. Vitamin C aids in the absorption and retention of iron. Vitamin E may be needed to help maintain the health of red blood cells.

NUTRIENTS THAT MAY BE BENEFICIAL IN TREATMENT OF ANEMIA

Body Member	Nutrients	Quantity*
Blood/Circulatory system	Vitamin B complex	
	Vitamin B_1	50-100 mg
	Vitamin B_6	
	Vitamin B_{12}	20-50 mcg
	Folic acid	0.5-5 mg
	PABA	Up to 50 mg
	Pantothenic acid	Up to 100 mg
	Vitamin C	500 mg
	Vitamin E	Up to 1,000 IU

*See note, p. 169.

[2]Phyllis Sullivan Howe, *Basic Nutrition in Health and Diseases* (Philadelphia: W. B. Saunders Co., 1971), p. 96.

Body Member	Nutrients	Quantity
	Calcium	
	Iron	10 mg
	Copper	
	Protein	

abling more blood to flow through the circulatory system.[3]

NUTRIENTS THAT MAY BE BENEFICIAL IN TREATMENT OF ANGINA PECTORIS

Body Member	Nutrients	Quantity*
Blood/Circulatory system	Vitamin A	25,000 IU
	Vitamin B complex	
	Vitamin B$_{12}$	25 mcg
	Choline	
	Pangamic acid	
	Vitamin C	3,000 mg
	Vitamin E	200 IU daily; gradually work up to 1,600 IU daily
	Iodine	
	Potassium	
	Protein	

*See note, p. 169.

ANGINA PECTORIS

Angina pectoris is a condition characterized by severe pain in the heart area. It is due to insufficient supply of blood to the heart tissue which results in a lack of oxygen in these tissues. The most frequent cause of this insufficient blood supply is atherosclerosis of the arteries that supply the heart with blood. This condition is most commonly found in males over age forty-five.

Attacks are brought on by a heavy meal, unaccustomed physical exertion, stress, emotional tension, or exposure to cold. The frequency and duration of attacks vary and may range from several attacks per day to one attack every few years.

The pain varies greatly in severity from a mild pressure to an intolerable agony. It usually starts in the upper chest or throat and radiates to the left shoulder and down the left arm. The patient is pale, sweaty, and very apprehensive. These symptoms are similar to those of a heart attack but can be differentiated in that the pain lasts only for minutes and can be relieved by rest. However, if the blood supply is insufficient enough, angina pectoris can progress to a heart attack.

In the treatment of angina pectoris, effort should be made to obtain rest and to decrease the workload of the heart. Because the workload of the heart increases after meals, the diet should consist of small, frequent feedings that are salt-free and low in saturated fat and calories. Cold fluids should be avoided because they may trigger irregularities in the heart function. Protein intake should be adequate to replace protein lost from the damaged heart cells.

Preventive measures for angina pectoris include avoidance of smoking, alcohol, exposure to cold, and overweight. The B-complex vitamins and vitamin C may be helpful in maintaining the integrity and health of the heart and circulatory system in the atherosclerosis victim. Some authorities state that vitamin E and iodine may prove helpful because they open the arteries, en-

ARTERIOSCLEROSIS AND ATHEROSCLEROSIS

A thickening and hardening of the walls of the arteries is known as arteriosclerosis. Arteriosclerosis occurs in two forms. The first type of hardening is caused by a gradual deposit of calcium in the artery walls, restricting the flow of blood to the body cells. A second, more advanced type of hardening, called atherosclerosis, is due to the buildup of cholesterol or fatty deposits in the artery walls and contributes to the degeneration of the arteries involved. Atherosclerosis usually affects the aorta, heart, and brain arteries as well as the other blood vessels of the body and extremities. It usually occurs in older people and is still considered the number one cause of death in the United States.

There are several theories as to the cause of atherosclerosis. It is often thought to be a metabolic defect involving fats. Fat molecules are normally absorbed through the artery walls. When an excess of fatty material starts to restrict blood flow, fatty streaks begin to appear on the interior of the arteries. As more and more

[3]Wilfrid E. Shute and Harold J. Taub, *Vitamin E for Ailing and Healthy Hearts* (New York: Pyramid House, 1969), p. 44.

of this fat is introduced, the artery walls thicken and plaques of cholesterol narrow the arteries. The artery walls then lose their elasticity and become hard and brittle. Hemorrhages from small vessels located in the arterial wall beneath the plaques may cause the cholesterol deposits to break free from the wall, or a clot may form as blood passes over the rough edge of a plaque. The plaques, clots, or a combination of these may cause a total block in the vessel, resulting in death.

Symptoms of atherosclerosis are hypertension, cramping or paralysis of muscles, a sensation of heaviness or pressure in the chest, and pains that radiate from the chest to the left arm and shoulder. Factors that enhance the tendency to develop atherosclerosis are obesity, lack of exercise, hypertension, smoking, heredity, stress, and poor diet. Males over forty years of age are highly susceptible, but women do not usually suffer from it until after menopause. Some researchers believe that a high intake of carbohydrates is a factor that predisposes toward atherosclerosis.[4]

Prevention and treatment measures for the disease include reducing the percentage of fat in the diet to no more than 30 to 35 percent with the ratio of unsaturates to saturates being 2 to 1 and limiting the cholesterol intake to 300 milligrams daily. If obesity is present, weight should be reduced to a normal level. Physical exercise is necessary for stimulating circulation and strengthening the heart muscles. Reducing salt intake is important if hypertension is present.

The B complex helps in the prevention of atherosclerosis by reducing blood cholesterol levels. Vitamin C is necessary to help maintain health of the arteries and prevent hemorrhaging. Some researchers indicate that vitamin E may help prevent clot formation.[5]

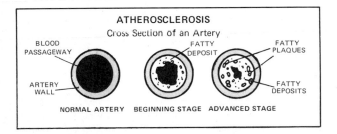

ATHEROSCLEROSIS
Cross Section of an Artery

BLOOD PASSAGEWAY   FATTY DEPOSIT   FATTY PLAQUES

ARTERY WALL   FATTY DEPOSITS

NORMAL ARTERY   BEGINNING STAGE   ADVANCED STAGE

[4] J. I. Rodale, *The Encyclopedia for Healthful Living* (Emmaus, Pa.: Rodale Books, 1970), p. 733.

[5] Linda Clark, *Get Well Naturally* (New York: Devin-Adair, 1963), p. 325.

NUTRIENTS THAT MAY BE BENEFICIAL IN TREATMENT OF ARTERIOSCLEROSIS AND ATHEROSCLEROSIS

Body Member	Nutrients	Quantity*
Blood/Heart	Vitamin A	20,000-100,000 IU
	Vitamin B complex	
	Vitamin B₆	50 mg
	Vitamin B₁₂	
	Choline	500 mg
	Folic acid	
	Inositol	500 mg
	Niacin	100-500 mg under doctor's supervision
	Vitamin C	Up to 3,000 mg
	Vitamin E	600-1,200 IU
	Bioflavonoids	300-600 mg
	Calcium	500 mg
	Chromium	
	Zinc	

*See note, p. 169.

ARTHRITIS

Arthritis results in inflammation and soreness of the joints. Osteoarthritis and rheumatoid arthritis are the two main types of the disease.

Osteoarthritis, usually found in elderly people, develops as a result of the continuous wearing away of the cartilage in a joint. Cartilage, which is a smooth, soft, pearly tissue, covers the ends of the bones at the joints. It provides a smooth surface for the bones to slide against, allowing easy movement of the joints. As a result of injury or years of use, cartilage becomes thin and may disappear. When enough cartilage has worn away, the rough surfaces of the bones rub together, causing pain and stiffness. Osteoarthritis usually affects the weight-bearing joints, such as the hips and knees. Symptoms of osteoarthritis include body stiffness and pain in the joints, especially during damp weather, in the morning, or after strenuous activity.

Rheumatoid arthritis affects the entire body instead of just one joint. Onset of the disease is often associated with physical or emotional stress and usually occurs between the ages of thirty and forty. Rheumatoid arthritis destroys the cartilage and tissues in and around the joints and often the bone surfaces themselves. The body replaces the damaged tissue with scar tissue, causing the spaces between the joints to become narrow and fuse together. This causes the stiffening and crippling onset of the disease. Symptoms of rheumatoid arthritis include swelling and pain in the joints, fatigue, anemia, weight loss, and fever. These symptoms often disappear and recur at a later date.

Exercise is important in both the prevention and treatment of arthritis because unused joints tend to stiffen. Good posture is also important to prevent stiffness and crippling. Poor posture can cause body weight to be distributed unevenly, placing more stress on certain joints, thus resulting in unnecessary pain for the arthritic person.

Many nutritional cures for arthritis have been claimed, upon which research still continues. It is recommended that the arthritic have a well-balanced diet in order to provide his body with all the nutrients it needs for repair. If the arthritic is overweight he or she should lose weight in order to reduce the stress on weight-bearing joints.

Vitamin C is necessary to prevent the capillary walls in the joints from breaking down and causing bleeding, swelling, and pain. Folic acid, vitamin B_{12}, and iron may be helpful in treating the anemia that can accompany arthritis. The frequency of liver disorders in arthritic patients may deter the conversion of carotene into vitamin A. Difficulty in assimilating carbohydrates suggests vitamin B deficiency. Treatment involves a diet high in raw fruits and vegetables low in sodium (salt).

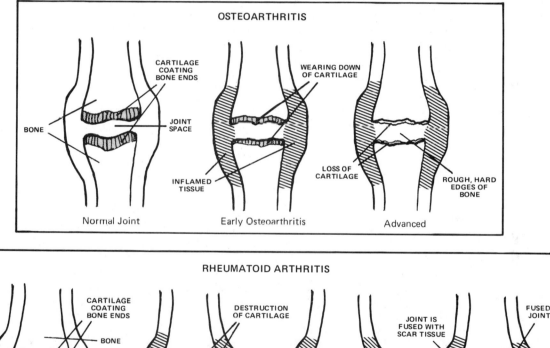

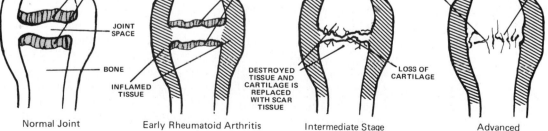

NUTRIENTS THAT MAY BE BENEFICIAL IN TREATMENT OF ARTHRITIS

Body Member	Nutrients	Quantity*
Joints	Vitamin A	
	Vitamin B complex	
	Vitamin B$_2$	1,000 mg under doctor's supervision
	Vitamin B$_6$	50-100 mg
	Vitamin B$_{12}$	30-900 mcg per week
	Folic acid	
	Niacin	Up to 1,000 mg under doctor's supervision
	Pantothenic acid	100 mg
	Vitamin C	3,000-5,000 mg; children, 600 mg
	Vitamin D	
	Vitamin E	600-1,000 IU
	Vitamin F	
	Bioflavonoids	3,000 mg
	Calcium	500 mg
	Iodine	
	Lecithin	
	Magnesium	500 mg
	Phosphorus	
	Potassium	500 mg
	Sulfur	
	Protein	

*See note, p. 169.

ASTHMA

Asthma is a chronic respiratory condition characterized by difficulty in breathing, frequent coughing, and a feeling of suffocation. An attack of asthma is often precipitated by physical or emotional stress, respiratory infections, air pollution, changes in temperature or humidity, and exposure to fumes such as those of gasoline or paint. It may also be related to low blood sugar, disorders of the adrenal glands, or specific allergies.

Symptoms of asthma are tightness in the chest and difficulty in breathing, usually accompanied by a wheezing or whistling sound. Violent coughing often occurs as the lungs attempt to expel mucus. An attack can last from several minutes to several days depending on individual situations and causative agents.

Skin tests are often given to pinpoint the patient's allergic tendencies. Common offenders are pollen, animal hair, dust, and certain foods. Proper nutrition is necessary, and the asthmatic should eliminate from the diet those foods that may bring on an attack. A high fluid intake and the inhalation of steam may help to liquefy mucus and make it easier to expel it from the air passages. Vitamin A is necessary for general health of the lungs and, together with vitamin E, guards against visible and invisible air pollutants. The person should have a diet sufficient in the vitamin B complex to avoid deficiency symptoms of nervousness, which might bring on an asthma attack. The need for vitamin C is increased by stress and exposure to hot or cold weather, cigarette smoking, and industrial air pollution.

NUTRIENTS THAT MAY BE BENEFICIAL IN TREATMENT OF ASTHMA

Body Member	Nutrients	Quantity*
Lungs/ Respiratory system	Vitamin A	Up to 50,000 IU
	Vitamin B complex	
	Vitamin B$_6$	50 mg
	Vitamin B$_{12}$	30 mcg
	Choline	
	Inositol	
	Pangamic acid	
	Pantothenic acid	100 mg
	Vitamin C	600 mg
	Vitamin D	800 IU
	Vitamin E	600 IU; 32 IU for children
	Vitamin F	
	Manganese	5 mg twice daily for 10 weeks

*See note, p. 169.

ATHLETE'S FOOT (TINEA PEDIS)

Athlete's foot is a fungus infection of the foot. It may occur as an inflammation, rash, or scaling of the skin. If the toenails are affected, they become brittle and discolored. Athlete's foot is most common in young adult males.

Athlete's foot is commonly transmitted from person to person through towels and locker room or bathroom floors because fungi thrive in these moist conditions. The frequent changing of socks and the use of foot powder are helpful in the prevention and treatment of athlete's foot. Vitamin A is necessary for the general health of the skin, and many enzymes that are effective in the healing of athlete's foot are activated by vitamin C.

NUTRIENTS THAT MAY BE BENEFICIAL IN TREATMENT OF ATHLETE'S FOOT

Body Member	Nutrients	Quantity
Skin	Vitamin A	
	Vitamin C	
	Vitamin E	

AUTISM

Autism is an illness that involves the personality of children who do not react to their environment. The children do not learn to talk, or if they have learned they soon stop. They are withdrawn and do not respond to other people.

A research psychologist in San Diego, California, Dr. Bernard Rimland, has had positive results in treating autism with megavitamin therapy. In his study, 50 percent of the children tested improved significantly by showing a reduction in tantrums, increased alertness, improved speech, better sleep patterns, and greater sociability. The vitamins that were most prominent were niacin, pantothenic acid, B_6, and C. For the children not responding to the treatment, the doctor suggested an increase in the dosage of vitamin B_6. Improvement was then noted. Three percent of the children in the study got worse with the treatment, with noticeable side effects such as extreme sensitivity to noise and bed-wetting. Because B_6 in large quantities can deplete magnesium from a person with a marginal supply of the mineral, the children were given a magnesium supplement and the side effects disappeared. When the vitamin treatment was discontinued, a regression of the illness resulted.

Prevention magazine, October 1978, reports information on pangamic acid and autism that was related by Dr. Allan Cott, a New York psychiatrist, during an informal talk at the International Academy of Preventive Medicine. An autistic seven-year-old child, who had never spoken, was given 200 milligrams of pangamic acid daily. He soon began to use single words, then pairs. He began to play games, tried to dress himself, and became more gregarious. Another nonverbalizing and hyperactive child, after administration of pangamic acid, began to talk and was able, for the first time, to sit still. When the supplement was withdrawn, he reverted to hyperactivity, gaze aversion, fright, and hostility. The child began to improve 24 hours after the administration of pangamic acid was resumed. In 72 hours, there was full recovery. After nine months, the child began to answer questions and talk to himself.

It must be noted that not all autism stems from vitamin deficiency. Some behavorial problems result from diseases of the brain. Allergies may be a possibility.

NUTRIENTS THAT MAY BE BENEFICIAL IN TREATMENT OF AUTISM

Body Member	Nutrients	Quantity*
General	Vitamin B complex	
	Vitamin B_6	450 mg daily
	Vitamin C	1–3 g daily
	Niacin	1–3 g daily
	Pangamic acid	
	Pantothenic acid	200 mg daily

*See note, p. 169.

BACKACHE

Backache may be a symptom of a variety of disturbances in the muscles, tendons, ligaments, bones, or underlying organs. "Lumbago" is a general term frequently used to describe pain in the lower back.

A few of the many underlying causes of backache, or lumbago, are arthritis, osteoporosis, infection and fever, tumor, peptic ulcer, emotional tension or stress, slipped disc or other spinal cord injury, and disorders of the urinary system. Muscle strain or sprain as a cause of backache is quite frequent and commonly results from excessive or improper physical exertion, incorrect posture, sleeping on soft beds, or incorrect lifting. A backache that is accompanied by fever or headache should receive medical diagnosis.

Nutritional therapy for backaches varies with the disorder, but certain nutrients are essential for maintaining a healthy back. Protein is necessary for firm supporting tissue. The B-complex vitamins, especially niacin, provide strength and health for nerve tissues. Backache prevention includes exercise, good posture, proper lifting (by bending at the knees instead of the waist), and avoidance of unnecessary physical or emotional stress or strain.

Vitamins C and D together with calcium are important in the development and maintenance of bones and nerve function.

NUTRIENTS THAT MAY BE BENEFICIAL IN TREATMENT OF BACKACHE

Body Member	Nutrients	Quantity*
Bones/Spine	Vitamin B complex	
	Niacin	
	Vitamin C	500 mg
	Vitamin D	
	Vitamin E	50 IU
	Calcium	1-2 g
	Magnesium	50 IU
	Phosphorus	
	Protein	

*See note, p. 169.

BALDNESS (ALOPECIA)

Baldness is the partial or complete loss of hair, most commonly in the scalp, resulting from heredity, hormonal factors, aging, or local or systematic diseases. Hair loss and thinning not due to scarring is most frequently found in males but may occur in females. No satisfactory treatment is known, but transplants from hairy areas are popular.

NUTRIENTS THAT MAY BE BENEFICIAL IN TREATMENT OF BALDNESS

Body Member	Nutrients	Quantity*
Hair/Scalp	Vitamin B complex	
	Vitamin B$_2$	
	Vitamin B$_6$	50 mg
	Biotin	25 mg
	Choline	500-1,000 mg
	Folic acid	1 mg
	Inositol	500-1,000 mg
	Niacin	50 mg

Body Member	Nutrients	Qualtity
	PABA	50 mg
	Pantothenic acid	50 mg
	Vitamin C	1,000 mg
	Vitamin E	Up to 1,200 IU
	Bioflavonoids	50-100 mg
	Copper	

*See note, p. 169.

BEDSORES

A bedsore forms when pressure on a bony area of the body, such as the elbow, heel, or hip, cuts off the blood supply to that area. The affected area is thus deprived of essential nutrients, and therefore tissue is destroyed.

The most effective prevention for bedsores is relieving pressure on the vulnerable areas of the body by using protective padding, massaging the skin to stimulate circulation, and keeping the skin dry and clean. Treatment for bedsores includes a well-balanced diet high in protein, calories, and vitamins. In some cases, direct applications of vitamins C and E to the wound have been beneficial.[6] Ointments containing vitamins A and D are also often used in treating bedsores.

NUTRIENTS THAT MAY BE BENEFICIAL IN TREATMENT OF BEDSORES

Body Member	Nutrients	Quantity*
Skin	Vitamin A	
	Vitamin B complex	
	Vitamin B$_2$	5 mg daily
	Vitamin C	
	Vitamin D	
	Vitamin E	
	Copper	
	Protein	

*See note, p. 169.

BELL'S PALSY (SEE ALSO "NEURITIS")

Bell's palsy is a type of paralysis characterized by distortion of the face due to a lesion of the facial nerve. It is accompanied by pain, weakness, and a sensation of pricking, tingling, or creeping on the skin, which may be

[6]J. I. Rodale, *The Complete Book of Vitamins* (Emmaus, Pa.: Rodale Books, 1968), pp. 355 and 651.

a result of injury or irritation of a sensory nerve or nerve root.

NUTRIENTS THAT MAY BE BENEFICIAL IN TREATMENT OF BITOT'S SPOTS

Body Member	Nutrients	Quantity*
Eyes	Vitamin A	50,000 IU
	Vitamin D	
	Protein	

*See note, p. 169.

NUTRIENTS THAT MAY BE BENEFICIAL IN TREATMENT OF BELL'S PALSY

Body Member	Nutrients	Quantity*
Brain/Nervous system	Vitamin B complex	
	Vitamin B$_1$	100-200 mg
	Vitamin C	
	Protein	

*See note, p. 169.

BERIBERI

Beriberi is a disease caused by a deficiency of thiamine. The disease seldom occurs outside the Far East, where the principal diet consists mainly of polished rice, which does not supply sufficient thiamine. Rare cases of beriberi in the United States are usually associated with stressful conditions, such as hypothyroidism, infections, pregnancy, lactation, and chronic alcoholism, which increase the body's need for thiamine.

Symptoms of beriberi in infants are convulsions; respiratory difficulties; and gastrointestinal problems, such as nausea, vomiting, constipation, diarrhea, and abdominal discomfort. Adult symptoms are fatigue, diarrhea, appetite and weight loss, disturbed nerve function causing paralysis and wasting of the limbs, edema, and heart failure.

The administration of thiamine will prevent and cure the disease. Because of the diarrhea that accompanies beriberi, the diet must be rich in all nutrients.

NUTRIENTS THAT MAY BE BENEFICIAL IN TREATMENT OF BERIBERI

Body Member	Nutrients	Quantity
General	Vitamin B complex	
	Vitamin B$_1$	
	Vitamin C	

BITOT'S SPOTS

Bitot's spots are characterized by white, foamy, elevated, and sharply outlined patches on the white of the eyes, caused by a deficiency of vitamin A.

NUTRIENTS THAT MAY BE BENEFICIAL IN TREATMENT OF BITOT'S SPOTS

Body Member	Nutrients	Quantity*
Eyes	Vitamin A	50,000 IU
	Vitamin D	
	Protein	

*See note, p. 169.

BOIL (FURUNCLE)

A boil, or furuncle, is an infected nodule on the skin with a central core of pus surrounded by inflamed and swollen tissue. A boil forms when skin tissue is weakened by chafing, lowered resistance due to disease, or inadequate nutrition. Boil symptoms include itching, mild pain, and localized swelling.

Proper hygiene is essential for the treatment of boils. The infected areas should be washed several times daily and swabbed with antiseptic. Hot compresses can relieve pain and promote healing. The person should receive adequate rest and pay special attention to eating a well-balanced diet. Vitamins A, C, and E are necessary for health of the skin.

NUTRIENTS THAT MAY BE BENEFICIAL IN TREATMENT OF BOILS

Body Member	Nutrients	Quantity
Skin	Vitamin A	Applied locally
	Vitamin C	
	Vitamin E	

BRONCHITIS

Bronchitis is an inflammation of the tissues lining the air passage leading to the lungs. Factors that increase susceptibility to bronchitis are asthma and other respiratory diseases, air pollution, cigarette smoking, fatigue, chilling, and malnutrition. Symptoms of bronchitis are a slight fever, back and muscle pain, and sore throat. A dry cough is followed by the coughing up of mucus as the inflammation becomes more severe.

Treatment for bronchitis includes rest, adequate fluid intake, and a well-balanced diet high in vitamins A and C. Vitamin A is essential to the health of the lung tissues; vitamin C helps fight infection and promotes healing. If the bronchitis victim is suffering from mal-nutrition, special attention should be paid to the adequate intake of protein and all other nutrients.

NUTRIENTS THAT MAY BE BENEFICIAL IN TREATMENT OF BRONCHITIS

Body Member	Nutrients	Quantity
Lungs/Respiratory system	Vitamin A	
	Vitamin C	
	Vitamin D	
	Vitamin E	
	Vitamin F	
	Protein	
	Water	

BRUISES

A bruise is an injury that involves the rupture of small blood vessels, causing discoloration of underlying tissues without a break in the overlying skin. Bruises are frequently the result of falling or bumping into objects.

Factors that make one susceptible to bruising are overweight, anemia, and time of menstrual period. Frequent bruising without apparent cause may signal that the materials needed for clotting may not be present in the blood. Leukemia and excessive doses of anticlotting drugs can also cause frequent or large bruises.

Excessive bruising may indicate a lack of vitamin D, a natural blood-clotting agent. Also, vitamin C and bioflavonoid deficiencies may be characterized by a weakening of the small blood vessels, resulting in easier bruising. If the cause of bruising is anemia, there should be an increased intake of iron in the diet. If obesity appears to be a cause of bruising, a well-balanced reducing diet is indicated. Frequent bruising with no apparent cause, or a bruise that applies pressure to a neighboring portion of the body, requires medical attention.

NUTRIENTS THAT MAY BE BENEFICIAL IN TREATMENT OF BRUISES

Body Member	Nutrients	Quantity
Blood/Circulatory system	Vitamin B complex	
	Folic acid	
	Vitamin C	
	Vitamin D	

Body Member	Nutrients	Quantity
	Vitamin K	
	Bioflavonoids	
	Iron	

BRUXISM (TOOTH-GRINDING)

Bruxism usually occurs during sleep, and results in teeth that are loosened in their sockets, which causes tooth loss and gum recession. Two University of Alabama doctors believe that bruxism is a nutritional problem that can be helped with increased dosages of calcium and pantothenic acid.

Calcium is effective for treating involuntary movement of muscles, and pantothenic acid is important for maintaining proper motor coordination. Both nutrients are also antistress formulas. Another reported cause of bruxism, as expressed by a Swiss dental scientist, is a change in the central nervous system due to nervous tension or a conflict situation.

NUTRIENTS THAT MAY BE BENEFICIAL IN TREATMENT OF BRUXISM

Body Member	Nutrients	Quantity
General	Vitamin A	
	Vitamin B_1	
	Vitamin B_2	
	Vitamin B_6	
	Vitamin C	
	Vitamin E	
	Niacin	
	Pantothenic acid	
	Calcium	
	Iodine	
	Protein	

BURNS

A burn is a tissue injury caused by heat, electricity, radiation, or chemicals. There are three degrees of burn severity. A first-degree burn appears reddened, a second-degree burn includes blister formation, and a third-degree burn involves destruction of the entire thickness of skin and possibly of the underlying muscle.

Because of tissue destruction, massive losses of body fluids, proteins, sodium, potassium, and nitrogen can occur. Because large amounts of fluids are lost in extensive burns, the possibility of shock exists. Infection is another threat to the burn victim.

Immediate treatment measures for burns include cold applications to reduce pain and swelling and cleansing and covering of the burn to minimize the possibility of bacterial infection. Ointments, salves, or butter should not be applied to burns. They tend to promote infection and prevent circulation of air to the wound by retaining heat within the body. Treatment of chemical burns may include application of an antidote specific to the offending agent.

Diet is very important to burn victims, especially to those with extensive burns. The diet should be high in calories for energy and high in protein for tissue repair. Adequate intake of fluids in proportion to the amount of fluids lost is also essential. Vitamin C may be helpful for healing the wound, and the B vitamins are necessary to meet the body's increased metabolic demands. Intake of vitamin A, necessary for the health of the skin, should be increased, as well as intake of potassium. Some authorities indicate that vitamin E relieves pain and promotes healing in burns.[7]

NUTRIENTS THAT MAY BE BENEFICIAL IN TREATMENT OF BURNS

Body Member	Nutrients	Quantity*
Skin	Vitamin A	
	Vitamin B complex	
	PABA	
	Vitamin C	
	Vitamin D	
	Vitamin E	200 IU after each meal; ointment
	Vitamin F	
	Potassium	
	Zinc	
	Protein	
	Water	

*See note, p. 169.

[7]Evan Shute, *The Heart and Vitamin E* (London: Shute Foundation for Medical Research, 1963), pp. 96-97.

BURSITIS

Bursitis arises from an inflammation of the liquid-filled sac, called a bursa, found within the joints, muscles, tendons, and bones, which helps to promote muscular movement and reduce friction. The affliction is commonly found in the hip or shoulder joints, elbows, or feet and is more commonly known as "frozen shoulder," "tennis elbow," or bunion.

Bursitis may be caused by stretched muscles, shoes that are too tight, injury such as a bump or bruise, or irritation from calcium deposits found in the bursa wall. Bursitis symptoms include swelling, tenderness, and agonizing pain in the affected area which frequently limits motion. Treatment involves removing the cause of the injury, clearing up any underlying infection, and possibly, surgically removing calcium deposits. Other measures include rest and immobilization of the affected part.

Vitamin B_{12} is beneficial to the normal functioning of body cells in the bone marrow. Vitamin E has also been found to be beneficial in the treatment of bursitis. The need for protein and vitamins A and C increases during infection, and extra amounts of these nutrients are required for bursitis victims.

NUTRIENTS THAT MAY BE BENEFICIAL IN TREATMENT OF BURSITIS

Body Member	Nutrients	Quantity*
Bones/ Muscles/ Joints	Vitamin A	
	Vitamin B complex	
	Vitamin B_{12}	1,000 mcg daily for first 7-10 days; three times per week for next 2-3 weeks; one to two times per week for next 2-3 weeks
	Vitamin C	
	Vitamin E	
	Protein	

*See note, p. 169.

CANCER

Cancer cells appear as young, rapidly growing cells that do not fulfill their natural functions and invade surrounding tissue. These cells rob neighboring normal cells of their essential nutrients, causing a severe wasting away of the cancer patient. Cancer cells are capable of migrating and planting themselves in any part of the body, causing abnormal growths or tumors. Cancers are categorized according to the type of tissue they invade.

The importance of early detection in treatment of cancer cannot be overemphasized. This is the only chance for successful treatment of the disease. One must be always alert to the American Cancer Society's seven warning signs: unusual bleeding or discharge, appearance of a lump or swelling, hoarseness of cough, indigestion or difficulty in swallowing, change in bowel or bladder habits, a sore that does not heal, or a change in a wart or mole. Symptoms and their severity vary with the type and location of the cancer.

For the treatment of cancerous growths or tumors, surgery, radiation, amygdalin or laetrile, and certain drugs have proved beneficial. Surgical operations remove the original growth and any secondary ones. Drugs, although unable to completely cure cancer, are used to reduce the growth or to delay the appearance of secondary growths. Radiation is often used to destroy cancer cells and to prevent them from spreading.

The following vitamins and minerals have been found to possess properties that promote protection against cancer and aid in its healing. Vitamin A is essential because a deficiency can definitely contribute to cancer development. Vitamin C is a potent antitoxin that can neutralize or minimize the effect of many chemical carcinogens in food and in the environment. Vitamins E and C help to inhibit the activity of a growth substance, or catalyst, which is found in cancerous tissue. Vitamin E increases oxygen-holding abilities of cells. The B vitamins are important for prevention of cirrhosis of the liver, which carries a 60 percent greater risk of developing cancer than does a normal liver. Riboflavin, niacin, and pantothenic acid help tissues resist the effects cancer produces.[8] Potassium deficiency is thought by some to be a contributing cause of cancer.

For the terminally ill cancer patient, the specific food needs depend on the location of the tumor. Generally, however, a high-protein, high-calorie diet is necessary to maintain and help restore normal cells. Iron is essential to the diet in order to prevent anemia, which is a frequent complication of cancer.

[8]J.I. Rodale, *The Encyclopedia of Common Diseases* (Emmaus, Pa.: Rodale Books, 1969), p. 239.

Vitamin K has been found to protect against certain cancer-causing substances.

NUTRIENTS THAT MAY BE BENEFICIAL IN TREATMENT OF CANCER

Body Member	Nutrients	Quantity*
General	Vitamin A	50,000 IU
	Vitamin B complex	
	Vitamin B_2	
	Laetrile	
	Niacin	100 mg
	Pangamic acid	50 mg twice daily
	Pantothenic acid	50 mg
	Choline	500-1,000 mg
	Vitamin C	Up to 5,000 mg
	Vitamin D	
	Vitamin E	Up to 1,200 IU
	Vitamin K	
	Iron	
	Phosphorus	
	Potassium	
	Protein	

*See note, p. 169.

CANKER SORES

Canker sores are shallow open sores found anywhere on the mouth. They are usually located on the mucous membrane inside the lips and cheeks.

A canker sore is identified by a sensation of burning and tingling and a slight swelling of the mucous membrane. The sore, a white center surrounded by a red border, is tender to pressure and is painful when acids or spicy foods are eaten. The sore lasts from 4 to 20 days and heals spontaneously, leaving no scar.

The specific cause of canker sores is unknown, although they appear to be brought on by anxiety, other emotional stress, or sensitivity to various foods and substances that produce allergic-type reactions. Because canker sores heal spontaneously, there is no prescribed treatment for them. Application of a mild astringent and avoidance of foods that further irritate the canker sores can be useful for providing relief from the accompanying pain. Vitamin A is necessary for maintaining the condition of mouth tissue. Niacin helps in the general condition of the skin, tongue, and digestive system. A well-balanced diet that provides adequate amounts of these vitamins protects against the formation of canker sores.

NUTRIENTS THAT MAY BE BENEFICIAL IN TREATMENT OF CANKER SORES

Body Member	Nutrients	Quantity*
Mouth	Vitamin A	Applied locally
	Vitamin B complex	
	Niacin	100 mg after each meal
	Vitamin C	
	Vitamin D	

*See note, p. 169.

CARBUNCLE

A painful, localized infection producing pus-filled areas in the deeper layers of the skin tissues under the skin is known as a carbuncle. It commonly appears as a group of boils but is usually more painful, deeper, and slower-healing than an ordinary boil. Carbuncles are formed when bacteria enter lesions in the skin, causing infection. Symptoms of carbuncles include fever and chills, fatigue, and weight loss.

Treatment for carbuncles demands proper hygiene, including frequent washing of the infected area with soap and water, and application of an antiseptic. Hot compresses can relieve pain and promote healing. Bed rest is beneficial, and a well-balanced diet is essential. Vitamins A and C are necessary for health of the skin. If a fever is present, vitamin E may reduce scarring. Calorie and nutrient levels should be increased.

NUTRIENTS THAT MAY BE BENEFICIAL IN TREATMENT OF CARBUNCLES

Body Member	Nutrients	Quantity
Skin	Vitamin A	Applied locally
	Vitamin C	
	Vitamin D	
	Vitamin E	

CATARACTS

A leading cause of blindness, a cataract is a condition in which the lens of the eye, that part of the eye which focuses and allows us to see objects both near and far, becomes clouded or opaque. Cataracts may occur at any time in life but are usually associated with the degenerative changes that occur with age. Cataracts in young people are usually congenital but may be caused by a nutritional disorder or inflammatory condition in the eye. There is a high incidence of cataracts among diabetics.

Symptoms of cataracts include painless, progressive blurring and loss of vision, sensitivity to bright light, and the appearance of halos around lights. Surgical removal of the lens is necessary to restore normal vision and prevent blindness.[9]

Research has shown that a reduction of vitamin C and riboflavin in the lens of the eye may contribute to the development of cataracts. High blood sugar levels, as in diabetes, can cause cataract formation. Low levels of calcium in the blood can also cause cataracts. Maintaining an adequate intake of vitamin C, riboflavin, and calcium may be useful in preventing cataract formation.

NUTRIENTS THAT MAY BE BENEFICIAL IN TREATMENT OF CATARACTS

Body Member	Nutrients	Quantity*
Eye	Vitamin A	100,000 IU
	Vitamin B complex	
	Vitamin B_2	
	Pantothenic acid	
	Vitamin C	500-15,000 mg
	Vitamin D	
	Vitamin E	400-600 IU
	Calcium	
	Protein	

*See note, p. 169.

CELIAC DISEASE

Celiac disease is an intestinal disorder caused by the intolerance of some individuals to gluten, a protein in

[9]David Holvey, *The Merck Manual*, 12th ed. (Rahway, N.J.: Merck and Co., 1972), p. 1015.

wheat, rye, and barley. Ingestion of gluten irritates the intestinal lining, interfering with the absorption of nutrients and water.

Symptoms of celiac disease are weight loss, diarrhea, gas, abdominal pain, and anemia. Malnutrition often accompanies this disorder because of the greatly reduced absorption of nutrients.

Treatment for celiac disease includes eating a well-balanced, gluten-free diet that is high in calories and proteins and normal in fats. The diet excludes all cereal grains except rice and corn. Common nutrient deficiencies that occur with celiac disease and that should be corrected include deficiencies in calcium, vitamin B complex, and vitamins A, C, D, K, and E. Iron, folic acid, and vitamin B_{12} can be used to correct the anemia that usually accompanies celiac disease.

NUTRIENTS THAT MAY BE BENEFICIAL IN TREATMENT OF CELIAC DISEASE

Body Member	Nutrients	Quantity*
Intestine	Vitamin A	
	Vitamin B complex	
	Vitamin B_6	30 mg
	Vitamin B_{12}	
	Folic acid	
	Vitamin C	
	Vitamin D	
	Vitamin E	
	Vitamin K	
	Calcium	
	Iron	
	Magnesium	
	Proteins (no gluten)	

*See note, p. 169.

CEREBROVASCULAR ACCIDENT (CVA, OR STROKE)

A stroke, or cerebrovascular accident, occurs when the blood supply of an area of brain cells is cut off for a long period of time, resulting in the death of the deprived cells due to lack of oxygen and nutrients essential for the proper function of the brain. The blood vessels may be blocked by atherosclerosis, clotting, or hemorrhaging. The process is similar to that of a heart attack, the difference being cell death in the brain during a stroke.

Typical symptoms include impaired memory and attention span, tingling or lack of feeling in limbs, a feeling of heaviness in the limbs, and loss of movement. Symptoms are often restricted to one side of the body, as seen in the frequent right- or left-sided paralysis. Strokes may be so small that they are not even noticed or so severe as to be fatal. It is difficult to tell the extent of injury or cell death at the time the stroke occurs, and the long-term outlook therefore depends upon the area and extent of the brain damage. Physical and speech therapy are often helpful in rehabilitating the patient.

Predisposing factors are prolonged high blood pressure, atherosclerosis, diabetes, old age, obesity, and cigarette smoking. Preventive dietary measures include restricting sodium intake to reduce high blood pressure and reducing cholesterol intake to prevent further cholesterol buildup in blood vessels. The diet should be well balanced, with special emphasis on B vitamins and vitamin C because they are needed for general health of the

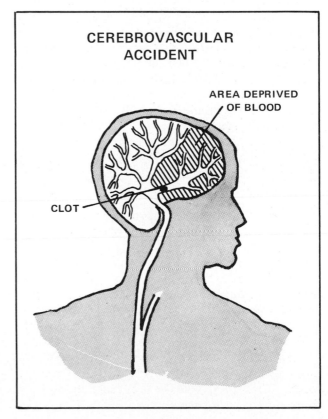

CEREBROVASCULAR ACCIDENT

AREA DEPRIVED OF BLOOD

CLOT

blood vessels. Vitamin E can be of help to prevent clots. Reduction of overweight by sensible dieting is of the utmost importance.

The diet for a patient recovering from a stroke should be well balanced and easily digested. Easily digested meals are usually light and low in roughage and gas-producing foods. Roughage comes from the carbohydrate cellulose. Caloric intake should be adjusted to the altered activity of the person.

NUTRIENTS THAT MAY BE BENEFICIAL IN TREATMENT OF CEREBROVASCULAR ACCIDENT

Body Member	Nutrients	Quantity*
Blood	Vitamin B complex	
	Choline	
	Inositol	
	Vitamin C	
	Vitamin E	300 IU
	Bioflavonoids	
	Lecithin	
	Potassium	
	Low sodium (salt)	
	Low cholesterol	
	Protein	

*See note, p. 169.

CHICKEN POX

Chicken pox is a highly contagious viral disease in which the chief symptom is generalized skin eruptions. One attack usually protects against the disease for life.

About 24 to 36 hours before the first series of eruptions, the patient may have a headache and a low fever. The rash appears as red bumps containing drops of clear fluid, usually on the face and trunk of the body. The fluid breaks out, forming a crust, and the eruptions continue in cycles for three or four days. Soothing lotions may be applied for relief of itching, and fingernails should be cut short to prevent scratching. The patient should be kept clean and should be frequently bathed with soap and water.

Fevers increase the body's need for calories and vitamins A and C. Extra protein is needed for the repair of tissues. The patient should be isolated for 10 to 14 days to prevent the spread of the infection.

NUTRIENTS THAT MAY BE BENEFICIAL IN TREATMENT OF CHICKEN POX

Body Member	Nutrients	Quantity
Skin	Vitamin A	
	Vitamin C	
	Protein	

CHOLESTEROL LEVEL, HIGH

Cholesterol is a fatty substance manufactured by the liver. It is found only in animal fat; it is not contained in vegetable fat. Cholesterol is needed to form sex and adrenal hormones, vitamin D, and bile salts. It also has a vital function in the brain and nerves.

Some researchers believe that when cholesterol levels in the blood become abnormally high, fatty deposits composed of cholesterol and calcium tend to accumulate in the arteries, including those of the heart, increasing the susceptibility to heart attacks. Cholesterol deposits occur mostly in parts of the blood vessels which have been weakened by high blood pressure or undue strain. Cholesterol in the blood must be kept in solution to prevent deposits from forming; lecithin seems to help the bile do this. Lecithin is contained in many fatty foods, but when these fats are hydrogenated, the lecithin is lost. Adequate supplies of unsaturated fatty acids (vitamin F, especially linoleic acid) and vitamin E seem to help control the cholesterol level of the blood and prevent atherosclerosis.

Many factors besides saturated fat affect the cholesterol level of the blood, including stress, anxiety, cigarette smoking, overeating, lack of exercise, and high consumption of refined carbohydrates. Choline, vitamin B_{12}, biotin, lecithin, pangamic acid, and possibly inositol are lipotropic substances—substances that must be present to prevent accumulation of fat in the liver. Since the liver regulates cholesterol, these vitamins may be essential. Deficiencies of magnesium, potassium, manganese, zinc, vanadium, chromium, or selenium, or of vitamins C, E, niacin, folic acid, or B_6 may also be significant.[10]

Several studies have confirmed the fact that pectin can limit the amount of cholesterol the body absorbs, thereby controlling the level of cholesterol accumulation in the

[10]Carl C. Pfeiffer, *Mental and Elemental Nutrients* (New Canaan, Conn.: Keats Publishing, 1975), p. 79.

bloodstream. Pectin is found in many fruits and berries, notably apples.

NUTRIENTS THAT MAY BE BENEFICIAL IN TREATMENT OF HIGH CHOLESTEROL LEVEL

Body Member	Nutrients	Quantity*
Blood	Vitamin B complex	
	Vitamin B_6	
	Choline	
	Inositol	
	Niacin	
	Pangamic acid	
	Vitamin C	500 mg
	Vitamin D	
	Vitamin E	
	Vitamin F	4-5 tbsp
	Bioflavonoids	
	Lecithin	
	Magnesium	500 mg
	Zinc	

*See note, p. 169.

CIRRHOSIS OF THE LIVER

Cirrhosis of the liver is a chronic disease characterized by degeneration and hardening of liver cells. Scarring of the liver tissue causes improper functioning and may result from alcoholism, malnutrition, viral hepatitis, or chronic inflammation or obstruction of certain ducts in the liver.

Early signs of the disease include fever, indigestion, diarrhea or constipation, and jaundice. Later symptoms include edema, anemia, and bleeding disorders characterized by the presence of spider-shaped bruises. A deficiency of the B complex and vitamins A, C, and K may also occur.

Optimal nutrition provides the key to recovery from the disease. A high-protein diet (1 gram of protein per kilogram of body weight, or approximately 75 to 100 grams of protein per day) is prescribed to promote regeneration of the liver cells. In the case of coma, however, protein should be restricted. A high-calorie (2500 to 3000 calories per day) and high-carbohydrate (300 to 400 grams per day) diet is needed to increase the storage of glycogen, to ensure that protein is used for regeneration, and to compensate for weight losses caused by

fever. If nausea is present frequently, small meals are better tolerated than three large meals.

A common complication of cirrhosis is the failure of the liver to make vitamins available in an active form in the body. For this reason, the diet should be high in the B complex and vitamins A (not in the form of carotene), C, D, and K. If jaundice is present, special attention should be paid to the fat-soluble vitamins, A, D, E, and K, because some kinds of jaundice interfere with the absorption of these nutrients. If edema is present, sodium, which causes the body to retain water, should be restricted. All alcohol should be strictly avoided.

NUTRIENTS THAT MAY BE BENEFICIAL IN TREATMENT OF CIRRHOSIS OF THE LIVER

Body Member	Nutrients	Quantity*
Liver	Vitamin A	50,000 to 100,000 IU
	Vitamin B complex	
	Vitamin B_{12}	
	Choline	1-5 g
	Inositol	
	Pangamic acid	
	Vitamin C	
	Vitamin D	
	Vitamin E	
	Vitamin F	
	Vitamin K	
	Magnesium	
	Zinc	
	Carbohydrates	
	Protein	

*See note, p. 169.

COLITIS

Colitis is a disease in which the lining of part of the colon, or large intestine, is inflamed. There are several types of colitis, all of which are determined by the extent of the inflammation, the amount of the colon involved, and the degree of severity of the colitis symptoms. Although the cause of the disease is unknown, there is usually always a correlation between colitis and depression or anxiety. The degree of a person's emotional stress will often indicate the severity of his colitis.

In early stages, colitis is characterized by abdominal

cramps or pain, diarrhea, and the need to eliminate several times daily. These symptoms are accompanied by rectal bleeding as the condition becomes more severe. Instead of being absorbed by the body, water and minerals are rapidly expelled through the lower digestive tract, resulting in a loss of weight and, possibly, dehydration or anemia. Because of this rapid expulsion and decreased absorption of water and nutrients, the entire nutritional status of the colitis patient is in jeopardy.

A therapeutic diet for colitis should be bland and high in protein and vitamin F to restore lost or worn-down tissues. Foods high in roughage, such as raw fruits and vegetables, should be avoided to prevent further intestinal irritation. Milk is also frequently not tolerated; therefore a calcium supplement may be necessary. Iron is necessary to deter the development of anemia and vitamin C to aid in the absorption of iron.

NUTRIENTS THAT MAY BE BENEFICIAL IN TREATMENT OF COLITIS

Body Member	Nutrients	Quantity*
Bowel/Intestine/Colon	Vitamin A	
	Vitamin B_6	50 mg
	Vitamin C	
	Vitamin E	
	Vitamin F	
	Calcium	
	Iron	
	Magnesium	
	Phosphorus	
	Potassium	
	Protein	
	Low cellulose	

*See note, p. 169.

COMMON COLD

The common cold is a general inflammation of the mucous membranes of the respiratory passages caused by a variety of viruses. Colds are highly contagious. On the average, Americans contact two or three colds per year. Factors that lower the body's resistance to virus infection are fatigue, overexposure to cold, recent or present infections, allergic reactions, and inhalation of irritating dust or gas.

The virus is spread about two days before the symptoms appear. Symptoms include nose and throat irritations, watery eyes, headaches, fever, chills, muscle aches, and temporary loss of smell and taste.

Prevention of colds includes adequate sleep and a well-balanced diet. Treatment includes adequate fluid and protein intake to sustain the losses that occur with fever. Vitamin B_6 helps in the production of antibodies that defend the body against infection. Vitamin A is necessary to maintain the health of the mucous membrane of the respiratory passages. Some individuals have found that vitamin D is also helpful in the prevention of colds.[11] Vitamin F, or unsaturated fatty acids, reduces the incidence and duration of colds.

Reports on the role of vitamin C in the treatment of the common cold are contradictory. However, many authorities claim that the intake of vitamin C in amounts from 1 to 2 grams daily is effective in preventing a cold.[12] Another source indicates that at the onset of a cold, vitamin D taken in amounts of 600 to 625 milligrams every three hours may be successful for treatment.[13] The amount of vitamin C recommended for the prevention and treatment of a cold varies from individual to individual.

NUTRIENTS THAT MAY BE BENEFICIAL IN TREATMENT OF COMMON COLDS

Body Member	Nutrients	Quantity*
General	Vitamin A	50,000-150,000 IU for one month; then reduce to 25,000 IU daily
	Vitamin B complex	
	Vitamin B_6	100 mg
	Vitamin C	600-625 mg every three hours first three or four days, then 375-400 mg daily

*See note, p. 169.

[11]Harriet Coston Moidel (ed.) et al., *Nursing Care of the Patient with Medical-Surgical Disorders* (New York: McGraw-Hill Book Co., 1971), p. 520.
[12]Helen A. Guthrie, *Introductory Nutrition*, 2d ed. (St. Louis: C. V. Mosby Co., 1971), p. 225.
[13]"Summer Cold? Vitamin C...," *Prevention*, July 1970, p. 49.

Body Member	Nutrients	Quantity
	Vitamin D	
	Vitamin E	600 IU
	Vitamin F	
	Bioflavonoids	200-600 mg
	Calcium	
	Protein	
	Water	

CONGESTIVE HEART FAILURE

A heart that is weakened or damaged by diseases such as rheumatic fever, heart attack, hypothyroidism, arteriosclerosis, or beriberi is unable to properly pump the blood through the body. This inefficient circulation, which leads to congestion of many organs with blood and other tissue fluids, is congestive heart failure.

Early symptoms of congestive heart failure are abnormal fatigue and shortness of breath following work or exercise. Swelling, particularly in the ankles and feet, is a further symptom. Congestion of the abdominal organs causes nausea, lack of appetite, and gas. Fluid in the lungs impairs breathing and in some cases causes a persistent cough.

Medical treatment for congestive heart failure includes prescription of drugs that strengthen the heartbeat and reduce the amount of excess water in the body. Bed rest is necessary to lessen the heart's workload. The diet should be divided into frequent small meals of easily digested foods. Calories, fats, gas-forming foods, and sodium (salt) are restricted.

Because sodium is found in so many foods, a heart patient on a sodium-restricted diet should take particular care that all his nutritional needs are met. The diet should be adequate in potassium and thiamine.

NUTRIENTS THAT MAY BE BENEFICIAL IN TREATMENT OF CONGESTIVE HEART FAILURE

Body Member	Nutrients	Quantity
Heart	Vitamin A	
	Vitamin B complex	
	Vitamin E	
	Potassium	
	Low fat	
	Low sodium	

CONJUNCTIVITIS

Conjunctivitis is an inflammation of the mucous membrane that lines the eyelids and covers the white portion of the eye. Symptoms of conjunctivitis include redness, swelling, itching, and pus in the membrane. The condition may be caused by allergy, bacteria, virus, smoke, dust, or chemical irritants.

Deficiency of vitamin A, vitamin B_6, or riboflavin may cause conjunctivitis symptoms. The diet should be adequate in these vitamins to help prevent the condition.

NUTRIENTS THAT MAY BE BENEFICIAL IN TREATMENT OF CONJUNCTIVITIS

Body Member	Nutrients	Quantity
Eye	Vitamin A	
	Vitamin B complex	
	Vitamin B_2	
	Vitamin B_6	
	Niacin	
	Vitamin C	
	Vitamin D	

CONSTIPATION

Constipation is a disorder causing decreased frequency of bowel movements, resulting in waste matter remaining in the colon and becoming dry and difficult to expel. Constipation may stem from a variety of causes. Insufficient muscle tone in the intestinal or abdominal wall due to a lack of exercise; repeated failure to heed the signal to eliminate; or excessive fatigue, nervousness, anxiety, or excitement may result in constipation. A poor diet or a diet lacking in fluids or roughage can bring about constipation. The continued use of laxatives as a substitute for proper exercise, rest, and diet may result in dependency and merely perpetuate the problem.

Laxatives, stool softeners, or lubricants such as mineral oil may be prescribed medically for the treatment of constipation. Mineral oil should not be taken along with meals because it interferes with the absorption of fat-soluble vitamins. The diet should provide adequate fluids and roughage in the form of fruits and vegetables high in water content. Foods containing fats may be useful in the treatment of constipation because of their lubricating effect on the mucous walls of the colon.

NUTRIENTS THAT MAY BE BENEFICIAL IN TREATMENT OF CONSTIPATION

Body Member	Nutrients	Quantity*
Intestine	Vitamin A	25,000 IU
	Vitamin B complex	
	Vitamin B$_1$	100 mg
	Choline	500 mg
	Inositol	500 mg
	Niacin	
	Vitamin C	1,000 mg
	Vitamin D	
	Vitamin E	
	Vitamin F	
	Carbohydrates (in the form of cellulose)	
	Calcium	
	Potassium	
	Fats	
	Water	

*See note, p. 169.

CROUP

Croup encompasses a variety of conditions in which there is a high-pitched cough and difficulty in breathing. Fever may or may not accompany the disorder. Croup usually affects children under the age of five. Conditions that may bring on the symptoms of croup are virus, diphtheria, a foreign body in the throat, and swelling due to a throat infection.

Croup may vary greatly in severity depending upon its cause. Any underlying infections should be treated, and any obstruction in the throat should be removed. The breathing of warm moist air from a humidifier often brings relief from cough.

Nutritional treatment for croup involves a well-balanced diet high in protein to promote the growth and repair of tissues. If fever is present, the need for vitamins A and C is increased. Increased fluid intake is also essential, especially when croup occurs in very small children or infants.

NUTRIENTS THAT MAY BE BENEFICIAL IN TREATMENT OF CROUP

Body Member	Nutrients	Quantity
Lungs/Respiratory system	Vitamin A	
	Vitamin C	
	Protein	

CYSTIC FIBROSIS

Cystic fibrosis is a hereditary disease affecting certain glands in the body, such as the gallbladder, pancreas, and sweat glands. The disease usually begins during infancy, though symptoms may manifest themselves later in life.

The greatest danger at the onset of the disease is malnutrition due to an underproduction of digestive juices. As a result, all foods, especially fats, are poorly digested and absorbed, and a deficiency in all nutrients, particularly in the fat-soluble vitamins, occurs. In addition, the sweat glands produce an unusually salty perspiration, draining the body of salt and making the patient susceptible to heat exhaustion. The mucous glands in the lungs, which normally aid in moistening the air passages, produce a thick mucus that blocks the passages and promotes the growth of harmful bacteria.

Treatment for the malnutrition that occurs with cystic fibrosis may include medication to compensate for the lack of digestive juices. The recommended diet is 25 percent higher than normal in calories, the majority being in protein, which is easier to digest than fats, and starches, which are nutritionally better than sugars. The intake of fluids and salt should be increased, particularly during hot weather. Because of the poor absorption of nutrients, additional vitamins—A, the B complex, C, D, E, and K—should be included in the diet.

A New Zealand physician, Dr. Robert B. Elliot, who based his treatment of the fact that persons afflicted with cystic fibrosis have abnormally low blood levels of linoleic acid, gave periodic infusions of soy oil, which contains a large amount of linoleic acid, to several groups of children. Oral supplementation was not effective. The results showed at least one of the characteristic biochemical abnormalities of the disease improved in all children tested. This treatment is still in the experimental stage, so complete confirmation is yet to be received.

At the University of Pennsylvania School of Medicine and the Wistar Institute, researchers gave 13 children afflicted with cystic fibrosis dietary supplements of corn oil, vitamin E (to prevent oxidation), and pancreatic enzymes. After a year on the diet, all the children gained weight, grew taller, and seemed healthier and happier. In individual cases, the supplements relieved symptoms such as diarrhea, sodium loss, and general problems associated with poor nutrition. Running and walking exercises were also part of the program. Regular exercise helped the patients to keep their lungs clear of mucus and may be a factor in slowing the deterioration of lung function. The doctors stress that at this time the study is suggestive and not yet conclusive.

NUTRIENTS THAT MAY BE BENEFICIAL IN TREATMENT OF CYSTIC FIBROSIS

Body Member	Nutrients	Quantity*
Glands	Vitamin A	
	Vitamin B complex	
	Vitamin C	
	Vitamin D	
	Vitamin E	300-1,500 mg
	Vitamin K	
	Sodium (salt)	
	Protein	

*See note, p. 169.

CYSTITIS (BLADDER INFECTION)

Cystitis is an inflammation of the urinary bladder. It is most frequently caused by bacteria that ascend from the urinary opening, but it may also be caused by infected urine sent from the kidneys to the bladder. Cystitis most frequently occurs in females.

Symptoms of cystitis are pain in the lower abdomen and back and frequent, urgent, and painful urination in which the urine may contain blood or pus. Fever may possibly accompany these symptoms. Treatment for cystitis includes increasing the fluid intake and maintaining a well-balanced diet. Vitamin B complex helps to maintain the muscle tone in the gastrointestinal tract and liver. Vitamin C helps ward off and clear up the infection. Vitamin E maintains proper functioning of the liver.

NUTRIENTS THAT MAY BE BENEFICIAL IN TREATMENT OF CYSTITIS

Body Member	Nutrients	Quantity*
Bladder	Vitamin A	25,000-50,000 IU
	Vitamin B complex	
	Vitamin B$_6$	
	Pantothenic acid	
	Vitamin C	5,000-10,000 mg
	Vitamin D	
	Vitamin E	600 IU
	Fluids (water)	

*See note, p. 169.

DANDRUFF

Dandruff (seborrhea) is a covering of dead skin that prevents new hair from growing because it cannot break through the dead skin. Dandruff may be dry and scaly or, at times, oily and is due to a dysfunction of the sebaceous glands. It often occurs in persons with oily skin who are prone to develop superficial, acute and chronic bacterial skin conditions.

It is caused primarily by a vitamin A deficiency or constipation and may be corrected by proper nutrient supplementation and cleansing with a shampoo designed to aid in the control of dandruff.

NUTRIENTS THAT MAY BE BENEFICIAL IN TREATMENT OF DANDRUFF

Body Member	Nutrients	Quantity
Skin/Scalp	Vitamin A	
	Vitamin B complex	
	Vitamin B$_6$	
	Vitamin E	
	Vitamin F	

DEPRESSION (SEE "MENTAL ILLNESS")

DERMATITIS

Dermatitis is an inflammatory, usually recurring skin reaction. It is caused by contact with an irritating agent that is ingested or found in the environment. Dermatitis is usually associated with hereditary allergic tendencies and may be aggravated by emotional stress and fatigue.

A primary symptom of dermatitis is eczema. Eczema is a type of skin eruption characterized by tiny blisters that weep and crust. Chronic forms are characterized by scaling, flaking, and eventual thickening and color changes of the skin. Itching is almost always present.

If the irritating agent is a food item, it should be eliminated from the diet. Deficiency of any of the B vitamins can cause dermatitis, and these vitamins should, therefore, be present in the diet in adequate amounts. Linoleic acid (unsaturated fat) and vitamin B$_6$ have been found to cure infants who have dermatitis caused by a fat-free diet.[14] Vitamin A is also essential for maintaining healthy skin tissue. A protein deficiency can cause chronic eczema.

[14]Marie V. Krause and Martha A. Hunscher, *Food, Nutrition and Diet Therapy*, 5th ed. (Philadelphia: Saunders, 1972), p. 56.

NUTRIENTS THAT MAY BE BENEFICIAL IN TREATMENT OF DERMATITIS

Body Member	Nutrients	Quantity*
Skin	Vitamin A	50,000-75,000 IU for two to three months; then reduce to 25,000 IU after one month
	Vitamin B complex	
	Vitamin B$_2$	
	Vitamin B$_6$	
	Biotin	
	Niacin	300 mg
	Vitamin D	
	Vitamin F	
	Potassium	
	Sulfur (ointment form)	
	Protein	
	Zinc	

*See note, p. 169.

DIABETES

Diabetes is a metabolic disorder characterized by decreased ability, or complete inability, of the body to utilize carbohydrates. Carbohydrates are normally broken down within the body in the form of glucose, the body's main energy source. Insulin, a hormone produced in the pancreas, is essential for the conversion of this glucose into energy. In the diabetic, there is insufficient production of insulin and therefore glucose cannot be converted to energy but instead accumulates in the blood, resulting in symptoms ranging in severity from mental confusion to coma.

The major symptoms of diabetes are excessive thirst, frequent urination, increased appetite, and loss of weight. Other symptoms, though less characteristic of the disease, are muscle cramps, impaired vision, itching of the skin, and poorly healing wounds.

The tendency to develop diabetes frequently seems to be hereditary. Other conditions that contribute to its development are pregnancy, surgery, physical or emotional stress, and obesity. Weight control through proper nutrition is an important factor in the prevention of diabetes.

Methods of medical treatment for diabetes are used in conjunction with a specific diet. In mild cases of the disease, diabetes can be regulated by diet alone. In more severe cases, regulation of the diet is accompanied by oral medication or injections to increase the pancreatic output of insulin. Exercise is a factor in diabetes treatment because it determines insulin needs.

Unless a diabetic is overweight, his caloric intake may remain the same but his calorie sources must be regulated. Since the diabetic cannot properly utilize carbohydrates, their intake must be greatly restricted. Concentrated sources of carbohydrates, such as cakes, cookies, and candy, should be avoided. The diabetic may be allowed some fruits and vegetables because their carbohydrate content is not as great as that of these foods. However, depending upon the individual diet, fruits and vegetables that have the greatest carbohydrate content may have to be avoided also. High-complex carbohydrates, such as whole grains and beans, may be permitted. To maintain his normal caloric intake while restricting his carbohydrates, the diabetic eats a diet that is increased in amount of proteins and unsaturated fats.

Generally, a well-balanced diet rich in vitamins and minerals is one of the most important factors in the control of diabetes. Some authorities find that the diabetic is unable to convert carotene into vitamin A, while others deny such findings. It is advisable, however, for the diabetic to ingest at least the Recommended Dietary Allowance of vitamin A from a noncarotene source, such as fish-liver oil.[15] Because the diabetic, especially when on insulin therapy, loses vitamin C more readily than does the nondiabetic, daily supplementation of vitamin C is necessary. The minerals zinc, chromium, and manganese have been associated with the treatment of diabetes, although their specific effect on the disease has not yet been determined.

NUTRIENTS THAT MAY BE BENEFICIAL IN TREATMENT OF DIABETES

Body Member	Nutrients	Quantity*
Blood/	Vitamin A	5,000 IU

*See note, p. 169.

[15]Norman Jollife (ed.), *Clinical Nutrition*, 2d ed. (New York: Harper Bros., 1962), p. 489.

Body Member	Nutrients	Quantity
Circulatory system	Vitamin B complex	
	Vitamin B$_1$	10 mg
	Vitamin B$_2$	10 mg
	Vitamin B$_6$	50-100 mg
	Vitamin B$_{12}$	25 mcg minimum
	Niacin	Up to 100 mg
	Pangamic acid	
	Vitamin C	1,000-3,000 mg
	Vitamin D	400 IU
	Vitamin E	400-1,200 IU
	Vitamin F	Six capsules or 2 tbsp of cold-pressed vegetable oil
	Calcium	
	Chromium	2 mg for six months
	Iron	
	Magnesium	500 mg
	Maganese	
	Potassium	300 mg
	Zinc	
	Protein	

DIARRHEA

Diarrhea is a condition causing frequent elimination of stools abnormally watery in nature. The condition is fairly common and can exist alone or as a symptom of other diseases. Diarrhea is accompanied by increased thirst, abdominal cramps and bloating, intestinal rumbling, and loss of appetite.

Because of the decreased appetite associated with diarrhea and rapid expulsion of food through the lower digestive tract, an individual with diarrhea does not properly absorb nutrients and can therefore develop nutrient deficiencies. In addition, the change in consistency of the stool causes the body to lose a great amount of water, a loss that can cause dehydration as well as the loss of minerals and water-soluble vitamins.

The most frequent cause of diarrhea is the presence in the colon of bacteria foreign to the intestinal tract. Bacteria may come from poisoned, poorly refrigerated, undercooked, or partially rancid food. Emotional stress, such as anxiety, is another major cause of diarrhea. Diarrhea can also be brought about by some types of allergic reactions, the prolonged use of laxatives, or a diet that is overly abundant in roughage, which increases the movement of food through the intestines.

Medical treatment of diarrhea may include the prescription of antibiotics to combat bacterial infection or medication to relax the colon muscles. The diet of the diarrhea patient should be low in bulk to decrease the tendency for rapid expulsion but rich in protein, carbohydrates, vitamins, and minerals to compensate for the loss of all nutrients that occurs with the condition. The diet should be supplemented with the water-soluble B-complex vitamins and vitamin C as well as with sodium and potassium, which are bound closely to water and which the body always loses when it becomes dehydrated. An adequate fluid intake is the most essential aspect of the treatment for diarrhea, to replace the water that is lost in the stools, thereby preventing dehydration.

NUTRIENTS THAT MAY BE BENEFICIAL IN TREATMENT OF DIARRHEA

Body Member	Nutrients	Quantity*
Bowel	Vitamin A	25,000 IU
	Vitamin B complex	
	Vitamin B$_1$	200 mg daily reduced to 50 mg after two weeks
	Vitamin B$_2$	10 mg
	Vitamin B$_6$	50-100 mg
	Folic acid	
	Niacin	100 mg three times daily reduced to 100 mg daily after two weeks
	Pantothenic acid	100 mg
	Vitamin C	1,000-3,000 mg
Cells	Vitamin F	
	Calcium	2 g
	Chlorine	
	Iron	
	Magnesium	500 mg

*See note, p. 169.

Body Member	Nutrients	Quantity
	Potassium	
	Sodium	
	Carbohydrates (cellulose)	
	Protein	

DIVERTICULITIS

Diverticulitis is the inflammation of the small sacs (diverticula), or out-pouchings, that may be found along the small or large intestine (colon). When empty, the diverticula remain dormant and without complication. However, when food particles get trapped in the sacs and are digested by the bacteria normally present in the colon for this purpose, the digested food particles become stagnant, a situation that leads to inflammation and infection. Diverticulitis may be hereditary, or it may accompany old age, when the muscles of the colon are weakened from years of use.

As diverticulitis becomes more severe, the infection can spread out of the sacs to the rest of the colon and to other organs of the abdomen. In very severe cases, the disease can result in perforation of the wall of the colon, causing severe bleeding for which immediate surgical attention is necessary.

Diverticulitis can manifest itself in a short but severe attack or in a long-term, less severe problem. Symptoms of the disease include cramps and pain in the lower abdomen accompanying bowel movements, abdominal bloating, and the frequent urge to eliminate followed by constipation. If infection ensues, fever can develop.

The most effective prevention for diverticulitis is to avoid constipation. One of the best ways to accomplish this is by a marked increase in fluid intake, which helps to prevent dehydration of intestinal material. A diet moderate in roughage will prevent further accumulation of food in the diverticula. Fruits and vegetables in juice or puree form will provide the body with vitamins and minerals. Supplementing the diet with agar-agar, a seaweed derivative, can help to increase bulk for movement through the colon.

Because some of the B vitamins are manufactured by the intestinal bacteria, a deficiency may occur if these bacteria are destroyed by the infection. It is therefore necessary that the diet provide adequate amounts of the B vitamins, especially folic acid.

NUTRIENTS THAT MAY BE BENEFICIAL IN TREATMENT OF DIVERTICULITIS

Body Member	Nutrients	Quantity*
Intestine	Vitamin B complex	
	Folic acid	1 mg
	Vitamin C	
	All minerals	
	Carbohydrates (cellulose)	
	Water	

*See note, p. 169.

DIZZINESS/VERTIGO

Dizziness is characterized by a sensation of giddiness, unsteadiness, or light-headedness. The terms "vertigo" and "dizziness" are often used interchangeably, but true vertigo is a sensation of spinning or a feeling that the floors are sinking or rising. True vertigo is usually accompanied by nausea, vomiting, perspiration, and headache.

Dizziness and vertigo both may be caused by infections of or injuries to the inner ear, which normally helps to maintain the body's sense of balance. A physical injury such as a concussion or skull fracture may injure the inner ear; in this type of injury, dizziness may occur long after the injury is supposedly healed. Brain tumors, anemia, high or low blood pressure, lack of oxygen or glucose in the blood, psychological stress, or nutritional deficiencies may be other causes of vertigo.

A deficiency of vitamin B_6 or niacin may cause dizziness. Including these B-complex vitamins in the diet may prevent and alleviate the sensation.

NUTRIENTS THAT MAY BE BENEFICIAL IN TREATMENT OF DIZZINESS/VERTIGO

Body Member	Nutrients	Quantity
Brain/Nervous system	Vitamin B complex	
	Vitamin B_1	
	Vitamin B_2	
	Vitamin B_6	
	Vitamin B_{12}	
	Choline	
	Inositol	
	Niacin	
	Vitamin C	
	Vitamin E	
	Calcium	

DRUG ABUSE OR DEPENDENCY

The use or abuse of drugs, whether illegal or legal, resulting in dependency over a prolonged period may have several detrimental effects on the general state of health of an individual. Research shows that most drugs have definite side effects, including severe depletion of essential nutrients stored in the body.

Continued use of illegal drugs, such as narcotics, stimulants, barbiturates, and hallucinogens, may result in dependency and severe mental and physical deterioration. Prolonged use may result in damage to the cells, chromosome damage, male sterility, and increased risks of cancer.

Of nearly as great a concern is the problem of indiscriminate use of legal drugs, both prescription and patent medicines. The classic example is the common aspirin tablet. Although many people consider average doses of aspirin completely harmless, researchers invariably discover that when taken in daily doses such as those used to relieve the pain of arthritis, aspirin causes irritation to the stomach lining and varying amounts of internal bleeding. This bleeding may be extensive enough to cause slight anemia. Aspirin-induced irritation of the stomach and accompanying internal bleeding may be very dangerous to ulcer sufferers. There may also be instances of severe allergic reactions to aspirin itself.

Especially dangerous is the habitual use of combinations of drugs such as sleeping pills to go to sleep, stimulants to wake up in the morning, and alcohol to calm down in the midafternoon. A person following such a daily pattern may be just as "hooked" on drugs as any recognized addict. In fact, the taking of such substances as alcohol and sleeping pills (barbiturates) together may so severely depress the body functions as to cause death.

It should be stressed that drugs may produce dietary deficiencies by destroying nutrients, preventing their absorption, and increasing their excretion. Also, many drugs depress the appetite; therefore people who become reliant upon drugs tend to eat inadequately, thus depriving themselves of the essential nutrients necessary for good health.

EAR INFECTION

An ear infection can occur in any of the three sections within the ear. The outer ear is that section which is visible, plus the ear canal, a skin-lined tube that ends at a disk known as the eardrum. The middle ear is composed of three small bones that lie on the inward side of the eardrum. These bones connect with the inner ear, which changes sound waves into nerve impulses and sends them to the brain.

Infection in the outer ear is usually caused by swimming in contaminated water or by damage to the wall of the ear canal. A symptom of the infection is severe pain, possibly accompanied by fever.

Infection in the middle ear is most frequently due to the spread of bacteria to the ear from infection in the nose and throat. Symptoms include earache, a feeling of fullness in the ear, diminished hearing, and fever.

Infection in the inner ear usually arises from meningitis or from the spread of a middle-ear infection. Symptoms include loss of hearing, dizziness, nausea, vomiting, and fever. Severe ear infections may result in permanent scarring and partial or total loss of hearing.

Medical treatment for ear infection involves rest, warmth applied to the ear, antibiotics, and surgical draining of the infected area. Nutritionally, the body's needs for vitamins A and C are increased during a fever. A well-balanced diet adequate in protein is necessary to help the body fight infection and repair damaged tissue.

NUTRIENTS THAT MAY BE BENEFICIAL IN TREATMENT OF EAR INFECTION

Body Member	Nutrient	Quantity*
Ear	Vitamin A	50,000 IU
	Vitamin C	
	Protein	

*See note, p. 169.

ECZEMA

Eczema is a skin condition characterized by inflammatory itching and the formation of scales. Sometimes eczema is related to an allergic reaction. Vitamins A and C together with the B-complex vitamins are helpful in the prevention and healing of eczema.

NUTRIENTS THAT MAY BE BENEFICIAL IN TREATMENT OF ECZEMA

Body Member	Nutrients	Quantity*
Skin	Vitamin A	50,000-75,000 IU for two to three months; 25,000 IU for next few months if condition does not clear up

*See note, p. 169.

Body Member	Nutrients	Quantity
	Vitamin B complex	
	Vitamin B_6	
	Biotin	
	Choline	
	Inositol	500 mg
	Vitamin C	Up to 1,000 mg
	Vitamin D	800 IU
	Vitamin F	
	Sulfur	Ointment
	Zinc	

Body Member	Nutrients	Quantity
	Vitamin B_1	
	Vitamin B_6	50-200 mg
	Vitamin C	2,000-5,000 mg
	Vitamin E	
	Copper	
	Potassium	
	Protein	
	Low sodium	

EDEMA (SWELLING)

Edema is a condition in which excess fluid is retained by the body, either localized in one area or generalized throughout the body. This retention of fluids appears as swelling. Swelling is most often seen in the hands, in the feet, or around the eyes, but it may be located in any area of the body.

Disorders that can cause edema are poor kidney functioning, congestive heart failure, protein or thiamine deficiency, varicose veins, phlebitis, or sodium retention. Other factors that may cause edema are standing for long periods of time, pregnancy, premenstrual tension, the use of oral contraceptives, injury to an area of the body (such as a sprain), or allergic reactions (such as an insect bite).

If edema is the result of protein or thiamine deficiency, correction of the deficiency is essential. Sodium, as found in table salt, is often restricted in diets of individuals who are prone to edema because excess sodium causes the body to retain water. Individuals who are prone to edema should try to promote good circulation by elevating the legs while at rest, exercising regularly, avoiding restrictive clothing, and refraining from crossing the legs.

An increase in vitamin B_6 intake reduces fluid retention. The recommended supplemental source of B_6 is dessicated liver.

NUTRIENTS THAT MAY BE BENEFICIAL IN TREATMENT OF EDEMA

Body Member	Nutrient	Quantity*
General	Vitamin B complex	

*See note, p. 169.

EMPHYSEMA

Emphysema is characterized by abnormal swelling and destruction of the tiny air sacs of the lungs. These sacs become thin and stretch, thus losing their elasticity. This results in an accumulation of used air in the lungs and leads to a decreased ability to utilize fresh air.

Factors that may contribute to the onset of emphysema are exposure to various dusts, cigarette smoking, bronchitis, asthma, or other respiratory diseases. Symptoms of the condition include wheezing, shortness of breath and difficulty in breathing, and coughing often accompanied by mucus. Weight loss occurs as the condition progresses, and the victim may develop a characteristic "barrel chest."

Vitamins A and C provide some protection against emphysema for cigarette smokers by helping to maintain healthy tissues in the respiratory passage. The vitamin B complex and protein are necessary to strengthen the deteriorating tissue. Since the emphysema victim suffers from a lack of oxygen, many authorities suggest that vitamin E may be beneficial.[16]

NUTRIENTS THAT MAY BE BENEFICIAL IN TREATMENT OF EMPHYSEMA

Body Member	Nutrients	Quantity*
Lungs/ Respiratory system	Vitamin A	50,000 IU
	Vitamin B complex	
	Folic acid	
	Pangamic acid	50 mg three times daily
	Vitamin C	3,000-5,000 mg

*See note, p. 169.

[16]Spencer H. Robley, *Emphysema and Common Sense* (West Nyack, N.Y.: Parker Publ. Co., 1968), p. 144.

Body Member	Nutrients	Quantity
	Vitamin D	
	Vitamin E	Up to 16,000 IU
	Protein	

EPILEPSY

Epilepsy is a disease characterized by seizures. There are two forms of seizures. A sensory seizure involves only a change in sensation or a loss of consciousness, while a convulsive seizure (convulsion) involves abnormal muscular behavior. Epileptic seizures are caused by an electrical disturbance in the nerve cells in one section of the brain and may be the result of such factors as head injury or infection, rabies, tetanus, meningitis, rickets, malnutrition, hypoglycemia, or fever.

Epilepsy occurs in both sexes and at all ages. An individual may experience only one seizure in his lifetime or several seizures per day. Factors that may precipitate a seizure are fatigue, overeating or overdrinking, emotional tension or excitement, fever, new environmental stresses, or menstruation.

The epileptic should maintain a well-balanced diet and should avoid taking in excessive amounts of food or fluid at one time, because these may bring on an attack. Alcoholic beverages should also be avoided. Regular exercise and rest should be encouraged.

Anticonvulsive drugs are effective in preventing most seizures. However, for children with petite mal epilepsy—characterized by brief losses of consciousness lasting from 5 to 30 seconds, accompanied by twitching of the eyeballs—a ketogenic diet may be beneficial when there is no response to drug therapy. A ketogenic diet is used in less than 8 percent of all epilepsy cases and must be administered under medical supervision. It consists of restricting protein and carbohydrate intake and increasing fat intake, producing acid levels in the bloodstream which act to inhibit brain stimulation of seizures.

Dr. Yukio Tanaka of St. Mary's Hospital in Montreal, Canada, through recent research, has demonstrated a link between manganese deficiency and convulsions in humans. He also states that pregnant women with a deficiency of manganese may give birth to epileptic children. Pregnant rats maintained on a low-manganese diet delivered young with poorly coordinated movements and a susceptibility to convulsions.

NUTRIENTS THAT MAY BE BENEFICIAL IN TREATMENT OF EPILEPSY

Body Member	Nutrients	Quantity*
Brain/ Nervous system	Vitamin A	10,000 IU (one capsule)
	Vitamin B complex	
	Vitamin B$_6$	100 mg under doctor's supervision, up to 300 mg
	Vitamin B$_{12}$	25 mcg
	Folic acid	0.5 mg
	Niacin	50 mg
	Pangamic acid	50 mg twice daily
	Pantothenic acid	50 mg twice daily
	Vitamin C	2,000 mg
	Vitamin D	1,000 IU (one capsule)
	Vitamin E	Begin dosage at 300 IU; increase up to 2,000 IU
	Calcium	1,000 mg
	Magnesium	800 mg; for children 500 mg
	Manganese	
	Fats	
	Low carbohydrates	
	Low protein	

*See note, p. 169.

EYESTRAIN

The human eyes are marvelously adaptable and sensitive organs, but they can be abused by using them excessively in improper light. Too little light, glaring light and reflections, shadows on work areas, and flickering light such as that from some fluorescent tubes cause the eyes to make numerous unnecessary adjustments that may lead to eyestrain. Eyestrain may also be a result of uncorrected eyesight; eyes should be checked regularly by an eye specialist for any corrections or adjustments that should be made.

Frequent relaxation of the eyes, especially by changing the range of focus by looking up and away from your work towards a distant object, may alleviate strain caused by improper light and headaches caused by nervous tension.

Vitamin A, the B complex, and vitamin C are especially important in the maintenance of good eye health.

NUTRIENTS THAT MAY BE BENEFICIAL IN TREATMENT OF EYESTRAIN

Body Member	Nutrients	Quantity*
Eye	Vitamin A	
	Vitamin B complex	
	Vitamin C	Large doses
	Vitamin D	
	Vitamin E	

*See note, p. 169.

FATIGUE

Fatigue is a feeling of physical and mental weariness which may be caused by a variety of conditions, such as anemia, physical exertion, nutrient deficiency, weight loss, obesity, boredom or emotional tension, or almost any disease process. In addition to a feeling of weariness, symptoms of fatigue include headache, backache, irritability, and indigestion.

Adequate rest, exercise, and a well-balanced diet can prevent fatigue. Reducing to a normal weight is necessary when overweight is present. Deficiencies of the vitamin B complex, vitamins C and D, or iron may cause fatigue and therefore should be corrected.

NUTRIENTS THAT MAY BE BENEFICIAL IN TREATMENT OF FATIGUE

Body Member	Nutrients	Quantity
General	Vitamin A	
	Vitamin B complex	
	Folic acid	
	Vitamin C	
	Vitamin D	
	Iron	
	Manganese	
	Carbohydrate (cellulose)	

FEVER

Fever is the elevation of body temperature above normal. Normal temperature varies from individual to individual, although normal is generally considered to be within the range of 97° to 99°F. When the body temperature is raised not more than 5°, the rise does not completely interfere with bodily functions. However, when fever reaches 106°F, convulsions are common, and if fever should reach 108°F, irreversible brain damage frequently results.

Fever accompanies a wide variety of diseases ranging from mild to severe and can be considered a warning that something is wrong within the body. Symptoms associated with fever include flushed face, headache, nausea, body aches, little or no appetite, and occasionally, diarrhea or vomiting. The skin may be either hot and dry or warm to the touch with some degree of perspiring. Perspiration is the natural result of the body's attempt to lower its temperature.

Because fever increases the body's use of energy, the caloric needs are greatly increased and intake should be adjusted accordingly. Additional protein is needed to replace and rebuild the damaged body tissue and to form antibodies, substances manufactured by the body to fight infection. A high fluid intake is necessary to compensate for the loss that occurs with fever. Sodium and potassium are lost when fluid is lost; therefore their replacement is also necessary during fever. The increased energy expenditure that occurs during fever increases metabolism; because vitamin A, the B complex, and vitamin C are involved in the process of metabolism, deficiencies of these nutrients may arise also. The vitamin B complex especially should be increased during an extended fever since these vitamins may stimulate the appetite. Additional calcium may also be required because of its decreased absorption during fever.

NUTRIENTS THAT MAY BE BENEFICIAL IN TREATMENT OF FEVER

Body Member	Nutrients	Quantity
General/Head	Vitamin A	
	Vitamin B complex	
	Vitamin B_1	
	Vitamin C	
	Vitamin D	
	Calcium	
	Phosphorus	
	Potassium	
	Sodium	
	Protein	

FRACTURE (BROKEN BONE)

A fracture is any break in a bone. When the bone breaks but the skin remains intact, the fracture is called "closed" or "simple." When the bone breaks through the skin, an opening for bacteria is created and the fracture is called "open" or "compound."

Most fractures occur as the result of an accident, but some occur because of tumors, osteoporosis, or deficiencies of vitamin D or calcium. Fracture symptoms include limb deformities, limited limb functioning, shortening of the limb in fractures of long bones, pain, a grating sensation if the broken bone ends rub against each other, and swelling and discoloration of the skin overlying the fracture area.

First aid treatment for fractures should include covering any wound and immobilizing or splinting the broken part in the position it was found. Medical treatment involves replacing the bone pieces into their normal position.

In the healing process, a bridge of tissue composed largely of protein fibers grows across the ends of the broken bones. Calcium and phosphorus then deposit among these protein fibers to form a new bone. The diet must therefore be high in protein and adequate in calcium and phosphorus. However, calcium intake should not be unusually high because a high calcium intake may promote kidney stone formation during the immobile period while the cast is on. Vitamin D intake must be adequate because it is essential for the absorption of calcium and phosphorus. Potassium is required for cell formation, vitamin C is necessary for the maintenance and development of bones, and vitamin A helps to increase the rate of bone growth. The diet should be high in calories to provide the energy necessary for new bone cell formation.

NUTRIENTS THAT MAY BE BENEFICIAL IN TREATMENT OF FRACTURE

Body Member	Nutrients	Quantity*
Bones	Vitamin A	
	Pantothenic acid	
	Vitamin C	
	Vitamin D	
	Calcium	
	Phosphorus	
	Potassium	

*See note, p. 169.

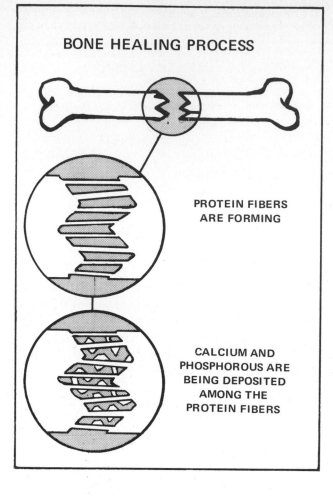

BONE HEALING PROCESS

PROTEIN FIBERS ARE FORMING

CALCIUM AND PHOSPHOROUS ARE BEING DEPOSITED AMONG THE PROTEIN FIBERS

Body Member	Nutrients	Quantity
	Magnesium	500 mg
	Protein	160 g

GALLSTONES

Gallstones develop when deposits of cholesterol or calcium combine with bile. Bile is a secretion produced by the liver to emulsify fats so that they can be digested. Most of the bile manufactured by the liver is stored in the gallbladder until the small intestine calls for it when fat has been ingested. However, some bile travels directly from the liver to the small intestine. Gallstones may form in the passages between liver and gallbladder, between liver and intestine, or in the gallbladder itself.

Gallstones are more frequently found in diabetics,

obese persons, elderly people, and females, especially those who have had children. Although the exact reason for this stone formation is still unknown, there are certain predisposing conditions, such as any infection in the body and long periods of inactivity or bed rest.

Nearly half of all gallstone patients are without symptoms. It is when a stone obstructs any of the bile passages that symptoms occur. These symptoms characteristically include nausea, vomiting, and severe right upper abdominal pain that may radiate to the right shoulder or back. The symptoms commonly occur a few hours after eating a heavy meal of fatty or fried foods. If the stone totally obstructs one of the bile passages, jaundice (a yellowish cast to the skin and eyeballs), dark urine, clay-colored stools, and itching of the skin may also occur.

Medical treatment for gallstones may involve a modification of diet or surgery. Persons suffering from gallstones should avoid large meals, fats, and other foods that aggravate the conditions. This type of diet is helpful in avoiding the abdominal discomfort (bloating, belching, heartburn) that commonly occurs several hours after eating. A diet high in protein and carbohydrates and low in fats is generally recommended to meet the person's nutritional needs. Fluid intake should be frequent. Since the gallstone patient may have impaired absorption of fats, particular attention to the adequate ingestion of the fat-soluble vitamins A, D, E, and K is imperative to avoid their depletion and deficiency.

prolonged, the stomach walls become very thin, secreting almost entirely mucus and very little digestive acid. In this condition the stomach is unable to produce the intrinsic factor, a substance necessary for the absorption of vitamin B_{12}, which the body needs for the formation of red blood cells. Thus the gastritis patient is in danger of developing pernicious anemia.

Symptoms of gastritis include dyspepsia or indigestion, vomiting, headache, coated tongue, and abnormal increase or decrease in appetite. Diarrhea and abdominal cramps also may occur.

Although the specific cause of gastritis is unknown, it appears to result from overindulgence in alcohol, coffee, or highly seasoned or fried foods, all of which increase the activity of the stomach, thereby irritating it more. Eating rancid foods can cause bacterial infection, which may cause gastritis. Recurring cases of gastritis may be the result of ulcers or of the buildup of poisonous body wastes due to such diseases as chronic uremia or cirrhosis of the liver.

The diet in treating gastritis should be bland. Roughage, fried foods, and highly seasoned foods should be avoided. Alcohol, coffee, aspirin, and other substances that irritate the stomach lining must be eliminated. Frequent small meals are easier for the stomach to digest than fewer large meals. If gastritis is severe, iron supplements and injections of vitamin B_{12} may be helpful for preventing pernicious anemia.

NUTRIENTS THAT MAY BE BENEFICIAL IN TREATMENT OF GALLSTONES

Body Member	Nutrients	Quantity
Gallbladder	Vitamin A	
	Vitamin B complex	
	Vitamin C	
	Vitamin D	
	Vitamin E	
	Vitamin K	
	High carbohydrates	
	High protein	
	Low fat	

NUTRIENTS THAT MAY BE BENEFICIAL IN TREATMENT OF GASTRITIS

Body Member	Nutrients	Quantity
Stomach	Vitamin A	
	Vitamin B complex	
	Vitamin B_6	
	Vitamin B_{12}	
	Folic acid	
	Inositol	
	Pantothenic acid	
	Vitamin D	
	Vitamin E	
	Lecithin	
	Linoleic acid	
	Iron	
	Low cellulose (a carbohydrate)	

GASTRITIS

Gastritis is a disease in which the mucous lining of the stomach becomes irritated and inflamed. If gastritis is

GASTROENTERITIS (STOMACH FLU)

Gastroenteritis, or stomach flu, is the inflammation of the lining of the stomach. The inflammation has a variety of causes, such as food poisoning, certain viruses, alcohol intoxication, sensitivity to drugs, and allergies. Symptoms of gastroenteritis include diarrhea, vomiting, possible fever, chills, and abdominal cramps that vary in severity, but recovery is usually within one or two days.

Treatment for stomach flu includes bed rest and abstention from food until the stomach can tolerate it. A regular well-balanced diet should then be introduced as soon as possible. Repeated vomiting and diarrhea can cause potassium and fluid loss, which should be corrected as soon as possible. If fever is present, intake of vitamins A and C should be increased.

NUTRIENTS THAT MAY BE BENEFICIAL IN TREATMENT OF GASTROENTERITIS

Body Member	Nutrients	Quantity
Stomach	Vitamin A	
	Vitamin C	
	Potassium	

GLAUCOMA

Glaucoma is characterized by an increase in pressure of the fluid within the eyeball and a hardening of the surface of the eyeball. The cause of glaucoma is currently unknown, but usually it occurs after age forty and it may be due to tumor, trauma, infection, and in one type, heredity. Glaucoma is often associated with anxiety and stress, allergy, or hormone disorders. Symptoms include eye discomfort or pain, especially in the morning, blurred vision, halos around lights, inability to adjust to a darkened room, and loss of vision at the sides. Early detection of glaucoma can substantially reduce the incidence of blindness resulting from it.

Glaucoma cannot be cured, but it can be controlled through the use of prescribed eye drops. The diet of those affected should be rich in vitamin A, essential for eye-tissue health. If the symptoms of anxiety are related to a deficiency of the B vitamins, then correction of this deficiency would decrease the susceptibility of an individual to glaucoma. Alcohol, tobacco, coffee, and tea should be avoided.

NUTRIENTS THAT MAY BE BENEFICIAL IN TREATMENT OF GLAUCOMA

Body Member	Nutrients	Quantity*
Eye	Vitamin A	25,000 IU
	Vitamin B complex	
	Vitamin B_2	
	Choline	Up to 2 g
	Inositol	
	Vitamin C	60-250 mg per lb of body weight
	Vitamin D	
	Bioflavonoids	

*See note, p. 169.

GOITER

A goiter is an enlargement of the thyroid gland. The thyroid gland is located at the base of the neck. Its chief function is to regulate the rate of metabolism. Goiter may be caused by a lack of iodine in the diet, inflammation of the thyroid gland due to infection, or under- or overproduction of hormones by the thyroid gland.

Symptoms of goiter are a swelling at the base of the neck, hoarseness, change in the rate of metabolism, and in extreme cases, difficulty in swallowing and breathing. Treatment of goiter varies with the cause. If goiter is due to an iodine deficiency, increasing the intake of iodine will prevent further enlargement of the gland and, in some cases, reduce its size. The use of iodized salt has helped to eliminate goiter in many places where iodine does not occur naturally in foods.

NUTRIENTS THAT MAY BE BENEFICIAL IN TREATMENT OF GOITER

Body Member	Nutrients	Quantity
Thyroid	Vitamin A	
	Vitamin C	
	Calcium	
	Iodine	

GOUT

Gout is a metabolic disturbance characterized by an excess of uric acid in the blood and deposits of uric acid salts in the tissue around the joints, especially in the fingers and the toes. It can also occur in the heel, knee, hand, ear, or any joint in the body.

Gout results when certain crystals are formed as an end product of improper protein metabolism. These crystals are deposited in a joint, forming a bump or growth that irritates the joint, causing it to become inflamed; thus an attack of gout occurs.

A gout attack begins with pain in the inflamed joint which may spread to other joints of the body. Pain is greatest in the early morning and finally abates later in the day. An attack usually lasts from 5 to 12 days and may recur months later.

Although the exact cause of gout is unknown, it most often appears to be hereditary. However, factors such as obesity, increasing age, and improper diet increase an individual's susceptibility to gout. Alcohol, a large meal, or any physical or emotional stress also may bring on an attack of gout.

Medical treatment for gout involves prescription of drugs to decrease the inflammation and pain, and encouragement of regular patterns of exercise, rest, and diet. A therapeutic diet should be moderate in protein and low in fats. Foods that have a high content of purine, forerunner of uric acid, should be avoided. One such type of food is organ meats. Because a low-purine diet is normally lacking in the vitamin B complex and vitamin E, special attention should be paid to including these vitamins in the diet. Emphasis should be placed on including adequate intake of fluids to prevent the buildup of the gout-producing crystals in the kidneys. A gradual weight-reduction program for overweight individuals will help prevent gout attacks, while a rapid weight loss may bring on attacks, due to the stressful effect on the body. Pantothenic acid especially aids in the metabolic functioning of the cells.

NUTRIENTS THAT MAY BE BENEFICIAL IN TREATMENT OF GOUT

Body Member	Nutrient	Quantity*
Joints	Vitamin A	
	Vitamin B complex	
	Pantothenic acid	
	Vitamin C	Up to 5,000 mg
	Vitamin E	
	Calcium	

*See note, p. 169.

Body Member	Nutrients	Quantity
	Iron	
	Magnesium	
	Phosphorus	
	Potassium	Two tablets

HAIR PROBLEMS

Hair is composed primarily of protein. A deficiency of protein in the diet can result in a temporary change of hair color and texture, resulting in dull, thin, dry hair. If the protein deficiency is corrected, the hair will return to its normal condition.

A deficiency of vitamin A may cause hair to become dull, dry and lusterless and eventually to fall out. However, an excess of vitamin A may cause similar problems. Deficiencies of the vitamin B complex and vitamin C have also been associated with poor appearance of hair.[17]

A well-balanced diet is important to maintain healthy hair, although hereditary graying and balding cannot be completely prevented by nutritional means.

Good hygiene is also important for healthy hair. This includes brushing the hair properly and washing it with mild shampoo. Exposure to wind and sun may cause brittle, broken hair.

NUTRIENTS THAT MAY BE BENEFICIAL IN TREATMENT OF HAIR PROBLEMS

Body Member	Nutrients	Quantity
Hair	Vitamin A	
	Vitamin B complex	
	Vitamin C	
	Iodine	
	Protein	

HALITOSIS

Halitosis is an unpleasant odor of the breath. It may be caused by improper diet, poor mouth hygiene, nose or throat infections, extensive teeth or gum decay, excessive smoking, or the presence of bacteria that are foreign to the mouth.

Treatment for halitosis involves proper mouth hy-

[17]Ruth Adams and Frank Murray, *Body, Mind and the B Vitamins* (New York: Larchmont Books, 1962), pp. 227-228.

giene, including regular tooth brushing. Often the use of dental floss is recommended. A carefully balanced diet is essential for the prevention of halitosis. Avoiding excessive consumption of carbohydrates may help prevent tooth decay that can cause bad breath. Vitamin C is needed to prevent scurvy, which can cause the gums to bleed and become infected. Vitamin A is necessary for the overall development and health of the gums and teeth.

NUTRIENTS THAT MAY BE BENEFICIAL IN TREATMENT OF HALITOSIS

Body Member	Nutrients	Quantity*
Mouth	Vitamin A	
	Vitamin B complex	
	Vitamin B_6	50 mg
	Niacin	
	Vitamin C	1,000 or more mg

*See note, p. 169.

HAY FEVER (ALLERGIC RHINITIS)

Hay fever is a reaction of the mucous membranes of the eyes, nose, and air passages to seasonal pollens and dust, feathers, animal hair, and other irritants. Hay-fever symptoms include itching in the eyes, nose, and throat, a clear, watery discharge from the nose and eyes, frequent sneezing, and nervous irritability. Alcoholic beverages and stressful situations may precipitate an attack of hay fever.

The most effective treatment for hay fever is to avoid the irritant. Vitamin A is essential for the general health of the respiratory system. Some authorities believe that vitamin C in doses of 200 or more milligrams daily can relieve hay-fever symptoms.[18]

NUTRIENTS THAT MAY BE BENEFICIAL IN TREATMENT OF HAY FEVER

Body Member	Nutrients	Quantity*
Lungs/ Respiratory system	Vitamin A	100,000 IU for four months
	Vitamin B complex	
	Vitamin C	100-1,000 mg daily
	Vitamin E	

*See note, p. 169.

[18]Guthrie, *Introductory Nutrition*, p. 225.

HEADACHE

A headache is a pain or ache in any portion of the head. It is a symptom rather than a disease in itself. Headache is most frequently a sign of emotional stress or tension. However, there are many other possible causes of headache, such as diseases of the eye, nose, or throat; trauma to the head; air pollution or poor ventilation; drugs; alcohol; tobacco; fever; generalized body infections; disturbances of the digestive tract and circulatory system; brain disorders; anemia; low blood sugar; niacin or pantothenic acid deficiency; an overdose of vitamin A; or allergies.

A migraine is a particular type of headache due to the alternating constriction and dilation of the blood vessels in the brain. The exact cause of migraine is unknown, although as in the case of most headaches, emotional stress usually plays a large role. The symptoms of migraine include either generalized or one-sided head pain and possibly nausea, vomiting, and visual disturbances. A migraine attack may last for hours or days.

Treatment for headache depends upon the underlying cause. Repeated headaches may be a symptom of a serious disorder and therefore deserve attention, or they may be the result of stress. Learning better ways of coping with stress and relieving nervous tension is often the most effective treatment for headaches and migraine. Special attention should be paid to prevent deficiencies of iron, niacin, and pantothenic acid. Vitamin A may also prove helpful to some headache victims. Treatment for migraine may include pain-relieving drugs and the entire B complex for health of the nerves.

NUTRIENTS THAT MAY BE BENEFICIAL IN TREATMENT OF HEADACHE

Body Member	Nutrients	Quantity*
Head	Vitamin A	
	Vitamin B complex	
	Vitamin B_1	
	Vitamin B_2	10 mg per meal
	Vitamin B_6	50 mg
	Niacin	100 mg three times daily
	Pangamic acid	100 mg
	Pantothenic acid	100 mg
	Vitamin C	Up to 1,000 mg
	Vitamin E	Up to 1,200 IU
	Calcium	
	Potassium	

*See note, p. 169.

HEART DISEASE

The heart is the chief organ of the circulatory system; it is the most delicate and yet the most durable because it is made of the toughest muscle fibers of the body. The heart is a very efficient pump, but over a million Americans die of heart disease each year.

Some of the major ailments connected with the heart are the following: A *coronary thrombosis* is the formation of a blood clot that blocks the artery leading to the heart. Although this type of heart disease is the greatest single killer in the world today, 50 percent of the victims of coronary thrombosis survive. Those who survive usually have damaged heart muscle because there is no replacement for the artery that flows into the heart. If a blood clot slips into the coronary artery and partially blocks the main artery, the attack is not fatal; complete blockage is fatal.

A *coronary occlusion* results if the clot blocks a small branch artery and the part of the heart that receives nourishment from that branch dies. The heart and brain are the only two organs susceptible to occlusion.

Coronary sclerosis, a restriction of the coronary blood supply to the heart muscle due to thickening and hardening of the blood vessels (sclerosis), results in the severe pain *angina pectoris*. This pain develops whenever the working demand exceeds the supply of oxygen to the heart. High blood pressure generally is an accompanying condition of coronary sclerosis.

A *stroke* occurs when the blood supply to the brain, or to some portion of it, is cut off. This usually takes place in the cerebrum, that part of the brain where nerve centers controlling sight, hearing, speech, and body movements are located. If a blockage stops blood flow to one of these control zones or to nerve fibers leading from the zones, the activity controlled by the zone will be impaired.

Some physicians believe that emotional stress is the main cause of *arteriosclerosis* (hardening of the arteries) because stress raises blood pressure. It is not normally high blood pressure, but the characteristic fluctuations in pressure caused by stress and strain, which damage the artery walls.

A nutritionally balanced diet is important for efficient operation of the heart. Protein foods, fresh vegetables and fruits, and whole grains should be substituted for high intake of refined starches, sweets, and hydrogenated fats. Protein is essential to the strength of all muscles, including the heart. An overconsumption of fat is believed to be detrimental because it may weaken arteries, reduce their elasticity, and clog them with cholesterol. Supplementary intake of vitamin E is needed as an anticoagulant to reduce arterial clots and as an oxygen conserver to keep oxygen in the blood. Vitamin E, through interaction with vitamin F, also allows for the reduction of cholesterol. This will prevent the metabolic imbalance that causes cholesterol to collect in the arteries. A deficient operation of the thyroid gland may be involved in some cases of faulty fat metabolism. Vitamin C and the B vitamins are necessary to maintain arterial health.

A pulse rate of about 70 beats per minute for men and 80 beats per minute for women is best for the heart. A pulse rate of 100 is usually considered abnormally high, although there are variations in normal rates. To lower a pulse rate, reduce the intake of food, avoid emotional stress, and curtail use of drugs, alcoholic drinks, and tobacco products. It should be remembered that substances to which one is allergic will raise the pulse rate and thus produce further stress on the heart.

Overweight can be a contributing factor to both high pulse rate and high blood pressure: excess pounds greatly tax the heart and the circulatory system in general. A properly balanced diet will lead to reduction of pounds without the adverse symptoms experienced when eating only one or two foods as is common in many fad diets.

Stress may raise blood pressure as well as pulse rate. Fluctuations of blood pressure against artery walls contribute to arterial injury and hardening. Exercise is an excellent way to deal with stress and improve muscle tone of the heart and entire body. Unless otherwise advised by your physician, begin walking for ten minutes a day and gradually increase up to one hour. Walking should be at a brisk pace but must be begun slowly. Strenuous exercise (work or recreation) to which one is not accustomed should be avoided because the heart may not be able to meet the unusual requirements made upon it. (See also "Arteriosclerosis" and "Cerebrovascular Accident.")

NUTRIENTS THAT MAY BE BENEFICIAL IN TREATMENT OF HEART DISEASE

Body Member	Nutrients	Quantity*
Heart/Blood/ Circulatory system	Vitamin B complex	
	Vitamin B$_6$	100 mg
	Choline	
	Inositol	

*See note, p. 169.

Body Member	Nutrients	Quantity
	Niacin	100 mg
	Pantothenic acid	
	Vitamin C	
	Vitamin E	300-400 IU
	Vitamin F	
	Calcium	1,000 mg
	Iodine	
	Lecithin	
	Magnesium	500 or more mg
	Phosphorus	

HEMOPHILIA

Hemophilia is a hereditary blood disease characterized by a prolonged coagulation time. The blood fails to clot, and abnormal bleeding occurs. Hemophilia is a sex-linked hereditary trait, transmitted by normal females carrying the recessive gene. This disease occurs almost exclusively in males. There is no known cure for hemophilia. Transfusion of fresh whole blood or plasma is required in emergencies to provide the necessary coagulation factors.

NUTRIENTS THAT MAY BE BENEFICIAL IN TREATMENT OF HEMOPHILIA

Body Member	Nutrients	Quantity
Blood/Circulatory system	Niacin	
	Vitamin C	
	Bioflavonoids	
	Vitamin T	
	Calcium	

HEMORRHOIDS (PILES)

Hemorrhoids are ruptured or distended veins located around the anus. The most common cause of hemorrhoids is strain on the abdominal muscles due to factors such as heavy or improper lifting, pregnancy, overweight, constipation, or an extremely sedentary life. Symptoms of hemorrhoids are local itching, pain, and the passage of bloody stools.

Treatment for severe hemorrhoids may involve surgical removal. Individuals with hemorrhoids should maintain a diet with large amounts of fluid to avoid constipation. Preventive measures include adequate exercise to strengthen abdominal muscles and avoidance of constipation.

NUTRIENTS THAT MAY BE BENEFICIAL IN TREATMENT OF HEMORRHOIDS

Body Member	Nutrients	Quantity*
Intestine	Vitamin A	25,000 IU
	Vitamin B complex	
	Vitamin B$_6$	25 mg after each meal
	Vitamin C	1,000-2,000 mg
	Vitamin E	600 IU
	Bioflavonoids	
	Calcium	
	Fluids (water)	
	Low cellulose (a carbohydrate)	

*See note, p. 169.

HEPATITIS

Hepatitis is an inflammation of the liver caused by infection or toxic agents. It begins with flulike symptoms of fever, weakness, drowsiness, abdominal discomfort, and headache, possibly accompanied by jaundice.

Infectious hepatitis is excreted in the feces two to three weeks before and up to one week after the appearance of jaundice, although many patients, particularly children, never develop jaundice. Toxic hepatitis may be caused by a wide variety of chemicals taken into the system by injection, ingestion, or skin absorption. The extent of the damage is related to the dose of the substance.

NUTRIENTS THAT MAY BE BENEFICIAL IN TREATMENT OF HEPATITIS

Body Member	Nutrients	Quantity*
General/Liver	Vitamin A	
	Pangamic acid	
	Vitamin C	10 g
	Vitamin F	

*See note, p. 169.

HYPERTENSION (HIGH BLOOD PRESSURE)

Hypertension is an abnormal elevation of blood pressure. The cause is generally unknown, but hypertension often accompanies arteriosclerosis or kidney diseases.

Symptoms of hypertension may be nonexistent, or they may include headache, nervousness, insomnia, nosebleeds, blurred vision, edema, and shortness of breath. Factors associated with the onset of hypertension are heredity, obesity, physical or emotional stress, high salt intake, cigarette smoking, and excessive use of stimulants such as coffee, tea, or drugs.

Stress is an important factor to be considered in hypertension. Many people drive themselves too hard and consequently become hypertensive. These people must learn to avoid stressful conditions by changing their lifestyle. They should take regular, unhurried meals, try to avoid worry, allow themselves plenty of leisure time, take vacations, and generally use moderation in all things. If their occupation involves excessive emotional and physical stress, they may have to consider changing it or adjusting it to make it less stressful.

Sodium is a primary cause of hypertension because it causes fluid retention, which adds additional stress to the heart and circulatory system. Increasing the potassium intake will cause the body to excrete more sodium. Vitamin C can help to maintain the health of the blood vessels that are strained by the greater pressure placed on them by hypertension.

Regular exercise is essential in preventing high blood pressure because it keeps the circulatory system healthy. Promoting a tranquil outlook on life is of primary importance in reducing and preventing hypertension.

NUTRIENTS THAT MAY BE BENEFICIAL IN TREATMENT OF HYPERTENSION

Body Member	Nutrients	Quantity*
Blood/ Circulatory system/ Heart	Vitamin B complex	
	Choline	
	Inositol	
	Niacin	
	Pangamic acid	
	Vitamin C	1,000-3,000 mg
	Vitamin E	100-600 IU
	Bioflavonoids	100-300 mg

*See note, p. 169.

Body Member	Nutrients	Quantity
	Calcium	8 g three times daily
	Lecithin	
	Magnesium	500 mg
	Protein	
	Low sodium	Less than 300 mg daily

HYPERTHYROIDISM

Hyperthyroidism is overproduction of hormones by the thyroid gland. Symptoms of the condition are nervousness, irritability, fatigue, weakness, loss of weight, goiter, and rapid pulse. Hyperthyroidism can be caused by hereditary factors, emotional stress, or other unknown factors.

The excess production of thyroid hormones speeds up all body processes. As a result, all nutrients in the body are used up at a greater rate. The diet should therefore be increased in all nutrients. If weight loss has been great, additional protein may be necessary to replace muscle tissue that may have been lost. Particular attention should be paid to the adequate intake of the vitamin B complex because it is needed for the metabolism of the extra carbohydrates and protein. Coffee and tea containing caffeine should be avoided because caffeine increases the metabolic rate, thereby resulting in more calories being expended. Nicotine and the initial effects of alcohol also increase the metabolic rate and should be avoided.

NUTRIENTS THAT MAY BE BENEFICIAL IN TREATMENT OF HYPERTHYROIDISM

Body Member	Nutrients	Quantity*
Gland, thyroid	Vitamin A	100,000 IU
	Vitamin B complex	
	Choline	
	Inositol	
	Vitamin C	
	Vitamin E	1,000 IU
	Calcium	
	Iodine	4-6 mg
	Carbohydrates	
	Protein	

*See note, p. 169.

HYPOGLYCEMIA (LOW BLOOD SUGAR)

Hypoglycemia is an abnormally low level of glucose, or sugar, in the blood caused by too much sugar in the diet, tumors in the pancreas causing an overproduction of insulin, or disorders of the liver interfering with the storage and release of sugar. An overconsumption of carbohydrates causes the blood sugar level to rise rapidly, stimulating the pancreas to secrete an excess of insulin. This excess insulin removes too much sugar from the blood, resulting in an abnormally low blood sugar level.

Symptoms of hypoglycemia include fatigue, weakness in legs, swollen feet, tightness in chest, constant hunger, eyeache, migraine, pains in various parts of the body, nervous habits, mental disturbances, and insomnia. Rapid fluctuations in blood sugar level give rise to many bizarre symptoms that may suggest mental disorder; however, a glucose tolerance test will ascertain the amount of sugar in the blood at a given time.

The therapeutic diet for hypoglycemia is high in protein, low in carbohydrates, and moderate in fat. The diet may be supplemented with high-protein between-meal snacks. Heavily sugared foods should be avoided, and foods with high natural sugar content should be restricted. When carbohydrates are unavoidable, only those that are slowly absorbed, such as fruits, vegetables, and whole-grain products, should be eaten, so that the change in the blood sugar level will be gradual. Coffee, strong tea, and cocoa should be avoided because they are capable of precipitating an attack of hypoglycemia.

There are no known drugs that specifically elevate the blood sugar. Several authorities suggest that daily ingestion of vitamin C can help prevent low blood sugar attacks.[19]

NUTRIENTS THAT MAY BE BENEFICIAL IN TREATMENT OF HYPOGLYCEMIA

Body Member	Nutrients	Quantity*
Blood/ Circulatory system	Vitamin B complex	
	Vitamin B$_6$	50 mg
	Vitamin B$_{12}$	25-50 mcg
	Pantothenic acid	100 mg
	Vitamin C	2,000-5,000 mg
	Chromium	
	High protein	

*See note, p. 169.

[19]Irvin Stone, *The Healing Factor* (New York: Grosset & Dunlap, 1972), p. 149.

Body Member	Nutrients	Quantity
	Low carbohydrates	
	Moderate fats (vitamin F)	

HYPOTHYROIDISM

Hypothyroidism is the underproduction of hormones by the thyroid gland. The condition may be hereditary, or it may result from a deficiency of iodine. Symptoms of hypothyroidism are fatigue; decreased appetite; dull, dry hair and skin; constipation; lack of mental and physical vigor; and sleeplessness.

Treatment for hypothyroidism may include administration of thyroid hormone or increased intake of iodine.

NUTRIENTS THAT MAY BE BENEFICIAL IN TREATMENT OF HYPOTHYROIDISM

Body Member	Nutrients	Quantity
Gland, thyroid	Iodine	

IMPETIGO

Impetigo is a skin disease caused by bacterial infection. The disease occurs primarily in children, especially in those who are undernourished.

Impetigo is characterized by pus-filled skin lesions located mainly on the face and hands. These lesions rupture and form a honey-yellow crust over the infected area. The disease is spread by scratching the lesions and contaminating other skin areas with the fingers.

Strict hygiene is essential to prevent spread of the infection to other parts of the body or to other people. Neglected impetigo in adults may result in boils, ulcers, or other complications. Vitamin A is necessary for the health of skin tissue and may be helpful in aiding the skin in its recovery from impetigo.

NUTRIENTS THAT MAY BE BENEFICIAL IN TREATMENT OF IMPETIGO

Body Member	Nutrients	Quantity
Skin	Vitamin A	
	Vitamin C	
	Vitamin D	
	Vitamin E	

INDIGESTION (DYSPEPSIA)

Dyspepsia is imperfect or incomplete digestion, manifesting itself in a sensation of fullness or discomfort in the abdomen accompanied by pain or cramps, heartburn, nausea, and large amounts of gas in the intestines. Dyspepsia may be a symptom of a disorder in the stomach or small or large intestine, or it may be a complaint in itself. If indigestion occurs frequently and with no recognizable cause, medical investigation is advised.

The most common causes of dyspepsia are overeating or eating too rapidly; improper diet, such as a diet overabundant in carbohydrates at the expense of other nutrients; or overconsumption of stimulants such as coffee, tea, or alcohol. Lack of niacin in the diet may result in a decrease in the amount of hydrochloric acid in the stomach, consequently leading to indigestion. Smoking before or during a meal or swallowing too much air with meals, as in periods of nervousness or anxiety, can also bring about indigestion.

Dyspepsia can be prevented by avoidance of foods that produce its symptoms, especially highly seasoned foods, which tend to irritate the stomach lining, and fatty foods, which remain in the stomach longer than most foods. In treating dyspepsia, the diet should be bland and nutritionally well balanced. Special attention should be paid to the adequate intake of B vitamins, for without them carbohydrate combustion cannot take place and symptoms of indigestion can result.

NUTRIENTS THAT MAY BE BENEFICIAL IN TREATMENT OF INDIGESTION

Body Member	Nutrients	Quantity*
Stomach	Vitamin B complex	
	Vitamin B_1	50 mg
	Vitamin B_6	50 mg
	Folic acid	
	Niacin	100 mg
	Pantothenic acid	
	Low fat	

*See note, p. 169.

INFLUENZA (FLU)

Influenza is an acute viral infection of the respiratory tract. It is highly contagious and easily spread by sneezing and coughing. Symptoms of influenza include chills, high fever, sore throat, headache, abdominal pain, hoarseness, cough, enlarged lymph nodes, aching of the back and limbs, and frequent vomiting and diarrhea. Serious complications, such as pneumonia, sinus infections, and ear infections, can develop.

Influenza vaccines are available which help the body become immune to the virus. Many doctors recommend that elderly persons, pregnant women, and persons with heart, kidney, or lung disease have these vaccinations.

There is no specific treatment for influenza other than to treat its symptoms and try to prevent complications. The fever that usually accompanies influenza requires additional calories in several small feedings and additional vitamin B complex to metabolize these calories. Protein is needed for repair of tissue destroyed by fever. Infections accompanied by fever also increase the need for vitamins A and C. Vitamin A is especially important in influenza for the health of the lining of the throat. Increased fluid intake is also important in the event of fever.

NUTRIENTS THAT MAY BE BENEFICIAL IN TREATMENT OF INFLUENZA

Body Member	Nutrients	Quantity*
Lungs/	Vitamin A	
Respiratory tract	Vitamin B complex	
	Vitamin B_1	50-200 mg
	Vitamin B_2	10 mg
	Vitamin B_6	50-100 mg
	Vitamin C	300-500 mg
	Niacin	50-100 mg
	Pantothenic acid	25 mg
	Protein	

*See note, p. 169.

INSOMNIA (SLEEPLESSNESS)

Insomnia is the inability to sleep soundly. It is a disturbance in the amount and depth of sleep. The need for sleep varies from person to person, but in general, it tends to decline as one grows older. The main causes of insomnia are anxiety or pain. Vigorous mental activity late at night, excitement, headache, or tired and aching muscles may also cause insomnia. In addition, caffeine, a stimulant found in coffee, tea, and cola drinks, is often responsible for keeping people awake.

Sleeplessness may be a symptom of a serious disease,

but often it is a result of an individual's faulty reactions to stress. Insomnia perpetuates itself, in that thinking about the inability to sleep creates further tension in the mind and body. Only by relaxing and ceasing to worry about insomnia can a person resume sleeping and thus relieve his anxiety and tension. In learning to change his patterns of thought associated with sleep, the insomniac must establish a new bedtime routine, which might include such muscle and mind relaxers as leisurely walks, warm baths, massages, hot milk, soft music, or quiet meditation.

The well-nourished person who enjoys good health and a feeling of well-being probably will be less troubled by insomnia than one who subsists on a diet deficient in some essential nutrients. Deficiencies in the B vitamins, particularly B_6 and pantothenic acid, have resulted in insomnia. In some cases, vitamin B_{12} has been helpful in treating anxiety in insomniacs. Vitamin C, protein, calcium, and potassium can also calm the nerves and promote sleep. Sleeping pills or barbiturates should be used only as a last resort because they may produce dependence and other serious side effects.

NUTRIENTS THAT MAY BE BENEFICIAL IN TREATMENT OF INSOMNIA

Body Member	Nutrients	Quantity*
Brain/Nervous system	Vitamin B complex	
	Vitamin B_6	10 mg
	Vitamin B_{12}	
	Inositol	
	Niacin	100 mg
	Pantothenic acid	
	Vitamin C	
	Vitamin D	
	Calcium	2 g taken before bedtime
	Magnesium	250 mg
	Phosphorus	
	Potassium	

*See note, p. 169.

JAUNDICE

Jaundice is a condition in which the skin, whites of the eyes, and urine become abnormally yellow because of the presence of pigments from worn-out red blood cells; the pigments accumulate in the blood because they are not being excreted as a waste product in the bile as they should be. Jaundice may indicate blood, kidney, or liver disorders; a doctor should be consulted in cases of jaundice.

NUTRIENTS THAT MAY BE BENEFICIAL IN TREATMENT OF JAUNDICE

Body Member	Nutrients	Quantity*
Blood	Vitamin A	
	Vitamin B_6	50 mg
	Vitamin C	1,000-1,500 mg every three hours in acute conditions, given even during fasting. In chronic conditions, 3,000-5,000 mg daily
	Vitamin D	
	Vitamin E	600 IU
	Vitamin F	
	Pantothenic acid	100 mg
	Calcium	
	Lecithin	Large amounts
	Magnesium	
	Phosphorus	
	Protein (sulfur-containing amino acids—eggs)	250 g

*See note, p. 169.

KIDNEY STONES (RENAL CALCULI)

Kidney stones are abnormal accumulations of mineral salts which form in the kidney but may lodge anywhere in the urinary tract. The stones are composed primarily of calcium. In the process of being filtered out of the blood by the kidneys, the calcium conglomerates into a stone. Stone formation may be due to overactivity of the parathyroid gland, which causes an elevated level of calcium in the blood. Additional conditions that increase the risk of kidney stone formation are dehydration, prolonged periods of bed rest, infections, and rarely, overingestion of vitamin D and calcium.

Symptoms of kidney stones include pain originating in the middle back which radiates around the abdomen toward the genitalia, increased urination that may contain blood or pus, nausea, and vomiting. Irritation by the stone may induce an infection in the urinary tract, giving rise to fever and chills and general discomfort.

Dietary therapy can not remove already formed kidney stones. However, to prevent further stone formation, calcium intake should be limited, although not excluded. A deficiency of vitamin B_6 and magnesium may cause stone formation; attention should therefore be paid to ensure their adequate intake. Persons whose diets are deficient in vitamin A tend toward kidney stone formation, so an adequate supply of this vitamin should be included in the diet.[20]

NUTRIENTS THAT MAY BE BENEFICIAL IN TREATMENT OF KIDNEY STONES

Body Member	Nutrients	Quantity*
Kidney	Vitamin A	
	Vitamin B_6	50 mg
	Vitamin C	
	Vitamin E	
	Magnesium	250-500 mg
	Restricted calcium	

*See note, p. 169.

KWASHIORKOR

Kwashiorkor is a severe malnutritional disease caused by a diet which supplies adequate calories through its carbohydrate content but which is seriously lacking protein. Kwashiorkor commonly develops in children who are between the ages of one and five and who are weaned from milk to a diet of primarily starches and sugars.

Symptoms of kwashiorkor include changes in the skin and hair, retarded growth, diarrhea, loss of appetite, nervous irritability, and edema. Severe infections and many vitamin deficiencies often accompany kwashiorkor.

The initial treatment for the disease is aimed at correcting the protein deficiency. Because of the patient's poor ability to tolerate fat, a skim-milk formula is often used in treatment. Gradually, additional foods are added until the patient progresses to a well-balanced diet. Vitamin deficiencies, if they exist, must be corrected.

[20]Krause and Hunscher, *Food, Nutrition and Diet Therapy*, p. 482.

NUTRIENTS THAT MAY BE BENEFICIAL IN TREATMENT OF KWASHIORKOR

Body Member	Nutrients	Quantity
Body	Vitamin A	
	Folic acid	
	Vitamin C	
	Vitamin D	
	Vitamin E	
	Chromium	
	Copper	
	Iron	
	Magnesium	
	Selenium	
	Protein	

LEG CRAMP, "CHARLEY HORSE"

A leg cramp is an involuntary contraction, or spasm, of a muscle in the leg or foot. Cramps most commonly occur at night, when the limbs are cool, particularly after a day of unusual exertion, and more frequently in the elderly, the young, and persons with arteriosclerosis. These cramps seem to be caused by unnatural positions, which impair the blood supply to the lower extremities causing the muscles to abnormally contract, thus bringing about cramps. A cramp usually lasts only a few seconds or minutes. If a cramp occurs while a person is walking, it may be a signal of seriously impaired circulation, but a cramp that occurs while a person is resting does not indicate this severity. Patients most susceptible to repeated leg cramps are those with advanced arteriosclerosis.

Leg cramps may signify a variety of nutritional deficiencies. The most common is lack of calcium, which is necessary for normal muscle contraction. Other deficiencies indicated are thiamine, pantothenic acid, biotin, and magnesium. Occasionally a sodium loss, such as occurs in heavy perspiration or diarrhea, may result in muscle cramps. A vitamin C deficiency also can be responsible for pains in the muscles and joints. Prevention and treatment for leg cramps should include an adequate diet containing sufficient amounts of these nutrients.

A "charley horse" is a pulled and bruised muscle that results in soreness and stiffness. It is usually due to a blow or to a forceful stretch of the leg during athletic activity. A person who has suffered a charley horse should have a high intake of protein to rebuild damaged tissues.

NUTRIENTS THAT MAY BE BENEFICIAL IN TREATMENT OF LEG CRAMP

Body Member	Nutrients	Quantity*
Leg	Vitamin B complex	
	Vitamin B_1	
	Vitamin B_2	
	Bioton	
	Pantothenic acid	100 mg
	Vitamin C	
	Vitamin D	
	Vitamin E	400-1,000 IU
	Vitamin F	
	Calcium	
	Magnesium	800 mg
	Phosphorus	
	Sodium	
	Protein	

*See note, p. 169.

LEUKEMIA

Leukemia is a fatal blood disease characterized by an overproduction of white blood cells. There are two basic types of leukemia. Acute leukemia usually occurs in children and young adults, and chronic leukemia is usually found only in adults.

Acute leukemia is marked by a sudden onset of symptoms. In chronic leukemia, symptoms develop more slowly. Symptoms of the disease include bleeding from the gums, nose, stomach, and rectum and abnormally easy, excessive bruising of the skin. Pain in the upper abdomen, anemia, fever, and increased susceptibility to infection are further leukemia symptoms.

The cause of leukemia is unknown. However, some theories suggest that excessive exposure to radiation, x-rays, or chemical pollution may cause the disease.

A well-balanced diet containing all vitamins is helpful in maintaining strength in the leukemia victim. Supplementing the diet with the vitamin B complex and iron may aid in the treatment of the anemia that accompanies the disease. Vitamin C may be helpful in fighting the infections that are often associated with leukemia.

NUTRIENTS THAT MAY BE BENEFICIAL IN TREATMENT OF LEUKEMIA

Body Member	Nutrients	Quantity
Blood	Vitamin B complex	
	Vitamin B_{12}	
	Folic acid	
	Vitamin C	
	Bioflavonoids	
	Copper	
	Iron	
	Zinc	

MEASLES

The two main varieties of measles are German measles and common measles. German measles is usually a mild illness with a rapid recovery period, alarming only to pregnant women. If a woman contracts German measles during the early months of her pregnancy, malformations such as heart defects, deafness, mental retardation, and blindness of the newborn commonly occur.

Symptoms of German measles may include fever, headache, and stiff joints, although most people seldom complain of any symptoms. A rash that lasts for about three days appears on the arms, chest, and forehead.

Since German measles is a virus that must run its course, there is little that can be done medically for its treatment. One attack of or vaccination for the disease will usually produce lifelong immunity against German measles. Lotions may be applied to the rash to relieve itching, and the patient should stay away from other people to avoid spreading the disease. A well-balanced diet rich in all nutrients is recommended.

Common measles is a highly contagious disease spread by droplets from the nose, throat, and mouth. The first symptoms of common measles are fever, cough, and inflammation of the eyes. Within 24 to 48 hours, small red spots with white centers appear on the inside of the cheeks. A rash which is first seen on the side of the neck and which then spreads to the rest of the body usually appears three to five days after the onset of the first symptoms. As the rash spreads, fever goes down. Common measles may have many serious complications, such as pneumonia, encephalitis, and injury to the nervous system.

The patient should be isolated in a well-ventilated room, which should be darkened if the patient is sensitive to light. Fevers increase the body's need for calories and vitamins A and C. Although the patient may not desire food for the first few days, he should be encouraged, but not forced, to eat. Frequent small meals and special foods may be beneficial. Increased fluid intake in any form, such as water, fruit juices, or milk, is essential to the measles patient.

NUTRIENTS THAT MAY BE BENEFICIAL IN TREATMENT OF MEASLES

Body Member	Nutrients	Quantity
General/Skin	Vitamin A	
	Vitamin C	
	Vitamin E	
	Protein	

MÉNIÈRE'S SYNDROME

Ménière's syndrome is a disease of the inner ear characterized by recurrent attacks of deafness, tinnitus, vertigo, nausea, and vomiting.

NUTRIENTS THAT MAY BE BENEFICIAL IN TREATMENT OF MÉNIÈRE'S SYNDROME

Body Member	Nutrients	Quantity*
Ear	Vitamin B complex	
	Vitamin B$_1$	10-25 mg four times daily for two weeks
	Vitamin B$_2$	10-25 mg four times daily for two weeks
	Niacin	100-250 mg four times daily for two weeks
	Vitamin E	
	Vitamin F	
	Calcium	

*See note, p. 169.

MENINGITIS

Meningitis occurs when the three layers of membranes lying between the skull and brain become infected by bacteria, viruses, or fungi. These infecting organisms are commonly spread via the bloodstream from acute infections of the nose and throat.

Meningitis is more commonly found in children than in adults. Symptoms include headache, stiff neck, high fever, chills, nausea, vomiting, changes in temperament, and drowsiness, which may develop into a coma.

Medical attention for meningitis should be sought promptly. The drug selected for treatment of the disease depends on the type of infecting organism. During the fever, the body's needs for vitamin A and C are increased. A well-balanced diet adequate in protein is necessary to help the body ward off infection and repair damaged tissue.

NUTRIENTS THAT MAY BE BENEFICIAL IN TREATMENT OF MENINGITIS

Body Member	Nutrients	Quantity
Brain	Vitamin A	
	Vitamin C	
	Vitamin D	
	Protein	

MENTAL ILLNESS

Mental illness is a serious disease that occurs when a person no longer is able to cope effectively with emotional or physical stress. The problems facing one person may not necessarily be more serious than the problems facing another person, but the mentally ill person has less ability to deal with problems and stress in a rational manner than does the mentally healthy person.

Mental illness may develop as a result of several factors. Inherited characteristics combined with certain environmental influences may trigger mental instability. Some types of mental illness may be a direct result of poor nutrition because the brain cells cannot function efficiently without proper nutrients. Deficiencies of B vitamins, ascorbic acid (vitamin C), and phosphorus are known to decrease the metabolic rate of the brain. Deficiency of niacin may cause symptoms of deep depression, often seen in psychosis. Symptoms of a severe vitamin B$_6$ deficiency are headache, irritability, dizziness, extreme nervousness, and inability to concentrate. Pantothenic acid is essential for the body's ability to handle stressful situations. Signs of a thiamine deficiency are lack of energy, constant fatigue, loss of appetite, and irritability. A prolonged thiamine deficiency may result in brain damage contributing to emotional upsets characterized by overreaction to normal stress. Irritability is also a symptom of vitamin C deficiency.

The proper phosphorus-calcium ratio (1 to 2) is essential for nourishment of the entire nervous system. Calcium deficiency results in tenseness, insomnia, and fatigue. The high copper level of many schizophrenics can be reduced by dietary intake of zinc and manganese.[21]

A lack of oxygen is involved in many cases of mental disturbance, since the brain is dependent upon an uninterrupted supply of oxygen not only to function properly but also to stay alive. Vitamin E is an oxygen conserver and increases the amount of oxygen available to the brain. An unbalanced blood sugar level and hypothyroidism (which leads to a deficiency of thyroxine in the blood) are acknowledged causes of emotional disturbances. Shortage of thyroxine (the iodine-carrying hormone) generally results in a slowdown of both physical and mental activity. Hyperthyroidism (overactive thyroid) is related to emotional disturbances, forgetfulness, slow thought processes, and irritability.

A person with a magnesium deficiency is apt to be uncooperative, withdrawn, apathetic, or belligerent. Defective adrenal function may contribute to depression and other forms of mental illness. These disorders may be alleviated by proper dietary habits and food supplementation.

Allergy specialists and psychiatrists have been successfully treating patients with psychiatric symptoms by isolating foods and chemicals in the environment that are causing the mental disturbances. The symptoms range from fatigue and dizziness to hyperactivity to catatonia (a complete loss of voluntary motion) and hallucinations. Allergic reactions may be a factor in criminal behavior. Allergens are able to get into the bloodstream and circulate through the brain. Besides immediate reactions that affect the brain, there is another response called "masked food allergy" that does not produce negative symptoms until hours after ingestion of the offensive food.

An example of a mental disorder that is caused by food allergies involves a patient of Dr. H.L. Newbold of New York who had spent nearly five years in a psychiatric hospital diagnosed as schizophrenic. The doctor placed the patient of a five-day spring water fast to cleanse her body of allergens. Her worst symptoms began to disappear. The doctor then began a refeeding program and watched for any foods that would cause a reaction. This particular patient was found to be allergic to certain foods, especially sugar, which rapidly brought back her previous illness. Many other patients were found to be allergic to such foods as wheat, corn, and milk and to cigarette smoke.

Many allergists feel that the typical modern diet, which is high in nonnutritive sugar and refined foods, does not provide optimal nutrition for the human body, and therefore lowers resistance to allergies. Food additives, preservatives, pesticide residues on food, air pollution, household cleaning items, and chlorine and fluorine in drinking water have been found to precipitate allergic reactions. Besides proper diet, supplementation (notably with vitamins A, B_6, C, and E) has been found to be effective in lessening or blocking allergic reactions.

Scientists at the Massachusetts Institute of Technology have found that choline has a direct and almost immediate effect on brain function. Because of this discovery, choline, a B vitamin, has been used successfully for the treatment of a neurological disease called tardive dyskinesia, and for manic-depressives. It may also be a factor in improving the memory of the aged.

Current research indicates that many of the schizophrenias, autism, abnormal behavior, and subsequent learning difficulties in children are caused by a biochemical imbalance within the body (e.g., too much copper or too much lead). Hyperactivity, perceptual changes involving any or all of the five senses, dyslexia, insomnia, and irritability—symptoms usually attributed to childhood schizophrenia—are manifestations of nutritional imbalances. Many members of the medical profession are treating these abnormalities with nutrient therapy. Because the nutrients work to correct the imbalance rather than to disguise it, the response is slow, taking three to six months at a minimum for maximal changes to become manifest. Carbohydrates, especially of the refined variety, and food additives can aggravate the above syndromes.[22]

NUTRIENTS THAT MAY BE BENEFICIAL IN TREATMENT OF MENTAL ILLNESS

Body Member	Nutrients	Quantity
Brain/Nervous system	Vitamin B complex	
	Vitamin B_1	
	Vitamin B_6	
	Vitamin B_{12}	
	Folic acid	
	Niacin	

[21]Pfeiffer, *Mental and Elemental Nutrients*, p. 253.

[22]Pfeiffer, *Mental and Elemental Nutrients*, pp. 411–412.

Body Member	Nutrients	Quantity
	Pantothenic acid	
	Vitamin C	
	Vitamin E	
	Vitamin F	
	Calcium	
	Magnesium	
	Phosphorus	
	Protein	
	Zinc	

MONONUCLEOSIS

Mononucleosis is an infectious disease, believed to be caused by a virus. It affects primarily the lymph tissues or glands that are located in the neck, armpits, and groin. The lymph glands remove many microscopic materials such as bacteria and viruses, thus helping to prevent the infection from spreading throughout the body. Symptoms of mononucleosis include sore throat, fever, chills, swollen glands, and fatigue.

Adequate rest, exercise, and nutrition are essential for the maintenance of general health and the prevention of mononucleosis. Protein is needed to stimulate the formation of antibodies, substances produced by the body to help protect it against other infections that may accompany or follow mononucleosis. Potassium and vitamin C supplements may be needed to compensate for the loss that occurs during fever. Vitamin A is needed for the health of the tissue lining of the throat. If there is a deficiency of thiamine, riboflavin, or biotin, supplementing these nutrients in the diet may be helpful in preventing fatigue and headaches.

NUTRIENTS THAT MAY BE BENEFICIAL IN TREATMENT OF MONONUCLEOSIS

Body Member	Nutrients	Quantity
Blood	Vitamin A	
	Vitamin B_1	
	Vitamin B_2	
	Vitamin B_6	
	Biotin	
	Choline	
	Pantothenic acid	
	Vitamin C	
	Potassium	
	Protein	

MULTIPLE SCLEROSIS

Multiple sclerosis is a chronic disease that causes the deterioration of the protective covering of the nerves in the brain and spinal cord, resulting in the hardening of various parts of the nervous system and the development of scars or lesions on the disturbed nerves. The cause of the disease is unknown, although it has been seen to follow malnutrition, emotional stress, and infections.

Multiple sclerosis usually occurs in persons between the ages of twenty-five and forty. The disease progresses slowly and may disappear for periods of time but returns intermittently, usually in a more severe form. Symptoms of the disease include visual and speech disturbances, dizziness, bowel and bladder disorders, weakness, lack of coordination, paralysis, loss of balance, and emotional instability.

Care should be taken to ensure adequate rest, exercise, and a well-balanced diet because all these are necessary for proper functioning of the nervous system. Vitamin B_{12} has been used to increase stability in standing and walking in some cases of the disease.[23] Vitamin B_{13} has been beneficial in treating multiple sclerosis.

A neurologist at the University of Oregon Health Sciences Center in Portland has been successfully treating MS patients with a daily high-potency vitamin supplement and minerals and a controlled diet. High-fat foods are eliminated and replaced with foods containing unsaturated fatty acids. Foods such as packaged cake mixes, cheeses, pastries, and other processed items are also not consumed, because they contain hidden or unknown quantities of saturated fat. The doctor also advises his patients to eat whole-grain breads and cereals and to take wheat germ or vitamin E to keep the unsaturated oils from being oxidized once inside the body. Observed results of the patients have been a reduction in relapses, more energy, the ability to continue walking and working, and an increase in life expectancy. Also, when the treatment was started in the early stages of the disease with little evident disability, 90 to 95 percent of the cases remained unchanged or improved during the following twenty years.[24]

[23]Rodale, *The Complete Book of Vitamins*, p. 257.
[24]Detailed information can be obtained from *The Multiple Sclerosis Diet Book*, by Dr. Roy Swank (New York: Doubleday, 1977).

NUTRIENTS THAT MAY BE BENEFICIAL IN TREATMENT OF MULTIPLE SCLEROSIS

Body Member	Nutrients	Quantity*
Brain/Nervous system	Vitamin B complex	
	Vitamin B_1	100 mg
	Vitamin B_2	150 mg
	Vitamin B_6	100-200 mg
	Vitamin B_{12}	
	Vitamin B_{13}	
	Choline	700-1,400 mg
	Niacin	100 mg
	Pangamic acid	
	Pantothenic acid	100 mg
	Vitamin C	Up to 1,000 mg
	Vitamin E	Up to 1,800 IU
	Vitamin F	Six capsules
	Lecithin	
	Magnesium	
	Manganese	
	Protein	

*See note, p. 169.

MUSCULAR DYSTROPHY

Muscular dystrophy is an inherited disease that causes wasting of the muscles. Some authorities believe muscular dystrophy to be nutritional in origin, but no direct link has been found. The major symptom is great weakness in the legs and back so that the patient has trouble walking. The weakness gradually progresses throughout the muscles of the body, creating partial, then total, paralysis.

Muscular dystrophy is marked by remissions, or periods in which the disease appears to be arrested, but the disease usually returns and is more severe. A varied diet that is high in protein, vitamins, and minerals is recommended in the early stages of the disease to help arrest the muscular wasting and to prolong the remissions.

NUTRIENTS THAT MAY BE BENEFICIAL IN TREATMENT OF MUSCULAR DYSTROPHY

Body Member	Nutrients	Quantity*
Muscles	Vitamin A	
	Vitamin B_6	

*See note, p. 169.

Body Member	Nutrients	Quantity
	Vitamin B_{12}	
	Choline	
	Niacin	
	Pantothenic acid	
	Vitamin C	
	Vitamin E	600 IU
	Potassium	
	Protein	

MYOCARDIAL INFARCTION (HEART ATTACK)

When the vessels leading to the heart, known as coronary arteries, become blocked by blood clots or by the fatty deposits of atherosclerosis, a myocardial infarction, or heart attack, occurs. If a blood clot partially blocks the main artery, the attack is not fatal and the individual survives with some degree of heart damage. Complete blockage results in death.

Symptoms may begin anytime. The most frequent complaint is an excruciating pain usually starting in the lower chest or upper abdomen. The pain often spreads to the neck and shoulders, down the arms, especially to the left side, and possibly to the back. The pain increases in severity and is not relieved by rest or nitroglycerin, a medication often prescribed for patients with mild angina pectoris. The pain causes the patient to appear very restless and anxious. In 15 percent of heart attack cases, however, no pain is experienced and the attack is known as a "silent coronary."[25]

Additional heart attack symptoms include perspiration and pale skin, a decrease in blood pressure, weak and rapid pulse, and, possibly, nausea and vomiting. A moderate fever usually appears 24 to 48 hours after the onset of the attack.

Immediate medical attention is necessary and can best be obtained at a coronary care unit in a hospital setting. Usually the patient will be given an electrocardiogram, or EKG, a test designed to detect changes in heart function or damage to some part of the heart. But often this test will not show the heart damage until hours or days after the attack. A blood test is also often done to help detect if a myocardial infarction has occurred.

[25]Lillian Brunner et al., *Medical Surgical Nursing* (New York: J.B. Lippincott Co., 1959).

Conditions that increase the risk of heart attack are lack of exercise, cigarette smoking, obesity, diabetes, prolonged high blood pressure, overabundance of salt in the diet, a family history of heart attacks, or prolonged emotional stress.

During the first three weeks of treatment, the patient runs a great risk of suffering further irregularities in heart function. The immediate effort in treatment is for the patient to obtain rest to decrease the workload of the heart. Pain medication and oxygen therapy are often applied. Because the workload of the heart increases after meals, the diet during the first few days often consists of six small feedings low in sodium. Cold fluids should be avoided because they may trigger irregularities in heart function. Protein intake must be adequate to replace protein lost in damaged heart cells. By six weeks the healing is almost complete and increased amounts of activity can be tolerated.

Dietary measures reducing the risk of heart attack include proper caloric intake to maintain or achieve normal weight and the use of unsaturated rather than saturated fats to help prevent further production of fatty deposits lining the blood vessels. Cholesterol intake should be restricted to 300 milligrams daily.[26] Many authorities suggest that refined carbohydrates, such as white sugar, play a large role in the development of heart disease and should therefore be restricted.[27] Vitamin C and the B complex help to maintain the integrity and health of the heart and circulatory system. Vitamin E may also help because of its anticlotting properties.

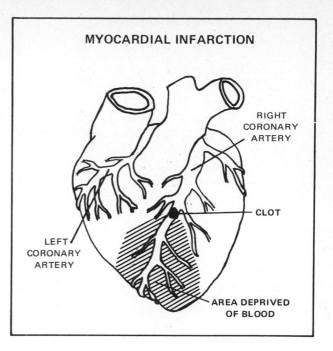

MYOCARDIAL INFARCTION

RIGHT CORONARY ARTERY

CLOT

LEFT CORONARY ARTERY

AREA DEPRIVED OF BLOOD

NUTRIENTS THAT MAY BE BENEFICIAL IN TREATMENT OF MYOCARDIAL INFARCTION

Body Member	Nutrients	Quantity*
Heart	Vitamin A	
	Vitamin B complex	
	Vitamin C	
	Vitamin E	Up to 1,600 IU
	Magnesium	
	Potassium	
	Protein	

*See note, p. 169.

[26]Alberta Dent Schackelton, *Practical Nurse Nutrition Education*, 3d ed. (Philadelphia: W.B. Saunders, 1972), p. 228.

[27]Stanley Davidson, R. Passmore, and J.I. Brock, *Human Nutrition and Dietetics*, 5th ed. (Baltimore: Williams and Wilkins Co., 1972), p. 324.

NAIL PROBLEMS

Nails are composed almost entirely of protein. Abnormal or unhealthy nails may be the result of a local injury, a glandular deficiency such as hypothyroidism, or a deficiency of certain nutrients.

A severe protein deficiency can cause opaque white bands to appear on the nails or cause them to become dry and brittle. A shortage of vitamin A or calcium in the diet may also cause dryness and brittleness. A lack of the B vitamins causes nails to become fragile, with horizontal or vertical ridges appearing. An iron deficiency can disturb the growth of the nails, causing dryness, brittleness, thinning, flattening, and eventually the appearance of moon-shaped nails.

NUTRIENTS THAT MAY BE BENEFICIAL IN TREATMENT OF NAIL PROBLEMS

Body Member	Nutrients	Quantity
Nails	Vitamin A	
	Vitamin B complex	
	Folic acid	
	Calcium	
	Iron	
	Protein	

NEPHRITIS (KIDNEY INFECTION)

Nephritis is the inflammation of one or both of the kidneys. The most common form of nephritis, pyelonephritis, occurs among females, especially during childhood or pregnancy. It is caused by bacteria from the stools being introduced into the urinary opening by wiping in a forward direction. The bacteria then travel to the bladder and finally to the kidney. Another form of nephritis, glomerulonephritis, occurs as a reaction to an infection elsewhere in the body, such as an infection in the throat.

Symptoms of nephritis may be nonexistent, or they may include blood and/or albumin in the urine, fatigue, lower back or abdominal pain, fever, chills, edema, nausea and vomiting, loss of appetite, and frequent urge to urinate. Anemia and high blood pressure may accompany severe nephritis.

Medical treatment of nephritis includes antibiotics, bed rest, and increased fluid intake. Sodium, potassium, and protein are restricted in the diet. If anemia is present, the nephritis patient should be receiving iron supplements. An adequate caloric intake is essential, and a multivitamin supplement of the water-soluble vitamins is recommended.

NUTRIENTS THAT MAY BE BENEFICIAL IN TREATMENT OF NEPHRITIS

Body Member	Nutrients	Quantity*
Kidney	Vitamin A	50,000-75,000 IU
	Vitamin B complex	
	Vitamin B$_2$	25 mg
	Choline	1,000 mg
	Vitamin C	
	Vitamin E	300-600 IU
	Calcium	250 mg
	Iron	
	Magnesium	
	Water	
	Restricted protein	
	Restricted sodium	
	Restricted potassium	

*See note, p. 169.

NEURITIS

Neuritis is the inflammation or deterioration of a nerve or group of nerves. Symptoms of neuritis vary with its cause. Some symptoms are pain, tenderness, tingling and loss of the sensation of touch in the affected nerve area, redness and swelling of the affected areas, and in severe cases, convulsions.

Causes of neuritis include injury to a nerve, such as in a direct blow or a nearby bone fracture; infection involving a nerve; diseases such as diabetes, gout, and leukemia; poisons such as mercury, lead, or methyl alcohol; and dietary deficiency of the vitamin B complex, especially thiamine. A thiamine deficiency results in the impairment of nerve tissue so that it cannot properly utilize carbohydrates for energy.

Treatment for neuritis also varies with the cause. If neuritis is caused by poisons, exposure to them should be ended, and if it is caused by a specific disease or trauma, treatment should be given. When a thiamine or vitamin B complex deficiency is responsible, administration of these vitamins will result in recovery within three to four days. Adequate intake of the B vitamins is necessary even when a deficiency does not exist, since they are needed for the general health of nerve tissue.

A well-balanced diet is important to the individual with neuritis for the maintenance and repair of muscles and nerves. If infection is present, protein, calorie, and fluid intake should be increased.

NUTRIENTS THAT MAY BE BENEFICIAL IN TREATMENT OF NEURITIS

Body Member	Nutrients	Quantity*
Nervous system	Vitamin B complex	
	Vitamin B$_1$	
	Vitamin B$_2$	
	Vitamin B$_6$	100-300 mg
	Vitamin B$_{12}$	
	Niacin	
	Pantothenic acid	
	Magnesium	
	Protein	

*See note, p. 169.

NIGHT BLINDNESS

Night blindness is the inability to see well in dim or dark light. The major cause of night blindness is deficiency of vitamin A. Vitamin A is necessary for the formation of visual purple, the substance in the eyes which enables them to adjust from bright light to darkness. Other causes of night blindness are fatigue, emotional disturbances, or hereditary factors.

Adequate intake of vitamin A will protect against night blindness. The Recommended Dietary Allowance of 5,000 units is necessary for normal and healthy vision. Riboflavin, niacin, thiamine, and zinc have been reported to relieve night blindness when vitamin A has not produced a response, and attention should therefore be paid to ensure their adequate intake.[28]

NUTRIENTS THAT MAY BE BENEFICIAL IN TREATMENT OF NIGHT BLINDNESS

Body Member	Nutrients	Quantity*
Eye	Vitamin A	
	Vitamin B complex	
	Vitamin B_1	
	Vitamin B_2	5 mg
	Niacin	
	Zinc	

*See note, p. 169.

OSTEOPOROSIS (BRITTLE BONES)

Osteoporosis is a reduction in the total mass of bone, with the remaining bone being fragile or "brittle." Symptoms of the disorder include increased incidence of fractures, pains in the hip and back, and reduced height. Osteoporosis is primarily a disease of the aged, usually beginning at about age fifty.

A major cause of osteoporosis is an inadequate intake of calcium over a period of years. Other causes are inability to absorb sufficient calcium through the intestine, calcium-phosphorus imbalance, lack of exercise, or lack of certain hormones.

A diet that is adequate in protein, calcium, phos-

[28]Krause and Hunscher, *Food, Nutrition and Diet Therapy*, p. 497.

phorus, and vitamin D is the best prevention and treatment for osteoporosis. Trace amounts of fluorides from foods or drinking water also protect against bone decomposition.

NUTRIENTS THAT MAY BE BENEFICIAL IN TREATMENT OF OSTEOPOROSIS

Body Member	Nutrients	Quantity*
Bones	Vitamin B_{12}	30-900 mcg
	Vitamin C	Up to 1,000 mg
	Vitamin D	Up to 5,000 IU
	Vitamin E	600 IU
	Calcium	500 mg
	Copper	
	Fluoride	
	Magnesium	500 mg
	Phosphorus	
	Protein	

*See note, p. 169.

OVERWEIGHT AND OBESITY

Overweight and obesity are one of the major nutritional problems in America today. Statistics show that people of average weight (see the "Desirable Height and Weight Chart," p. 246), have a longer life-span, have more energy, and usually feel better than those people who are overweight. Overweight and obesity precipitate such conditions as heart disease, kidney trouble, diabetes, high blood pressure, malnutrition, complications of pregnancy, and psychological problems. Glandular malfunction, malnutrition, emotional tension, boredom, habit, and love of food are the main causes of overweight.

Calories and exercise are essential considerations in losing weight. Fat is metabolically formed in the body when more food energy or calories are consumed than the body is able to use. One pound of fatty tissue is equal to 3500 calories. When the number of calories used during the day exceeds the amount consumed, the body oxidizes its supplies of fat to produce energy, and thereby a reduction of body weight results. A daily decrease of 1000 calories results in approximately two pounds of weight loss per week.

Calories may be burned up by the basal metabolism, which includes normal body functions such as breathing and digestion. All activity, such as walking, talking, working, or playing baseball, uses up additional energy and calories. For example, one hour of average office work probably uses up only 10 to 15 calories, whereas moderate housework may require 70 calories per hour more than basal metabolism requirements. Brisk walking uses up about 110 calories per hour; driving a car uses up about 40. Strenuous exercise and hard physical labor may require more than 400 calories per hour.

In order to lose weight safely, a person must set up a sensible long-range diet plan that includes all the essential nutrients and minerals. A high-protein, low-carbohydrate, low-fat diet is generally recommended for safe, gradual weight loss. Carbohydrates should be chosen from the best nutritional sources, such as whole-grain products and fruits that contain essential nutrients. Fat intake should come primarily from sources of unsaturated fatty acids and from such animal fats as butter and whole milk, which are good sources of fat-soluble vitamins. Excess fat is hard to metabolize and can upset liver and kidney functions. In general, losing weight is a matter of consciously curbing the amount of food eaten, regulating the types of food eaten, and increasing daily activity.

NUTRIENTS THAT MAY BE BENEFICIAL IN TREATMENT OF OVERWEIGHT AND OBESITY

Body Member	Nutrients	Quantity*
	Vitamin B complex	
	Vitamin B_6	Up to 100 mg
	Vitamin B_{12}	
	Inositol	500 mg
	Vitamin C	Up to 1,000 mg
	Vitamin E	Up to 600 IU
	Vitamin F	
	Calcium	500 mg
	Lecithin	2 tsp
	Magnesium	500 mg
	Protein	

*See note, p. 169.

PARKINSON'S DISEASE

Parkinson's disease is a slowly progressive disease of the nervous system in which an essential type of nerve cell is destroyed. The cause of the disease is unknown, although it usually begins after age fifty.

Symptoms of Parkinson's disease include muscular rigidity and cramping, involuntary tremors that include a characteristic pill-rolling movement of the thumb and forefinger as they rub against each other, impaired speech, a staring facial expression, drooling, and a short, shuffling gait. Despite these symptoms, sensation and mental activity are not impaired. There is often a loss of appetite and some weight loss, giving rise to the possibility of malnutrition developing. Chronic constipation may complicate the condition.

There is no cure for the disease, although drugs may be used to alleviate the symptoms. Modification of the diet and treatment of the constipation may also be helpful. Frequent small meals will increase the patient's nutrient and caloric levels, thus preventing malnutrition. The vitamin B complex is necessary for the health of the nerves; the person with Parkinson's disease should include adequate amounts of these vitamins in his or her diet. A marked increase in fluid intake is also necessary because the normal secretions of the intestines may be lessened by some of the prescribed drugs. High-residue food will assist in alleviating constipation.

NUTRIENTS THAT MAY BE BENEFICIAL IN TREATMENT OF PARKINSON'S DISEASE

Body Member	Nutrients	Quantity*
Brain/Nervous system	Vitamin B complex	
	Vitamin B_2	Up to 100 mg
	Vitamin B_6	10-200 mg
	Niacin	
	Vitamin C	Up to 100 mg
	Vitamin E	600 IU
	Calcium	
	Magnesium	500 mg
	Glutamic acid	
	Protein	

*See note, p. 169.

PELLAGRA

Pellagra is a disease caused by a deficiency of the B vitamins, particularly riboflavin, niacin, and thiamine. The disease occurs frequently in populations whose diets consist mainly of corn. Although the disease is seldom found in the United States, its rare occurrence affects persons with gastrointestinal disturbances or chronic alcoholism.

Symptoms of pellagra are diarrhea, loss of appetite and weight, reddened and swollen tongue, weakness, depression, and anxiety. Itchy dermatitis on the hands and neck is a prominent characteristic of the disease.

A diet that is adequate in the B vitamins and protein will prevent pellagra. A diet rich in the B vitamins niacin, thiamine, riboflavin, folic acid, and vitamin B_{12} will cure the disease.

NUTRIENTS THAT MAY BE BENEFICIAL IN TREATMENT OF PELLAGRA

Body Member	Nutrients	Quantity
Skin	Vitamin B complex	
	Vitamin B_1	
	Vitamin B_2	
	Vitamin B_{12}	
	Folic acid	
	Niacin	
	Protein	

PERNICIOUS ANEMIA

Pernicious anemia is a form of anemia resulting from a deficiency of vitamin B_{12}. It is a severe form of anemia in which there is a gradual reduction in the number of blood cells because the bone marrow fails to produce mature red blood cells. Pernicious anemia probably arises from an inheritable inability of the stomach to secrete a substance called the "intrinsic factor" which is necessary for the intestinal absorption of vitamin B_{12}.

Pernicious anemia occurs in both sexes. Its occurrence is rare in persons under the age of thirty, but susceptibility increases with age. Symptoms of pernicious anemia include weakness and gastrointestinal disturbances causing a sore tongue, slight yellowing of the skin, and tingling of extremities. In addition, disturbances of the nervous system, such as partial loss of coordination of the fingers, feet, and legs; some nerve deterioration; and disturbances of the digestive tract, such as diarrhea and loss of appetite, may occur.

Pernicious anemia may be fatal without treatment. Vitamin B_{12} injections together with a highly nutritious diet supplemented with large amounts of desiccated liver are the recommended treatment. Intake of the entire vitamin B complex will help maintain the health of the

nervous system, although folic acid should not be taken in amounts exceeding 0.1 milligram daily. Folic acid has the effect of concealing the symptoms of pernicious anemia, allowing the unseen destruction of the nervous system to continue until irreparable damage is done. A diet rich in protein, calcium, vitamin C, vitamin E, and iron is recommended.

NUTRIENTS THAT MAY BE BENEFICIAL IN TREATMENT OF PERNICIOUS ANEMIA

Body Member	Nutrients	Quantity*
Blood/ Circulatory system	Vitamin B complex	
	Vitamin B_6	50-100 mcg
	Vitamin B_{12}	50-100 mcg in injections
	Folic acid	
	Vitamin C	
	Vitamin E	
	Calcium	
	Cobalt	
	Protein	

*See note, p. 169.

PHLEBITIS

Phlebitis, the inflammation of a vein wall, is usually found in the legs and can be a complication of varicose veins. Symptoms of phlebitis include reddening and cordlike swelling of the vein, increased pulse rate, slight fever, and pain accompanying movement of the afflicted area.

A complication that may occur in individuals with phlebitis is thrombophlebitis, the formation of a clot in the inflamed vein. If this clot should break loose from the vein wall and lodge in a blood vessel that supplies some vital area with blood, serious and possibly fatal damage may occur. In some cases, the use of oral contraceptives has been related to the occurrence of thrombophlebitis.

Factors that seem to encourage the onset of the phlebitis are operations, especially in the lower abdomen, childbirth, and infections resulting from injuries to veins. Phlebitis can be prevented by the treatment of varicose veins so that inflammation does not set in. Infections in the legs or feet, especially fungus infections of the toes, should be given immediate attention as a safeguard against phlebitis. Regular exercise is a further preventive measure.

Supplementing the diet with niacin, part of the vitamin B complex, may be useful to help prevent clot formation.[29] Vitamin C can help strengthen the blood vessel walls. Some research indicates that vitamin E may dilate blood vessels, thus discouraging the formation of varicose veins and phlebitis.

NUTRIENTS THAT MAY BE BENEFICIAL IN TREATMENT OF PHLEBITIS

Body Member	Nutrients	Quantity*
Blood/Circulatory system/Legs	Vitamin B complex	
	Niacin	
	Pantothenic acid	100 mg
	Vitamin C	5-25 g
	Vitamin E	200-600 IU

*See note, p. 169.

PNEUMONIA

Pneumonia is an ailment in which the tiny air sacs in the lungs become inflamed and filled with mucous and pus. The primary causes of pneumonia are bacteria, viruses, chemical irritants, and allergies. Factors that contribute to the onset of pneumonia are colds, alcoholism, malnutrition, and foreign matter in the respiratory passages. Symptoms of the disease vary from mild to severe, but they usually include sharp pains in the chest, fever and chills, fatigue, rapid respiration, and cough.

Vitamin A is necessary for maintaining the health of the lining of the respiratory passages. A deficiency of the vitamin increases susceptibility to respiratory infections, which in turn can lead to pneumonia. Since protein loss accompanies high fever and because protein is necessary for the repair of body tissue, its intake should be increased during pneumonia. Water and fluid intake should be increased to prevent dehydration that can result from fever and perspiration. Vitamin C intake is required to fight infection. Because deficiency of the vitamin B complex usually occurs with pneumonia, an increased intake is necessary. Some research shows a correlation between vitamin E deficiency and lung disease.[30]

[29]Carlton Fredericks, *Eating Right for You* (New York: Grosset & Dunlap, 1972), p. 262.

[30]Martin Ebon, *The Truth about Vitamin E* (New York: Bantam Books, 1972), p. 34.

NUTRIENTS THAT MAY BE BENEFICIAL IN TREATMENT OF PNEUMONIA

Body Member	Nutrients	Quantity*
Lungs/ Respiratory system	Vitamin A	
	Vitamin B complex	
	Vitamin C	500 mg every 90 minutes
	Vitamin D	
	Vitamin E	
	Bioflavonoids	
	Protein	

*See note, p. 169.

POLIO

Polio is a virus infection of the spinal cord which destroys the nerves controlling muscular movement, resulting in paralysis of certain muscles. There are two stages of this disease: the infectious stage, when the virus is active, and the noninfectious, or recovery, stage. Symptoms of the infectious stage include fever, nausea, diarrhea, headache, and irritability.

During the infectious stage, the diet of the polio patient should be high in protein and potassium to replace that which is lost because of the rapid tissue destruction. Caloric intake should also be increased because of the increased energy expenditure during fever, and additional B vitamins are necessary to help metabolize the additional calories. Fever creates the need for additional sodium because of the loss that occurs with perspiration. Fluid intake should also be increased during fever to compensate for loss and to dilute the toxic substances produced by the virus. Fever and the accompanying increase in metabolism also increase the need for vitamins A and C, and attention should be paid to their intake. The intake of calcium and phosphorus should be lowered to reduce the risk of kidney or gallstone formation during prolonged periods of immobilization or bed rest.

NUTRIENTS THAT MAY BE BENEFICIAL IN TREATMENT OF POLIO

Body Member	Nutrients	Quantity
Brain/Nervous system	Vitamin A	
	Vitamin B complex	
	Vitamin C	

Body Member	Nutrients	Quantity
	Magnesium	
	Potassium	
	Sodium	
	Protein	

Body Member	Nutrients	Quantity
	Protein	
	Water	

PROSTATITIS

Prostatitis is the inflammation of the prostate, a male sex gland. The usual cause of prostatitis in young men is a bacterial infection from another area of the body which has invaded the prostate. Prostatic enlargement, which is usually found in older males, is often due to gradual enlargement over a period of several years.

Symptoms of acute prostatitis are pain between the scrotum and rectum, fever, frequent urination accompanied by a burning sensation, and blood or pus in the urine. Symptoms of long-term prostatitis are frequent and burning urination, lower back pain, and premature ejaculation, or loss of potency. As prostatitis becomes more advanced, urination becomes increasingly difficult.

Treatment for prostatitis involves increasing the fluid intake to meet the increased needs during infection and to stimulate urine flow, thus preventing retention of urine. Urinary retention can result in cystitis and possibly in a kidney infection. Increased protein and calories are needed during fever and infection, to replace lost body tissues and energy. A well-balanced diet rich in vitamin A, the B complex, and vitamin C is also important during fever and infection. Some sources advocate the avoidance of alcoholic beverages, spicy foods, and exposure to very cold weather if prostatitis is present.[31]

NUTRIENTS THAT MAY BE BENEFICIAL IN TREATMENT OF PROSTATITIS

Body Member	Nutrients	Quantity*
Gland, prostate	Vitamin A	
	Vitamin B complex	
	Vitamin B_6	
	Vitamin C	100-5,000 mg
	Vitamin E	600 IU
	Vitamin F	Six capsules
	Zinc	

*See note, p. 169.

PSORIASIS

Psoriasis, a recurring disease, is characterized by eruptions on the skin of red circular patches of all sizes covered with dry, silvery scales. The patches enlarge slowly, forming more extensive patches. Psoriasis appears mainly on the legs, arms, scalp, ears, and lower back. The cause is unknown, although its occurrence correlates highly with heredity.

Exposure to sunlight or ultraviolet light reduces the scaling and redness of psoriasis. An increased intake of animal protein can spread the disease, while a reduction in animal protein and fat intake can be useful for treating psoriasis. Vitamin A, the B complex, vitamin C, and vitamin D, all of which play a part in skin health, have been found to be useful in treating some cases of the disease. Some researchers have also found vitamin E to be effective in healing psoriasis.[32]

NUTRIENTS THAT MAY BE BENEFICIAL IN TREATMENT OF PSORIASIS

Body Member	Nutrients	Quantity*
Skin	Vitamin A	Up to 100,000 IU during first week; reduce to 25,000 IU for three months; repeat
	Vitamin B complex	
	Vitamin B_2	
	Vitamin B_6	100-200 mg
	Vitamin B_{12}	
	Folic acid	
	Pantothenic acid	
	Vitamin C	Up to 3,000 mg
	Vitamin D	
	Vitamin E	Up to 1,600 IU

*See note, p. 169.

[31]Robert E. Rothenberg, *Health in the Later Years*, rev. ed. (New York: Signet Books, 1972), p. 499.

[32]Rodale, *The Complete Book of Vitamins*, p. 389.

Body Member	Nutrients	Quantity
	Vitamin F	2 tbsp
	Bioflavonoids	
	Lecithin	3,500 mg
	Magnesium	
	Sulfur	Ointment
	Low fat	
	Low animal protein	

PYORRHEA (SORE GUMS)

Pyorrhea is an infectious disease of the gums and tooth sockets characterized by the formation of pus and usually by loosening of the teeth. Gum disorders such as puffiness, tenderness, soreness, and bleeding are often related to vitamin C and bioflavonoid deficiencies that cause increased capillary fragility. Sore gums may also indicate a niacin deficiency. One form of gum inflammation is gingivitis.

NUTRIENTS THAT MAY BE BENEFICIAL IN TREATMENT OF PYORRHEA

Body Member	Nutrients	Quantity*
Teeth/Gums	Vitamin A	
	Vitamin B complex	
	Vitamin B_6	
	Niacin	300 mg
	Vitamin C	300 mg
	Bioflavonoids	300 mg
	Calcium	

*See note, p. 169.

RHEUMATIC FEVER

Rheumatic fever is an infection, caused by streptococcal bacteria in the body, which occurs most frequently in children between the ages of four and eighteen. It affects one or more of the following body members: joints (arthritis), brain (chorea), heart (carius), tissues (nodules), and skin (erythema marginatum). Residual heart disease is a possible complication.

A salt-restricted diet containing all essential nutrients, together with a planned exercise program to relieve joint pain is recommended. Bioflavonoids have been found valuable for treating and preventing rheumatic fever.

NUTRIENTS THAT MAY BE BENEFICIAL IN TREATMENT OF RHEUMATIC FEVER

Body Member	Nutrients	Quantity*
General	Vitamin A	
	Pangamic acid	
	Vitamin C	1-10 g
	Vitamin D	
	Vitamin E	
	Bioflavonoids	

*See note, p. 169.

RHEUMATISM

Rheumatism is a general term referring to acute and chronic conditions characterized by stiffness of muscles and pain in the joints. Rheumatism includes such conditions as arthritis and bursitis, as well as other diseases.

NUTRIENTS THAT MAY BE BENEFICIAL IN TREATMENT OF RHEUMATISM

Body Member	Nutrients	Quantity
Muscles/Joints	Vitamin B_6	
	Pangamic acid	
	Vitamin C	
	Vitamin E	
	Bioflavonoids	
	Calcium	
	Phosphorus	
	Potassium	
	Protein	

RICKETS AND OSTEOMALACIA

Rickets is primarily a childhood disease of malnutrition in which there is a deficiency of vitamin D, calcium, and/or phosphorus. The chief symptom of rickets is an inability of the bones to retain calcium. This causes them to become soft, which results in deformities when the bones are called upon to support weight that they are too weak to support. Such deformities include bowlegs, knock-knees, protruding breast bone, narrowed rib cage, and bony beads along the ribs. Other symptoms of rickets include tetany and easily decaying teeth. However, weight gain and growth are generally normal in children with rickets.

The adult form of rickets is known as osteomalacia. It is most likely to occur at times of bodily stress such as pregnancy or during breast-feeding. Its causes may be a kidney defect or disease, a deficiency of calcium or phosphorus, or an inability to use vitamin D. In addition to the symptoms of rickets, aching of joints and generalized weakness occur. Vitamin D, calcium, and phosphorus work together to form strong bones; if one of these nutrients is missing, the result is rickets or osteomalacia. Vitamin D is needed for proper absorption and use of calcium and phosphorus, which hardens the bones. A deficiency of vitamin C can make the bones less able to retain calcium and phosphorus. Therefore the diet must be adequate in vitamin C, calcium, and phosphorus.

NUTRIENTS THAT MAY BE BENEFICIAL IN TREATMENT OF RICKETS AND OSTEOMALACIA

Body Member	Nutrients	Quantity
Bones	Vitamin A	
	Vitamin C	
	Vitamin D	
	Calcium	
	Magnesium	
	Phosphorus	

RHINITIS

Rhinitis is the inflammation of the nasal mucosa causing nasal congestion with increased secretion of mucus.

No specific treatment is known; general measures include rest, adequate fluid intake, and a well-balanced diet. Vitamin A has been used successfully in the treatment of rhinitis. Sulfonamides and antibiotics are of no value and should not be administered.

NUTRIENTS THAT MAY BE BENEFICIAL IN TREATMENT OF RHINITIS

Body Member	Nutrients	Quantity
Mucous membrane	Vitamin A	
	Protein	

SCIATICA

Sciatica refers to severely painful spasms along the sciatic nerve of the leg. This nerve runs from the back of the thigh, down the inside of the leg, to the ankle. Among the possible causes of sciatica are trauma or inflammation of the nerve itself, sprained joints in the lower back, rupture of a disk between the spinal bones, or neuritis.

Treatment for sciatica includes rest and hot, wet applications to the affected leg for the relief of pain and inflammation. The vitamin B complex is essential for the health of nerve tissue.

NUTRIENTS THAT MAY BE BENEFICIAL IN TREATMENT OF SCIATICA

Body Member	Nutrients	Quantity*
Leg/Nervous system	Vitamin B complex	
	Vitamin B_1	25 mg/cc (injections)
	Vitamin D	
	Vitamin E	

*See note, p. 169.

SCURVY

Scurvy is a malnutrition disease caused by a diet that is deficient in vitamin C. Symptoms of adult scurvy include swelling and bleeding of the gums, tenderness of joints and muscles, rough, dry, discolored skin, poor healing of wounds, and increased susceptibility to bruising and infection. Because vitamin C facilitates the absorption of iron, scurvy may be complicated by anemia.

An infant with scurvy experiences joint pain that causes him to assume a position called the "scrobutic pose" in which he is comfortable only when lying on his back with his knees partially bent and his thighs turned outward. The vitamin C deficiency makes the infant's bones less capable of retaining calcium and phosphorus, causing them to become weak and eventually brittle.

Scurvy responds dramatically, usually in two or three days' time, to the daily administration of 100 to 200 milligrams of vitamin C. In treating complications such as anemia and bone changes, a well-balanced diet high in protein and iron is also necessary to promote tissue repair.

NUTRIENTS THAT MAY BE BENEFICIAL IN TREATMENT OF SCURVY

Body Member	Nutrients	Quantity*
General	Vitamin A	
	Folic acid	
	Vitamin C	300-500 mg
	Bioflavonoids	
	Iron	
	Protein	

*See note, p. 169.

SENILITY

In many cases, as age advances, the blood vessels become narrow and reduce the supply of available oxygen to the brain tissues. The result is confusion, disorientation, and loss of memory. A New England hospital successfully treated patients with narrowed blood vessels by administration of niacin in combination with a high-potency multivitamin supplement. The doctors state that the positive results are due to the fact that niacin has a vasodilatory (opening of the blood vessels) effect on the system. A report in the *Journal of the American Geriatrics Society* (June 1971) stated that nutritional deficiencies were being recognized with increasing frequency in the practice of geriatric medicine. Heavy emphasis is placed on adequate intake of the B vitamins and vitamin C in addition to a change in dietary habits.

NUTRIENTS THAT MAY BE BENEFICIAL IN TREATMENT OF SENILITY

Body Member	Nutrients	Quantity
General	Vitamin B complex	
	Vitamin B_1	
	Vitamin B_{12}	
	Vitamin C	
	Vitamin E	
	Choline	
	Folic acid	
	Niacin	

SHINGLES (HERPES ZOSTER)

Shingles (herpes zoster) is an infection caused by a virus of the nerve endings in the skin. The disease is charac-terized by blister and crust formation and severe pain along the involved nerve which may last for several weeks. The infection commonly occurs on the chest or abdomen, although it may occur on the face around the eyes.

The B vitamins are necessary for the proper functioning of the nerves. Intramuscular injections of thiamine hydrochloride and vitamin B_{12} are sometimes used in the treatment of herpes zoster. Vitamins A and C help promote healing of the skin lesions characteristic of the disease.

NUTRIENTS THAT MAY BE BENEFICIAL IN TREATMENT OF SHINGLES

Body Member	Nutrients	Quantity*
Skin	Vitamin A	
	Vitamin B complex	
	Vitamin B_1	200-300 mg
	Vitamin B_6	
	Vitamin B_{12}	
	Vitamin C	
	Vitamin D	

*See note, p. 169.

SINUSITIS

Sinusitis is the inflammation of one or more of the sinus cavities, or passages. Sinusitis usually occurs in the nasal sinuses, which are located in the bones surrounding the eyes and nose. Symptoms of the inflammation include nasal congestion and discharge, fatigue, headache, earache, pain around the eyes, mild fever, cough, and an increased susceptibility to infection.

Sinusitis may be the result of a cold, sore throat, tonsilitis, or poor mouth hygiene. Recent studies indicate that a deficiency of vitamin A, which helps maintain the health of the mucous membrane of the nose and throat, may cause the condition. Smoking, damp weather, or the ingestion of spicy foods or alcohol may aggravate sinusitis.

Adequate intake of vitamin A may be useful in the treatment of sinusitis, especially if a deficiency exists. Vitamin C can help fight the infections that may occur with this condition, and protein will help restore damaged sinus tissues.

NUTRIENTS THAT MAY BE BENEFICIAL IN TREATMENT OF SINUSITIS

Body Member	Nutrients	Quantity
Sinuses	Vitamin A	
	Vitamin C	
	Vitamin E	
	Protein	

STOMACH ULCER (PEPTIC)

There are several conflicting views on dietary treatment for ulcer patients. Many physicians initially put patients with severe ulcers on a diet of milk and cream, given in hourly feedings, to reduce the acidity of the gastric juices. Other sources state that frequent small feedings of protein snacks or skim milk should be used but that cream should be avoided, particularly in patients with atherosclerosis or obesity. Further sources indicate that the patient himself should decide which foods seem to agree best with him.

Vitamin A is important for the ulcer patient for maintenance of the tissue that lines the stomach. Fruits and vegetables, sources of vitamins and minerals, should be served in puree form to eliminate hard-to-digest fiber from the diet. Citrus fruit juices, although acidic, are high in vitamin C content and may be used if they are diluted. Eggs and lean meats are good sources of iron, which the ulcer patient requires. A vitamin B complex deficiency may occur with peptic ulcers, and supplementation may therefore be necessary.

NUTRIENTS THAT MAY BE BENEFICIAL IN TREATMENT OF STOMACH ULCER (PEPTIC)

Body Member	Nutrients	Quantity*
Stomach	Vitamin A	25,000-50,000IU
	Vitamin B complex	
	Vitamin B_2	5 mg three times daily
	Vitamin B_{12}	
	Vitamin C	
	Vitamin E	600-1,200 IU
	Calcium	
	Iron	
	Protein	

*See note, p. 169.

STRESS

Stress is any physical or emotional strain on the body or mind. Physical stress occurs when an external or natural change or force acts upon the body. Extreme heat or cold, overwork, injuries, malnutrition, and exposure to drugs and poisons are example of physical stress. Emotional stress may be a result of fear, hate, love, anger, tension, grief, joy, frustration, and/or anxiety. Physical and emotional stress can overlap, as in special body conditions such as pregnancy, adolescence, and aging. During these times, body metabolism is increased or lowered, changing the body's physical functions, which, in turn, affect the person's mental and emotional outlook on life. A certain amount of stress is useful as a motivating factor, but when it occurs in excess or is of the wrong kind, the effect can be detrimental.

The metabolic response of the body to either physical or emotional stress is to produce more adrenal hormones. These adrenal hormones are secreted by glands that lie above the kidneys. When released into the blood, these hormones prepare the body for action by increasing blood pressure and heartbeat and by making extra energy available. These body responses are useful when physical action is needed, but in our modern civilization there is usually little physical outlet for them, and the body must react to stress by channeling the body's responses inward to one of the organ systems, such as the digestive, circulatory, or nervous system. When this happens, the system reacts adversely, and conditions such as ulcers, hypertension, backache, atherosclerosis, allergic reactions, asthma, fatigue, and insomnia often develop.

Anxiety, a fearful or distressful feeling, is responsible for the stress of many individuals. Anything that threatens a person's body, job, loved ones, or values may cause anxiety. If the person cannot cope with the situation, stress on the body is increased, resulting in many of the disorders associated with stress. Change in attitude or life-style may be necessary to eliminate the needless strain and allow the body to resume normal functioning.

The increase in the production of adrenal hormones which occurs with stress increases the metabolism of protein, fats, and carbohydrates, producing instant energy for the body to use. As a result of this increased metabolism, there is also an increased excretion of protein, potassium, and phosphorus and a decreased storage of calcium. Many of the disorders related to stress are not a direct result of the stress itself but a result of nutrient deficiencies caused by increased metabolic rate during periods of stress. For example, vitamin C is utilized by the adrenal gland during stressful conditions, and any stress that is sufficiently severe or prolonged will cause a depletion of vitamin C in the tissues.

People experiencing stress need to maintain a nutritious, well-balanced diet with special emphasis on replacing the nutrients that may be depleted during stress.

NUTRIENTS THAT MAY BE BENEFICIAL IN TREATMENT OF STRESS

Body Member	Nutrients	Quantity*
General	Vitamin A	
	Vitamin B complex	
	Vitamin B_1	
	Vitamin B_2	2 mg every three hours
	Vitamin B_6	2 mg every three hours
	Vitamin B_{12}	
	Folic acid	
	Niacin	
	Pantothenic acid	100 mg
	Vitamin C	500 mg every three hours
	Vitamin D	
	Vitamin E	
	Calcium	
	Phosphorus	
	Potassium	
	Carbohydrate	
	Fat	
	Protein	

*See note, p. 169.

SUNBURN

Sunburn is caused by excessive exposure to ultraviolet rays, which actually burn up surface skin and later the lower cells.

The amount of exposure to ultraviolet rays which causes burning depends basically on four things: the individual, place, time, and atmospheric conditions.

Caution should be used in exposing oneself to the sun for extended periods of time between 10:00 A.M. and 2:00 P.M., when most of the ultraviolet rays are present.

Reflections from water, metal, sand, or snow may double the amount of rays one absorbs.

Burns may be classified in three degrees. First-degree sunburn causes reddening of the skin and possibly slight fever. Second-degree sunburn causes reddening of the skin accompanied by water blisters. Third-degree sunburn causes lower cell damage and the release of fluid resulting in eruptions and breaks in the skin where bacteria and infection can enter.

Cold water soaking or cold water compresses, together with additional intake of vitamins A, C, and E, are recommended for treatment of sunburn.

NUTRIENTS THAT MAY BE BENEFICIAL IN TREATMENT OF SUNBURN

Body Member	Nutrients	Quantity*
Skin	PABA	1,000 mg plus ointment
	Vitamin E	
	Calcium	

*See note, p. 169.

SWOLLEN GLANDS

Swollen glands is a term commonly used to describe enlargement of the lymph nodes, or glands of the neck, on both sides of the throat. Technically, however, it can also describe enlargement of any of the lymph glands, such as those located in the armpit or groin. The enlargement of lymph glands is usually a signal of an infection in the area because the lymph glands function to filter out microscopic material, such as bacteria, in order to prevent the spread of infection.

Symptoms include enlarged or swollen glands that may be hard or soft. These symptoms may be accompanied by heat, tenderness, and reddening of the overlying skin, and fever.

Swollen glands may simply indicate a localized infection or may be a symptom of a more serious disease. Swollen gland conditions may occur with such disorders as mononucleosis, measles, chicken pox, leukemia, cancer, tuberculosis, and syphilis.

Treatment includes maintaining a well-balanced diet and fighting the particular infection that is causing the lymph node enlargement. In general, infection requires an increased intake of protein, fluids, and calories. If the infection is accompanied by fever, the diet should be rich in vitamins A and C and the B complex.

NUTRIENTS THAT MAY BE BENEFICIAL IN TREATMENT OF SWOLLEN GLANDS

Body Member	Nutrients	Quantity
Glands/Lymph nodes	Vitamin A	
	Vitamin B complex	
	Vitamin C	
	Protein	
	Water	

TONSILITIS

Tonsilitis is an inflammation of the tonsils, which are glands of lymph tissue located on either side of the entrance to the throat. Tonsilitis may be caused by virus infections when the body's resistance is lowered or by an improper diet that is high in carbohydrates and low in protein and other nutrients.

Symptoms of tonsilitis include pain, redness and swelling in the back of the mouth, difficulty in swallowing, hoarseness, and coughing. Headache, earache, fever and chills, nausea and vomiting, nasal obstruction and discharge, and enlarged lymph nodes throughout the body are additional symptoms of tonsilitis.

In cases of severe tonsil infection, surgical removal may be necessary. The most effective means of prevention for tonsilitis is maintaining a well-balanced diet that is adequate in protein, vitamins, and minerals. The regular intake of vitamin C may help prevent tonsilitis.[33]

NUTRIENTS THAT MAY BE BENEFICIAL IN TREATMENT OF TONSILITIS

Body Member	Nutrients	Quantity
Glands/Tonsil	Folic acid	
	Vitamin C	
	Protein	

TOOTH AND GUM DISORDERS

Cavities (dental caries) are the primary dental problem in the United States. Most cavities are caused by persistent eating of refined sugars and starches, which mix with saliva to form an acid that erodes tooth enamel. One can control cavities by avoiding refined carbohydrate

[33]Linus Pauling, *Vitamin C and the Common Cold* (New York: Bantam Books, 1970), p. 29.

foods, eating a nutritionally balanced diet, and properly cleansing the mouth, including brushing both teeth and gums and cleansing between the teeth with dental floss following meals and snacks.

Although cavities are the major dental disease, a condition known as periodontitis accounts for the loss of more teeth than do cavities. Periodontitis, an inflammation of the gums and the bones that surround and support the teeth, can accompany mouth and upper respiratory infections, or it may be caused by poor fillings, poorly fitting dentures, improper cleansing of teeth and gums, or inadequate diet. Periodontitis begins as a condition known as gingivitis, in which the gums redden, swell, and tend to bleed. If not treated, gingivitis can lead to pyorrhea (see p. 160), characterized by further gum inflammation accompanied by a continuous discharge of pus, gum recession, and loosening of teeth.

Although all vitamins and minerals are essential for the proper formation and continued health of the teeth, an adequate vitamin C intake is especially helpful for the prevention of gingivitis and pyorrhea, while a deficiency of it causes teeth to loosen and break down. Vitamin A seems to control the development and general health of the gums; a lack of this vitamin often results in gum infection. Vitamin A is also necessary for the formation and maintenance of tooth development in children. Minerals important for healthy teeth are sodium, potassium, calcium, phosphorus, iron, and magnesium.

A varied diet of fresh fruits, green leafy vegetables, meat, and whole-grain bread will provide the teeth and gums with needed exercise and supply the body with vitamins and minerals essential for dental health.

NUTRIENTS THAT MAY BE BENEFICIAL IN TREATMENT OF TOOTH AND GUM DISORDERS

Body Member	Nutrients	Quantity*
Teeth/Gums	Vitamin A	
	Vitamin B$_6$	
	Niacin	
	Vitamin C	
	Vitamin D	
	Vitamin F	1 tbsp vegetable oil
	Bioflavonoids	
	Calcium	
	Copper	
	Fluorine	

*See note, p. 169.

Body Member	Nutrients	Quantity
	Iron	
	Magnesium	
	Manganese	
	Phosphorus	
	Potassium	
	Sodium	
	Zinc	
	Protein	

TUBERCULOSIS

Tuberculosis is a contagious disease caused by bacterial infection. A person normally has some defense against the bacteria, but when the body is weakened or rundown, its susceptibility to infection is increased. Tuberculosis usually affects the lungs, but it may also involve other organs and tissues.

Many tuberculosis patients may exhibit mild symptoms from which they recover completely. This usually means that the body has successfully controlled the bacteria. Mild symptoms of the disease include fatigue and appetite and weight loss. As the disease becomes more severe, symptoms include fever, increased perspiration, and rapid loss of weight and strength. Coughing up blood is often the first indication of a severe form of the disease.

A tuberculosis patient should be isolated in a hospital for treatment during the contagious state. Antibiotics, adequate rest, and proper diet comprise the most effective therapy for tuberculosis.

Because malnutrition makes an individual more susceptible to tuberculosis, a patient is often treated with a high-protein, low-carbohydrate diet. Supplementation with vitamin A is necessary because the patient is less able to convert carotene to vitamin A.[34] Vitamin C may also be deficient in the tuberculosis patient; thus additional intake may be necessary. Extra vitamin D is needed for the absorption of additional calcium, which the patient needs in order to form a case, or wall, around the invading bacteria. If the patient is losing blood, increased iron intake is required to rebuild the red blood cells. A diet high in protein and the necessary vitamins and minerals will help a person maintain his ideal weight and thus help prevent tuberculosis from recurring.

[34]J.I. Rodale, *The Health Seeker* (Emmaus, Pa.: Rodale Books, 1967), p. 857.

NUTRIENTS THAT MAY BE BENEFICIAL IN TREATMENT OF TUBERCULOSIS

Body Member	Nutrients	Quantity*
Lungs/Respiratory system	Vitamin A	10,000-40,000 IU
	Vitamin B_6	2 mg six times daily
	Vitamin B_{12}	50 mcg six times daily
	Niacin	
	Pantothenic acid	
	Vitamin C	500 mg six times daily
	Vitamin D	
	Calcium	
	Iron	
	Phosphorus	
	Protein	
	Low carbohydrate	

*See note, p. 169.

ULCER

An open sore (not wound) on the skin or mucous membrane is called an ulcer. Ulcerated sores often form pus and are characterized by the disintegration of tissue and resistance to healing.

NUTRIENTS THAT MAY BE BENEFICIAL IN TREATMENT OF ULCERS

Body Member	Nutrients	Quantity*
Skin	Vitamin A	100,000 IU for three months; then reduce to 25,000 IU
	Vitamin B complex	
	Vitamin B_2	400 mg
	Vitamin B_{12}	
	Folic acid	5 mg three times daily
	Vitamin C	Up to 3,000 mg
	Vitamin E	800 IU
	Vitamin K	

*See note, p. 169.

Body Member	Nutrients	Quantity
	Bioflavonoids	
	Iron	
	Protein	

UNDERWEIGHT

A person is underweight when he is 10 percent or more under the desired weight for his body size and build (see "Desirable Height and Weight Chart," p. 246). Underweight develops when more calories are utilized by the body than are consumed. Underweight without a lack of nutrients may or may not be serious, depending upon the degree of underweight. The thin person is probably less apt to suffer from heart diseases and certain other ailments and will live longer than a person who is overweight. Malnutrition occurs when an individual is deficient in the nutrients necessary for life. Individuals with this problem are very susceptible to infections, lack nutrient reserves for times of stress, and are easily fatigued. When underweight and malnutrition are severe, there is starvation, the body's stores of nutrients and fats are depleted, and muscle tissue is broken down to provide energy for bodily functions.

Symptoms that may accompany underweight are weakness, fatigue, sensitivity to cold, hunger, dizziness, and loss of ambition. Underweight may be due to poor eating habits, a nervous condition, overactivity, illness, or metabolic and heredity problems. Underweight can be corrected by removal of the underlying causes and improvement of the diet. The diet should be well-balanced and higher in calories. Extra protein is needed to rebuild tissues. Frequent smaller feedings may be of help in weight gain. Exercise is important during weight gain, so that muscles, rather than fat, are formed. For the same reason, weight should not be gained at the rate of more than a pound a week. Any vitamin deficiencyis should be corrected as quickly as possible (see "Nutrient Allowance Chart," p. 247).

NUTRIENTS THAT MAY BE BENEFICIAL IN TREATMENT OF UNDERWEIGHT

Body Member	Nutrients	Quantity
Body	Vitamin F	
	Protein	

VAGINITIS

Vaginitis is an inflammation of the vagina, usually caused by bacterial or yeast infection, excessive douching, vitamin B deficiency,[35] or intestinal worms. Symptoms of vaginitis include a burning or itching sensation and an abnormal vaginal discharge that is white or yellow. Vaginitis is common in pregnant or diabetic women and in women using antibiotics or oral contraceptives.

Adequate rest, a healthful diet, and meticulous personal hygiene with frequent bathing are important for the treatment of vaginitis. White cotton underwear is sometimes recommended because it allows for free circulation of air. Vaginal itching may be prevented by the intake of vitamin A and the B complex if a deficiency is present.

NUTRIENTS THAT MAY BE BENEFICIAL IN TREATMENT OF VAGINITIS

Body Member	Nutrients	Quantity*
Reproductive system	Vitamin A	50,000 IU
	Vitamin B complex	
	Vitamin B_2	6 mg
	Vitamin B_6	
	Vitamin D	
	Vitamin E	

*See note, p. 169.

VARICOSE VEINS

Varicose veins are veins that have become enlarged, twisted, and swollen. They may be located anywhere in the body, but they are most commonly found in the legs.

Factors that inhibit blood circulation, such as obesity, certain hereditary conditions, tight clothing, crossing of legs, and a sedentary occupation, can increase susceptibility to varicose veins. A pregnant woman or a woman who has had several pregnancies is usually more prone to varicose veins than are most other women because pregnancy causes increased pressure on the legs.

It is essential that individuals who must sit for extended periods of time receive adequate exercise. Ele-

[35]Davis, *Let's Get Well*, p. 308.

vating the legs while resting is another preventive measure.

Adequate amounts of the B vitamins and vitamin C are necessary in the diet for the maintenance of strong blood vessels. Some research has indicated that vitamin E can dilate blood vessels and improve circulation, thus perhaps reducing the susceptibility to varicose veins.[36]

NUTRIENTS THAT MAY BE BENEFICIAL IN TREATMENT OF VARICOSE VEINS

Body Member	Nutrients	Quantity*
Leg	Vitamin B complex	
	Vitamin C	Up to 3,000 mg
	Vitamin E	600-1,000 IU
	Bioflavonoids	300-500 mg
	Protein	

*See note, p. 169.

VENEREAL DISEASE

Venereal disease is usually acquired through intimate contact with the sexual organs of an afflicted individual. The most frequent vehicle of the disease is the act of sexual intercourse or intimacy associated with sexual intercourse. Gonorrhea and syphilis are the two most common types of venereal disease.

Gonorrhea is transmitted through sexual intimacy or from the mother to the newborn infant as it passes through an infected birth canal. Within 3 to 14 days after contact, males experience burning, pain, and discharge of pus upon urination. Complications of gonorrhea in males may include prostatitis and testes infection. Females may have increased urinary frequency and a yellowish discharge from the vagina, but there are usually no immediate symptoms until the infection has included all of the reproductive organs of the pelvic region. Complications of gonorrhea may result in sterility in both sexes.

Syphilis is also most commonly spread through sexual intimacy, but it may also be received through a break in the skin that has come in contact with a chancre, or open sore, fresh blood, semen, or a vaginal discharge from an infected individual. Syphilis can also be trans-

mitted from the mother to the fetus via the bloodstream during pregnancy.

There are three distinct stages of syphilis. First, a chancre appears 10 to 28 days after contact at the point where the infecting organism entered the body, but it disappears in 2 to 5 weeks. Other possible symptoms of this stage include fever, weight loss, and anemia.

Six weeks to six months after appearance of the chancre, the second stage begins. It is characterized by skin rashes, hair loss, warts near the mouth or anus, fever, headache, sore throat, and possibly bone pain. The next one to several years may be without symptoms.

During the third stage the disease is no longer contagious. In this stage the organisms settle in specific body organs and destroy them. Commonly, the circulatory system and nervous system are attacked, often resulting in death.

Treatment for venereal disease includes massive injections of antibiotics, usually penicillin, to rid the body of the venereal organism. Early treatment is essential to prevent complicating tissue damage. To prevent the spread of venereal disease, an afflicted person should abstain from sexual intercourse and intimacy until the disease has been cured. In addition to obtaining medical treatment, an afflicted person should maintain a well-balanced diet high in protein to help repair the tissue damage that has occurred.

NUTRIENTS THAT MAY BE BENEFICIAL IN TREATMENT OF VENEREAL DISEASE

Body Member	Nutrients	Quantity
General	Protein	

VISION AND FOCUS DISORDERS

There are several disorders of the eyes, which may be due to hereditary factors, nutrient deficiencies, strain, or natural aging processes. Symptoms that indicate visual disorders are squinting, blurred vision, inability to see near or far, sensitivity to light, and itching and burning of the eyes and lids.

Vitamin A is essential to the health of the eyes. A deficiency of vitamin A can result in various conditions of poor sight. A riboflavin deficiency can result in sensitive and easily fatigued eyes, blurred vision, itching, and bloodshot eyes.

[36]Rodale, *The Complete Book of Vitamins*, p. 352.

NUTRIENTS THAT MAY BE BENEFICIAL IN TREATMENT OF VISION AND FOCUS DISORDERS

Body Member	Nutrients	Quantity*
Eyes/General	Vitamin A	
	Vitamin B complex	
	Vitamin B$_2$	50 mg daily
	Vitamin C	500-1,500 mg
	Vitamin D	
	Vitamin E	200 IU

*See note below.

WORMS

There are several types of parasitic worms which can live in human intestines, the most common being pinworms, tapeworms, hookworms, and roundworms. Worms irritate the intestinal lining and therefore cause poor absorption of nutrients. Signs of worms often include diarrhea, hunger pains, appetite loss, weight loss, and anemia. Diagnosis can be made by examining the stools or, occasionally, by inducing the vomiting of worms. The extent of the intestinal damage is then determined by the type of worm, the size of the worm, and the number of worms present.

Pinworms are the most common parasitic worm in the United States. The chief symptom of this small, threadlike worm is rectal itching, especially at night. Pinworms are transmitted when eggs, which lodge under the fingernails when a person scratches, contaminate food. Personal hygiene is most important for the control of pinworms.

Tapeworms can be contracted from eating insufficiently cooked meats, especially beef, pork, and fish. The most common tapeworm in the United States, beef tapeworm, grows to a length of 15 to 20 feet in the intestines.

Hookworms are often found in the soil or sand in moderate climates. They can enter the body by boring holes in the skin of the bare feet or can enter by mouth if food contaminated by dirty hands is eaten.

Roundworms are most common in children. These worms can leave the intestines and settle in different areas of the body, causing diseases such as pneumonia, jaundice, or periodontitis.

When a person is afflicted with worms, the body's supply of all nutrients is depleted to the point that supplementation of all nutrients is necessary to restore normal health. Nutrients of special importance are vitamin A; the B complex, especially thiamine, riboflavin, B$_6$, B$_{12}$, and pantothenic acid; vitamins C, D, and K; and calcium, iron, and protein.

NUTRIENTS THAT MAY BE BENEFICIAL IN TREATMENT OF WORMS

Body Member	Nutrients	Quantity
Body/Intestine	Vitamin A	
	Vitamin B$_1$	
	Vitamin B$_2$	
	Vitamin B complex	
	Vitamin B$_6$	
	Vitamin B$_{12}$	
	Pantothenic acid	
	Vitamin D	
	Vitamin F	
	Vitamin K	
	Calcium	
	Iron	
	Potassium	
	Sulfur (ointment form)	
	Protein	

NOTE: Quantities shown are not prescriptive; some are extremely high and represent therapeutic test dosages. Individual needs and tolerances will vary according to body size, metabolism, age, diet, and ailment. Consult a physician who is familiar with nutritional therapy before taking large quantities.

NORMAL LIFE CYCLE

PREGNANCY

Pregnancy is a stressful condition involving numerous physical and mental changes in the mother's body as the fetus develops. The tissues in the breasts and uterus increase, the blood supply increases, there is a frequent urge to urinate, there is slight nausea in the morning or even later in the day, the menstrual period is absent, and the need for sleep and fluids is increased. Because of these changes, all nutritional needs of the mother increase in preparation for the newborn baby.

A woman who has maintained a nutritionally balanced diet throughout her life has the best possible chance of bearing a healthy child. However, during pregnancy, nutritional needs are increased, and the condition of the mother and her child could be greatly improved by dietary supplementation. All known nutrients must be supplied to the expectant mother.

Protein, calcium, and iron are especially important to the development of bones, soft tissues, and blood of the body. Protein of both animal origin (meat, eggs, cheese, milk, fish, etc.) and plant origin (whole-grain cereals, nuts, peas, beans, soybeans, lentils, etc.) should be included in the diet because the body can make the fullest use of these products in combination. Protein is also needed to provide for the 20 percent increase in blood volume during pregnancy. An adequate supply of vitamin D is needed to ensure proper absorption and utilization of calcium and phosphorus.

Additional iron is essential to prevent anemia in both mother and baby and to guard the mother against excessive blood loss during birth. Adequate iron also guards against miscarriage and fetal malformation.

Vitamin C, vitamin K, and the bioflavonoids are necessary to strengthen blood vessels and to prevent excessive bleeding. In late pregnancy and postdelivery, thiamine requirements are greatly increased. Vitamin E may prevent miscarriage and toxemia. Iodine deficiency during pregnancy may cause mental retardation.[37]

In addition, the pregnant woman should take special care to ensure adequate intake of the vitamin B complex, protein, and calcium, which help to normalize emotional states that occur frequently during pregnancy. The B-complex vitamins, found in brewer's yeast or wheat germ, will also help relieve fatigue, insomnia, and nervous tension. Together with calcium, found in milk or bone meal, B vitamins may also help to relieve leg, back, and joint pains often associated with pregnancy. Nausea and morning sickness due to nervous conditions will probably respond to additional intake of B vitamins

[37] Adelle Davis, *Let's Have Healthy Children.* (New York: Harcourt, Brace and World, 1959), p. 47.

and vitamins C and K. The pregnant woman should not take baking soda or other common antacids for indigestion or heartburn because they contain sodium, which will increase fluid retention. Vitamin B_6 has been found to be effective in regulating fluid retention associated with the development of toxemia. The B-complex vitamins and enzyme supplements may relieve heartburn and digestive upsets.

Birth defects can be a disease of heredity, but they are just as likely to result from fetus-damaging drugs; environmental pollutants; viral, parasitic, or bacterial infections; and poor nutrition. Poor diets lacking in any vitamin, mineral, or enzyme for the mother will deprive the fetus of necessary building materials. There is growing evidence that the fetus must compete with the mother's body for vital nutrients. Any shortage can result in a stillbirth; a premature infant of low birth weight; a baby with brain damage, including impaired intelligence and psychological disturbances; or a baby with weak immunity to infections. Ingestion by the mother of nicotine, alcohol, chemical food additives, and drugs can interfere with the fetal enzyme system and growth factors. Any interference with the B-complex metabolism in the fetus will produce deformities or abnormalities.

A weight gain of 20 to 25 pounds is desirable and in most cases is in keeping with good health.

The end results of proper prenatal nutrition are a more comfortable pregnancy, an easier delivery, a healthier baby, and a greater chance of successfully nursing the baby.

LACTATION

Lactation is the secretion and yielding of milk by the mammary gland. Preparation for lactation begins during early pregnancy, when the increased production of the hormones estrogen and progesterone leads to the storage of maternal energy in the form of fat. After the baby is born, changes occur in the ductless glandular system of the mother's body which initiate the secretion of milk.

Human breast milk has a remarkably constant composition. It is the most nearly perfect food, but it is low in certain essential nutrients such as vitamin C, vitamin D, and iron. Efforts should be made to see that these nutrients are included in the diet, either through fortified formulas or through supplements.

Poor nutrition of a lactating mother tends to reduce the quantity rather than the quality of breast milk. The body maintains the quality of milk by drawing upon the mother's own store of nutrients.   Therefore, a lactating mother, besides her normal requirements, needs extra nutrients to replace both those lost at delivery through bleeding and those she provides in the milk for her infant.

The requirements for thiamine, riboflavin, and nicotinic acid are related to the caloric intake.   Since the lactating mother needs extra calories to meet the physiological cost of milk production, her needs for these vitamins become higher than at normal times. The best sources of these vitamins are whole-grain cereals, brewer's yeast, milk, meat, and eggs.

Since a lactating mother needs more calcium and vitamin D is necessary for the absorption of calcium, it is desirable that her diet contain an adequate supply of vitamin D.   The best sources of vitamin D are fish-liver oils, butter, and milk.   Adequate supply of iron is also needed.

INFANCY AND CHILDHOOD

The period of life from birth to maturity is one of intense growth and development.   Heredity, environment, and nutrition are the major determinants of a child's growth potential.   Nutrition, however, is the single most important factor in determining the healthy growth and development of a child.

Foods supply the chemicals necessary for forming all tissues, especially muscles, bones, blood, and teeth, and also for repairing tissues.   Children need extra calories to provide energy for this growth and for the increased activity and metabolic rate in youth.   Children require the same nutrients as adults for good nutrition, however, often in greater proportions.   See the "Nutrient Allowance Chart" on p. 247 for children's Recommended Dietary Allowances.

ADOLESCENCE

Adolescence is a period when profound physiological and emotional changes occur within a young person, signifying the onset of puberty and continuing until maturation.

The physical development and rapid growth associated with adolescence make this a time when good nutrition is vitally important for the building of a strong, healthy body.   The need for calories, protein, and other body-building elements increases during this period.   Adolescents need protein, calcium, phosphorus, and vitamin D for proper bone formation.   Protein is especially important for the development of new tissues and contains the amino acids vital for growth.

MENSTRUATION

Menstruation is the cyclical process that continuously prepares the uterus for pregnancy; it starts at puberty and continues through menopause.   Menstruation occurs on an average of every 28 days except during pregnancy and lactation.   It is characterized by a passing of the blood-rich uterine lining lasting approximately four or five days.   However, individuals may differ in time between periods and duration of menstrual flow.

Women whose general health and resistance are good are apt to have less premenstrual tension or cramping than those women suffering from poor nutrition and lack of physical exercise.   Symptoms of premenstrual tension include abdominal bloating, weight gain, breast tenderness, irritability, headache, depression, and, possibly, edema of the legs.   Edema may be helped by limiting the salt and fluid intake a short time before the onset of the menstrual period.   Vitamin A may relieve general symptoms associated with premenstrual tension.

The loss of blood which occurs during menstruation causes a loss of iron.   The diet should be adequate in iron and iodine to replace loss plus vitamin C to aid in iron absorption.   Cramping may be relieved with additional intake of calcium and niacin.   The vitamin B complex, especially vitamin B_6 and folic acid, may relieve some of the tension associated with menstruation.

Unusually frequent, heavy, or scanty periods of menstrual flow may warrant concern.   Medical attention should be sought to determine the cause.

SEX

Many people are not aware of the important role proper nutrition plays in improving sexual vitality.   Adequate nourishment is needed to stimulate the hormonal production of the endocrine glands; this increased hormone secretion results in increased sexual vigor.

Endocrine glands, such as thyroid, pituitary, testes, and ovaries, can be specifically nourished by certain nutrients. For example, the B-complex vitamins enter into the cellular and tissue construction of the thyroid gland and act as "energizers" to increase the hormonal flow. An excellent way of obtaining B factors is mixing two tablespoons of brewer's yeast and two tablespoons of wheat germ with vegetable juice and drinking it with the evening meal. This combination is assimilated by the body in about an hour.

An iodine-deficient thryoid gland may cause a decreased interest in sex, because of a decreased rate of hormone production.[38] One teaspoon of sea salt or kelp may increase the thyroid's metabolism and promote a flow of hormones. In addition, the amino acid tyrosine, from which the thyroid hormone thyroxine is made, helps activate sluggish thyroids. The combination of one tablespoon each of brewer's yeast, wheat germ, and blackstrap molasses mixed with fruit juices and taken three times daily may help the work of tyrosine.

The pituitary gland is responsible for the functioning of the male and female sex hormones, thus providing sex drive for body and mind. The B-complex vitamins are recommended to ensure against impotence and premature menopause.[39]

Zinc and vitamin E are also important in maintaining sexual powers. Zinc deficiency may cause retarded genital development (see "Zinc," p. 83). This mineral is found in highly concentrated form throughout the entire male reproductive system. Vitamin E is often referred to as the "sex vitamin." It may help restore the sexual organs, help stimulate the production of new sperm, and help rejuvenate the sex glands.

In the Italian medical journal *Rivista di Ostetrica e Genecologia* (May 1954), Dr. A. Narpozzi reported results of studies he conducted on the effects of certain vitamins on men who had varying levels of sperm deficiencies, some of which may lead to sterility. He found that vitamin A along with vitamin E restored sperm levels to normal. Similar studies have confirmed these findings. Dr. Thomas Moore of the Dunn Nutritional Laboratory in Cambridge, England, also discovered through experimentation with animals that female reproductive organs need vitamin A to ensure conception and to lessen the possibility of abortion.[40]

MENOPAUSE

Menopause is the period in a woman's life marked by glandular changes that denote the end of her menstrual cycle and reproductive years. Menopause usually results from a decreased production of the female sex hormones when a woman is between the ages of forty-two and fifty-two.

Poor diet, lack of exercise, and emotional stress may exaggerate the symptoms and discomfort of menopause. Some women experience severe nervous symptoms and become irritable, over excitable, or depressed. They may have headaches, abdominal pains, rushes of blood to the head and upper body known as "hot flashes," backaches, leg cramps, nosebleeds, frequent bruises, varicose veins, and even ulcers. Some women find themselves extremely fatigued or experiencing insomnia.

Usually within a period of months or a year or two, the body readjusts and the symptoms disappear. Although the menstrual periods cease, a woman's normal sexual needs remain after menopause, and she does not need to experience rapid aging.

Vitamin E (up to 1,200 IU) is especially important during menopause. The B complex, especially pantothenic acid and PABA, relieve nervous irritability. Vitamin C together with bioflavonoids increases capillary strength. The calcium-phosphorus balance should be carefully maintained during the mature years, and an increase in protein with reduction of carbohydrates is generally recommended. Adequate intake of vitamin D, iron, and magnesium is also important.

AGING

Aging refers to the changes of the body that are related to the passage of time and is characterized by a deterioration of organs in the body and a general lowering of the body's ability to deal with externally produced stress. Aging may begin in persons twenty years old, as soon as growth hormones present during the teen-age years are

[38]Carlson Wade, "How Nutrition Can Boost Your Sex Powers," *Bestways*, September 1974, p. 25.
[39]Wade, "How Nutrition Can Boost Your Sex Powers," p. 25.
[40]Rodale, *The Complete Book of Vitamins*, p. 143.

no longer being produced. These processes of aging are accelerated by illness or abuse of the body.

It is important to remember that a diet that may be sufficient for a young person may be deficient for an older person because the older person cannot utilize nutrients in the same capacity as the young person. Many of the diseases associated with aging may be prevented or retarded through proper nutrition, adequate rest, and exercise. The process of aging increases the need for vitamins and minerals because nutrients are not as well absorbed by the aging digestive organs.

Ailments often associated with aging include impaired mobility of joints, loss of coordination and sense of balance, lessened muscle tone, and increased mental instability. They may be due to a deficiency of the vitamin B complex, especially vitamin B_{12} and niacin. A B_{12} deficiency may also be related to the development of abnormal fatigue often found among older persons.

Vitamin C decreases the probability of blood vessel ruptures and strokes, promotes healing of wounds, and increases the aging person's ability to withstand the stress of injury and infections.

Brittleness and fragility of bones are caused by loss of weight and density of bones arising from the loss of calcium from the bones. Iron should be taken to prevent anemia.

Many of the conditions normally associated with aging may arise from increased oxidation of cells; therefore vitamin E, which is an effective antioxidant, may help retard aging.

Herbs

In meadows, prairies, and wildwoods, people for centuries have been collecting herbs to use as medicine. Vast amounts of information have been collected and tested; much of this information had never been written down, but had been passed on verbally instead. A disadvantage of most archaic theory is that it is permeated with magic, superstition, and dogma that is, for all practical purposes, irrelevant. Many Renaissance herbalists recorded information from ancient herbalists such as Pliny or Dioscorides without testing the ancients' claims, thus preserving statements that were to cast a suspicious light over the rest of the Renaissance findings about herbs.

In the *Journal of the Florida Medical Association,* August 1967, Drs. Max Michael, Jr. and Mark V. Barrow write, "It cannot be denied that folk remedies have yielded potent therapeutic weapons when one remembers the instances of digitalis and other drugs. That most of the remedies of the past and most of the present are without scientific foundation is probable. That there are traces of some compounds in many of the folk remedies which have appropriate pharmaceutical effects is also known. Before one closes his mind to all folk remedies and looks on them with derision, he must reckon with the fact that some indeed may be efficacious."[1]

Walter Lewis, Professor of Biology at Washington University in St. Louis, Missouri, states that the approach to research since the synthetic era, with little regard for past data, ". . . has served to delay the application of many potential benefits. For example, it is unfortunate that man's first cosmopolitan tranquilizer derived from rauvolfia did not come into general use until 1952, despite the long history of its use in Ayurvedic medicine in India, or that cromolyn, the miraculous prophylactic drug for asthma, has only recently been introduced, though its use in the form of ammi seeds was part of Bedouin folk medicine for centuries."[2]

Pharmaceutical companies have begun to search for plants that can cope with the diseases that are associated with our modern life-style. Stress, coronary disease, ulcers, rheumatism, and other ailments have already yielded to the power of plants. Even antitumor properties have been found in several species.[3]

There may be a word of caution to the chemist who first isolates the beneficial substance and leaves the rest of the root, bark, stem, leaf, or flower behind. This purified chemical may act favorably on a particular part of the body, but may also have deleterious effects on other parts of the body. Side effects may include rashes, dizziness, fainting, palpitations, blurred vision, diarrhea, or

[1]Max Michael, Jr., and Mark V. Barrow, *Journal of the Florida Medical Association,* vol. 54, no. 8, pp. 778–784, August 1967.

[2]Walter H. Lewis, *Medical Botany* (New York: John Wiley & Sons, 1977), p. vii.
[3]*Medical Botany,* pp. 127–132.

depression. The constituents of the plant that were discarded in the laboratory may have an inherent balancing or modifying mechanism that exerts control over the active principle. Both digitalis and rauvolfia have recently been shown to be of greater benefit when the whole part of the plant involved was taken.

The exact reason for the positive effect that herbs exert on the human body is not always known. It is evident, however, that the nutrients stored within the plants' cellular structure are in forms that are easily metabolized by the gastric juices, enzymes, and hormones of the body. The therapeutic action of herbs comes from *alkaloids,* organic nitrogenous compounds that cause certain chemical reactions within the body. Herbs also contain minerals, vitamins, and salts that help the body to resist disease, strengthen tissues, and improve the nervous system. They also contain glycosides, which are important sugars for the proper functioning of the heart and bloodstream. Tannins present in herbs aid recovery from illness by preventing passage of harmful bacteria. Plant mucilage can assist in the proper functioning of the intestines.

In order to receive the beneficial effects that can be obtained from herbs, the herbs must be consumed regularly for long periods of time, sometimes indefinitely. There are exceptions, such as golden seal, which if taken too long can retrogress the illness. Herbs should be kept in air-tight containers away from heat, light, and dampness to prevent deterioration of their active ingredients.

One very important note: Case histories of different allergies reveal the vast differences among individual metabolisms. If an herb does not agree with you or if you feel adverse effects, discontinue using the herb and find one that does agree with you. Herbs can be potent. Practice moderation. Adverse side effects are possible with many herbs when they are taken in overdoses. THE INFORMATION IN THIS SECTION IS NOT INTENDED TO REPLACE THE SERVICES OF PHYSICIANS.

Following is a summary of some of the most common herbs. There are hundreds of herbs available, about which information can be found in the many books written exclusively about this subject. Herbs can be obtained from health food stores, from herbalists who are listed in the yellow pages, from homeopathic pharmacies, and from some food markets.

ALFALFA (*Medicago sativa*)

Medicinal Use

Mild laxative, tonic, stomachic, diuretic.

Comments

Centuries ago, the Arabs used alfalfa as feed for their horses, because they claimed that it made the animals swift and strong. They then tried the herb themselves and became so convinced of its benefits to their health and strength that they named the grass "Al-Fal-Fa," which means "Father of All Foods."

The roots of the alfalfa plant burrow deep into the earth to reach minerals that are inaccessible to most other plants. Alfalfa contains vitamins A, E, K, B, D, and U. It is high in protein and it contains phosphorus, iron, potassium, chlorine, sodium, silicon, magnesium, and other trace elements. Alfalfa has eight enzymes known to promote chemical reactions that enable food to be assimilated properly within the body.

Alfalfa has been effective for aiding stomach ailments, gas pains, ulcerous conditions, dropsy, and pain and stiffness of arthritis. It may eliminate retained water, help cure peptic ulcers, and help in treating recuperative cases of narcotic and alcohol addiction and also in treating cases of overweight.

Alfalfa herb tea is said to possess no unfriendly components and may be given to children and adults of all ages. It is good for nursing mothers and for others who wish to abstain from beverages that contain caffeine. The tea is especially pleasant when it is combined with a mint-flavored herb.

ANGELICA (*Angelica archangelica*)

Medicinal Use

Aromatic, stimulant, carminative, diuretic, diaphoretic, emmenagogue, tonic, expectorant, stomachic.

Comments

It is thought by many that angelica derived its botanical name, *Angelica archangelica,* from its blooming date, May 8, which used to be the day of Michael the Archangel. In eighteenth-century Europe, giving a bouquet of angelica to one who was dearly loved meant "you are my inspiration."

Angelica has been used as a remedy for stomach problems such as sour stomach, heartburn, gas or colic, and for colds, coughs, shortness of breath, and fever. It may be good for sluggish liver and spleen, rheumatism, and nervous headache. It is useful for ulcers (taken internally and tea-dropped externally), because it restores normal tissues. Because of its unique ability to clear tiny passages, angelica has been used to relieve dimness of vision and of hearing by placing drops of the tea into the eyes and ears. Large doses may have a positive effect on blood pressure, heart action, and respiration. In Eurasia, angelica is considered a tonic to improve well-being and mental harmony. In England, the plant juice has been placed into carious teeth, and the oil has been used in dental preparations. Angelica salve applied externally is beneficial as a skin lotion and for relief of rheumatic pains. A decoction can be applied to the skin for itching and wounds. As a compress it is helpful for gout. Angelica has a tendency to increase the sugar in the urine, so those with diabetes or with diabetic tendencies should avoid it.

The dried leaf stalks of angelica are often preserved with sugar, thus forming a confection (also known as angelica) that is used in sweetmeats and cake decorations. The hollow stems of the plant can be added to stewed apples or rhubarb. In Iceland, both stems and roots are eaten raw with butter. The Norwegians make a bread with the roots, and in Lapland the stalks are regarded as a delicacy. As a bath additive, it is soothing to the nerves.

CHAMOMILE (*Anthemis nobilis*)

Medicinal Use

Stomachic, antispasmodic, tonic, emmenagogue, stimulant, tonic, aromatic, anodyne, vermifuge.

Comments

Chamomile is widely known for its applelike fragrance and flavor. It derives its name from the Greek *kamai* (on the ground) and *melon* (apple), for "ground apple."

Chamomile may relieve upset stomachs, colds, bronchitis, bladder troubles, dropsy, and jaundice. Intermittent and typhoid fever may be broken in the early stages through ingestion of the tea. It is helpful in regulating the menstrual cycle, rheumatic pains, headaches, and hysteria. It has been traditionally used as a sleep inducer and mild sedative. In Italy, a million cups of chamomile are drunk each day, and an Italian company now markets it under the slogan "cup of serenity." It is effective for colic in infants and is a good remedy for a child's fever and restlessness. The tea can be used as a wash for sore or weak eyes and for open sores and wounds, as a gargle, and as a poultice for pains and swellings. A chamomile poultice is helpful in preventing gangrene. When sponged over the body and left to dry, the tea acts as an insect repellant.

The dried leaves and flowers have for centuries been used as a hair rinse for blond hair, as an additive for baths, and as a scent among linen.

COMFREY (*Symphytum officinale*)

Medicinal Use

Demulcent, astringent, pectoral, vulnerary, mucilageneous, anodyne, emollient, hemostatic, refrigerant.

Comments

Comfrey is high in calcium, potassium, phosphorus, and other trace minerals. It contains protein and vitamins. The leaves are rich in vitamins A and C. It is a good source of the amino acid lysine, which is usually lacking in diets that contain no animal products. It is also one of the few vegetable sources of vitamin B_{12}. Chemical analysis has shown that comfrey contains the healing agent allantoin, which is known to promote granulation and formation of epithelial cells, thus increasing the speed at which nature can heal a wound, internal irritation, or broken bone. B_1, B_2, niacin, pantothenic acid, D, E, and choline are other vitamins found in the comfrey plant. Comfrey is recommended for all pulmonary complaints and hemoptysis. It is helpful for coughs; consumption; ulceration or soreness of the kidneys, stomach, or bowels; bloody urine; rheumatic pains; digestive disorders; and eczema and other skin disorders. It is useful for scrofula, anemia, dysentery, diarrhea, leucorrhea, colitis, gall and liver diseases, and hemorrhoids. Comfrey cleanses the entire system of impurities. In some parts of Ireland, it is eaten as a cure for defective circulation and used to strengthen the blood.

Bruises, sores, ulcerous wounds, and broken bones can be dressed externally with a poultice made from comfrey, which is also useful for boils and carbuncles. A little Vaseline may first be applied to avoid irritation from the prickly leaves. Fomentations or poultices can be used for any kind of inflammatory swelling. Comfrey ointment can be used for scratches, sores, itches, burns, and rashes. Fomentations relieve sore breasts and headache. A decoction makes a good gargle and mouthwash for throat inflammations, hoarseness, and bleeding gums. Dried comfrey can be ground and added to bread and muffins. It also tones the skin when it is added to the bath.

DANDELION (*Taraxacum officinale*)

Medicinal Use

Diuretic, tonic, slight aperient, hepatic, depurative, stomachic, cholagogue.

Comments

Dandelion has a high vitamin and mineral content. It is very useful for treating kidney and liver disorders, and helpful with jaundice, skin diseases, scrofula, and loss of appetite. It is useful for treating dropsy, fever, inflammation of the bowels, infectious hepatitis, edema resulting from liver problems, rheumatism, gout, and stiff joints. Dandelion increases the activity of the liver, pancreas, and spleen. Based on a compilation by Dr. Norman Farnsworth, Professor of Pharmacognosy at the University of Illinois in Chicago, dandelion has been shown to contain insulin substitutes that are needed by diabetics. The Chinese use a dandelion poultice for snake bites. The milky juice can be applied daily to warts.

Young dandelion leaves can be used in salads. The larger leaves can be cooked as a vegetable. Dandelion wine is made from the flowers, and the roots are dried and ground to make a coffee substitute.

EUCALYPTUS (*Eucalyptus globulus*)

Medicinal Use

Antiseptic, antispasmodic, stimulant, expectorant, aromatic.

Comments

The leaves and oil from this tree are an extremely potent but safe antiseptic, which results from the antimicrobial properties of one of their constituents, eucalyptol. An infusion is good for scarlet, typhoid, and intermittent fevers; and for indigestion. It is soothing to inflamed mucous membranes; thus it is a relief for asthma and croup. The oil may be applied locally for ulcers, growths, wounds, sores, neuralgic or rheumatic pains, pyorrhea, and burns. When inhaled, eucalyptus is valuable for treating asthma, diphtheria, sore throat, and stuffy nose. A solution of one teaspoon of oil to one half-pint of warm water may be rubbed into the skin as an effective insect repellent. The oil may be taken internally in small doses only. Excessive doses of eucalyptus may produce digestive disturbances, nausea, vomiting, diarrhea, kidney irritation, muscular weakness, and related effects.

Eucalyptus is a major ingredient in many commercial medicines such as cough and sore throat lozenges, nasal sprays, and chest rubs. A facial steam that is made with the leaves or oil in a pot of boiling water, and inhaled with a towel placed over the head, is effective for relieving congestion. This same water can be poured on sauna rocks. Eucalyptus tea or oil can also be put into the bath.

GINSENG (*Panax quinquefolium*)

Medicinal Use

Tonic, stimulant, demulcent, stomachic, anodyne, sedative, slight laxative, diaphoretic, carminative, alterative.

Comments

The Chinese have used ginseng for over 5,000 years. They composed the name "ginseng" from two words meaning "man-plant." Often the roots resemble the shape of a man, sometimes in detail. It was given the botanical name *Panax,* which means "all-healing" and is related to the word "panacea."

Ginseng strengthens the heart and nervous system. It builds up general mental and physical vitality and resistance to disease by strengthening and stimulating the endocrine glands that control all basic physiological processes, including the metabolism of minerals and vitamins. Dr. Keijiro Takagi, Dean of the Faculty of Pharmaceutical Sciences at the University of Tokyo, stated that "with the use of ginseng there is a significant anti-fatigue reaction in mice. We also learned that ginseng aids in the acceleration and acquisition of learning."[4] In a Chinese study, high blood sugar levels in animals were lowered with ginseng, and it was found to be effective for counteracting the deficiency of vitamins B_1 and B_2. Soviet researchers report that ginseng normalizes the level of arterial pressure and is effective in the treatment of both hypotension and hypertension.

Ginseng may be effective for treating colds, coughs, rheumatism, neuralgia, gout, diabetes, anemia, insomnia, stress, headache, backache, and double vision. Women find it helpful for normalizing menstruation and easing childbirth. It is believed to rejuvenate the entire system, to increase sexual energies, and to contain compounds that may exhibit antitumor value. In an experimental study in Eastern Europe, ginseng was used effectively as a mouthwash against periodontal disease, which is a progressive destruction of the supporting structures of the teeth. Ginseng's value is mainly as a preventative. It must be taken over a long period of time to stimulate rejuvenation and virility.

GOLDEN SEAL (Hydrastis canadensis)

Medicinal Use

Tonic, laxative, alterative, detergent, aperient, diuretic, antiseptic, astringent, deobstruent, antiperiodic.

Comments

Golden seal was one of the favorite herbs of the Cherokee Indians of North America. The name "golden seal" was given to the herb because of the seallike scars on the golden-yellow root. It has a very positive effect on the mucous membranes and body tissues. It is excellent for all catarrh conditions, whether of the throat, nose, bronchial passages, intestines, stomach, or bladder. It is a tonic for spinal nerves and is helpful for treating spinal meningitis. It is helpful with indigestion, biliousness, and liver disorders. It increases the secretion of bile and gastric juices. Golden seal is useful for treating typhoid fever, gonorrhea, leucorrhea, and syphilis. It is helpful with mouth sores, ulcerations of the stomach and bowels,

dysentery, and diarrhea. Golden seal shows experimental activity that is useful for diabetics. Small doses taken frequently will help to relieve nausea during pregnancy. It is an excellent nontoxic substitute for quinine. A douche that is made with an infusion of golden seal will soothe inflammations of the vagina and uterus. Golden seal will help to alleviate pyorrhea and sore gums when the teeth and gums are brushed with the tea. An infusion, cooled, can be applied to an inflamed eye.

An external wash is effective for skin diseases and sores. Sprinkle the powdered root on after washing with the tea. The powder may also be snuffed up the nostrils for nasal congestion or catarrh.

Golden seal should not be taken in large amounts during pregnancy. Persons with hypoglycemia and severe hypertension should avoid using it internally. It also has a tendency to retrogress an illness after use for too long a time.

HAWTHORN (Crataegus oxyacantha)

Medicinal Use

Tonic, antispasmodic, sedative, vasodilator.

Comments

A yellow substance from the hawthorn was isolated by Ullsperger (Pharmazie, 1951, p.141), who found that it caused the dilation of the coronary vessels. Fasshauer reported (Deutsche Med. Wchnschr., vol. 76, p. 211, 1951)[5] that one hundred heart patients who required continual therapy were given the liquid extract of hawthorn. The results were generally beneficial. Marked improvement was shown in patients with mitral stenosis and heart diseases of old age. For other patients who used hawthorn, digitalis could be either temporarily discontinued or considerably reduced. Scientific investigation has also found hawthorn to be helpful for insomnia, for alleviating irregular heart rhythm, and for a variety of other heart ailments, including angina pectoris. It has been used to treat high blood pressure when taken over a period of time, arteriosclerosis, inflammation of the heart muscle (myocarditis), arthritis, and rheumatism. It may be effective for alleviating nervous conditions and stress

[4]Dian Buchman, "Ginseng: An Oriental Panacea," The Herbalist, June 1977, p. 30.

[5]Richard Lucas, Nature's Medicines (N. Hollywood, Calif.: Wilshire Book Co., 1977), p. 189.

from daily pressure. Although hawthorn is nontoxic, large doses can cause dizziness.

LICORICE *(Glycyrrhiza glabra)*

Medicinal Use

Demulcent, pectoral, emollient, expectorant, laxative, diuretic.

Comments

Archeologists have found great quantities of licorice stored among other treasures in the 3,000-year-old tomb of King Tut-Ankh-Amen of Egypt. The practice of placing this herb in the tombs was instituted to enable the spirit of the deceased person to make a sweet drink in the next world.

Licorice has been used for centuries as a confection, and because of its saponin content, it is an effective soother of various internal pains. It is helpful for alleviating such ailments as inflamed stomach, bronchitis, sore throat, coughs, irritations of the bowel and kidney, and indigestion. In Denmark, experiments have shown licorice to be very effective for treating duodenal and peptic ulcers. It also contains a female hormone that has estrogenic action. Southern Europeans drink large amounts of licorice water, because they believe it to be a blood purifier. The Romans thought so highly of its medicinal value that it was included in the rations of the Roman legions. The licorice root has a substance known as glycyrrhizin, which is fifty times sweeter than sugar cane. Despite this fact, it alleviates rather than increases thirst.

Licorice can be added to other, less pleasant-tasting herbs to make them more palatable. Licorice root sticks can be sucked on by persons who wish to stop smoking. Excessive licorice intake can lead to cardiac dysfunction and hypertension.

PEPPERMINT *(Mentha piperita)*

Medicinal Use

Stimulant, stomachic, carminative, aromatic, vermifuge, anodyne, antispasmodic, cholagogue, tonic.

Comments

According to the Greek philosopher-scientist Theophrastus, 300 B.C., the botanical name *mentha* was derived from Greek mythology. Mintho was a beautiful nymph who was loved by Pluto, god of the underworld. Persephone, who had been abducted by Pluto to reign with him over his domain, became jealous of Mintho and changed her into a fragrant and lowly plant, the mint.

Peppermint is one of several mints within the mint family. All mints are said to strengthen the stomach and improve digestion. The pleasant aroma is soothing and invigorating. Peppermint is used against liver complaints, flatulence, nausea, seasickness, vomiting, chills, colic, fevers, dizziness, diarrhea, dysentery, cholera, influenza, and such heart problems as palpitations. It may be helpful in cases of insanity, convulsions and spasms in infants, and nervous headache. Peppermint cleanses and strengthens the entire system, including the nerves. It diffuses like alcohol and warms the whole body.

The herb tea is an excellent substitute for coffee or tea. The oil of peppermint when applied externally is useful for toothache, headache, neuralgia, burns, and rheumatism. A peppermint salve helps skin conditions. When placed in the bath, peppermint can have a calming and strengthening effect on the nerves and muscles. Peppermint enemas are excellent for cholera or for colon troubles.

ROSE HIPS

Comments

Hips are the fruit of the rose, or what is left after the flower has bloomed and the petals have fallen. The ancient Greeks used the fresh hips as a food, and 1,000 years before Christ, hips were referred to as the "Food of the Gods." "Gods" were believed to be men who lived so close to nature that nature whispered her secrets to them.

During World War II, the governments of England, Sweden, and Norway discovered that rose hips contained from ten to one hundred times more vitamin C than any other food. They also contain vitamins A, E, B_1, B_2, K, P, niacin, and the minerals calcium, phosphorus, and iron. Rose hip tea may be beneficial for the bladder and kidneys, and helpful in preventing colds.

SARSAPARILLA *(Smilax ornata)*

Medicinal Use

Alterative, diuretic, demulcent, stimulant, carminative, tonic.

Comments

Several years ago, researchers at Pennsylvania State College found three hormones in the sarsaparilla plant—testosterone, progesterone, and cortin. Scientists say that impotence generally results from the inability of the testicles to supply the body with a normal amount of the male hormone. Experiments have shown that testosterone tends to restore sexual power, mental alertness, and physical strength. However, the positive effects are only apparent so long as the hormone is taken. Testosterone has also been shown to improve the condition of patients with angina pectoris. Patients who used the hormone were able to tolerate more physical activity, and paroxysms were less frequent and less severe. Results have also been good when testosterone has been given for diseases of the blood vessels in the legs and feet.

The second hormone found in sarsaparilla, progesterone, is normally produced by the ovaries in the female and is essential for the development of the mammary and genital organs and for reproduction. It is also found in the corpus luteum, a yellow mass in the ovary, which aids in the preparation of the womb for pregnancy and also tends to prevent miscarriage. Progesterone has a calming effect on the womb muscles, and eases the spasmodic pains that sometimes follow childbirth.

The third hormone, cortin, is secreted by the adrenal glands. If too little cortin is secreted, the body becomes susceptible to infectious disease, nervous depression, and general weakness.

Dr. Eric Solmo, a Hungarian scientist, lived in Mexico for several years and became curious about a remedy used by the natives as a cure for physical debility, weakness, and sexual impotence. After extensive tests and studies of men and animals, he came to the same conclusion about the benefits of the hormones contained in sarsaparilla as the earlier researchers.

Philippsohn (*Derm. Wchnschr.*, vol. 93, p. 1220, 1931)[6] reported the use of a water extract of sarsaparilla in the treatment of psoriasis. One patient who previously had a very stubborn case took the treatment daily for 20 years without a single relapse. Sarsaparilla stimulates the body's defense mechanism, and is therefore a valuable treatment for syphilis. It has been used for rheumatism, gout, skin eruptions, ringworm, scrofula, internal inflammations, catarrhs, fever, colds, and dropsy. It is an excellent blood purifier. The tea may also be used as an eye wash.

[6] Lucas, *Nature's Medicines*, p. 55.

SKULLCAP (*Scutellaria laterifolia*)

Medicinal Use

Tonic, nervine, antispasmodic, slight astringent, diuretic, sedative.

Comments

Skullcap is a beautiful blue-helmeted flowery plant whose name is derived from the leather helmets worn by the early Romans. By its action through the cerebrospinal centers, it is one of the best nerve tonics ever discovered. It may be used for all disorders of the nervous system, including hysteria, convulsions, tremors, and palsy. It is also good for neuralgia, aches and pains, rheumatism, epilepsy, poisonous insect and snake bites, rabies, children's fever, female cramps caused by suppressed menstruation resulting from colds, fevers, functional heart troubles where cardiac action is irregular, insomnia, exhaustion, and lockjaw. It is helpful for alcoholics in delirium tremens, and relieves restlessness. It is an effective substitute for quinine. Skullcap must be taken regularly for a long period of time to be of permanent benefit.

STRAWBERRY (*Fragaria vesca*)

Medicinal Use

Mild astringent, diuretic, tonic.

Comments

Strawberry is excellent for children and for convalescents as a strengthening tonic for the entire system. It is helpful for diarrhea, dysentery, night sweats, liver complaints, gout, and jaundice. It is a good blood purifier. It may be effective against the bodily poisons that cause eczema. It should be taken internally and used as a wash externally. Strawberry is used internally for weak intestines and is also used as an enema. A gargle of the tea may be taken for sore mouth and throat. Strawberry leaves are rich in iron and also contain rutin and the minerals potassium, sodium, and magnesium.

YARROW (*Achillea millefolium*)

Medicinal Use

Diaphoretic, stimulant, tonic, astringent, alterative, vulnerary, diuretic.

Comments

Yarrow gets its botanical name *Achillea* from the legend that comrades of the Greek hero Achilles used yarrow to heal their wounds during the Trojan War. The name *millefolium* was taken because of yarrow's feathery leaves, which are so well divided that the plant appears to have a thousand leaves. Yarrow has a healing and soothing effect on the mucous membranes. It may be effective for treating bleeding from the lungs and urinary organs, diabetes, bleeding hemorrhoids, dysentery, and stomach disorders. It is helpful with typhoid and other fevers, colds, diarrhea, measles, smallpox, chicken pox, Bright's disease, colic, rheumatism, constipation, toothache, and earache. It is very good when applied externally as an ointment for cuts and wounds. Yarrow can also be used as a douche for leucorrhea and as an enema for hemorrhoids.

HERBAL PREPARATIONS

Decoction. Seeds, barks, roots, and other hard materials are prepared by decoction. Put 1 oz herb in $1^1/_2$ pints cold water. Cover and simmer for $^1/_2$ hour. Then cover and steep for 15–30 minutes. Honey or lemon can be added. Use porcelain or glass vessels.

Fomentation. Dip cloth in the infusion or decoction, wring it out, and apply locally.

Infusion. Leaves, flowers, and some roots are prepared as teas or as infusions. Take 1 tsp per cup or 1 oz per pint. Do not boil the herb. Bring water to boil and pour the water over the herb. Cover and steep for 10–15 minutes. Honey or lemon can be added. Use porcelain or glass vessels.

Oil. Mix 2 tablespoons minced or powdered herbs with $^1/_4$ pint of oil. Place in hot sun or heat daily in hot water. Shake daily. After three weeks, strain and use.

Ointment or salve. Take 4 parts Vaseline or like substance to 1 part herb. Stir and heat gently for 20 minutes.

Cool slightly and strain. This works best if herb has been ground.

Poultice. Bruise the herb, add enough boiling water to moisten it, then apply it to the affected part of the body, covering it with a cloth wrung out in hot water.

Syrup. Boil tea for 20 minutes, add 1 oz glycerin, and seal up in bottles as you would fruit.

Tincture. Add 1 oz powdered herb to 8 oz alcohol and 4 oz water. Shake daily. Let stand for two weeks, then strain.

HERB GLOSSARY

ALTERATIVE Gradually altering or changing a condition, also a blood purifier.

ANODYNE Relieving pain.

ANTIPERIODIC Preventing the periodic return of certain diseases.

ANTISEPTIC Destroying infection-causing microorganisms.

ANTISPASMODIC Relieving or preventing involuntary muscle spasms or cramps.

APERIENT Mild and gently acting laxative.

AROMATIC Substance with a spicy scent and a pungent but pleasing taste. Useful for fragrance, and often added to medicines to improve their palatability.

ASTRINGENT Temporarily tightening or contracting the skin or tissues. Checks the discharge of mucus and blood, etc.

CARMINATIVE Checking formation of gas and helping to dispel whatever gas has already formed.

CHOLAGOGUE Promoting the discharge of bile from the system.

DEMULCENT Mucilaginous substance that soothes the intestinal tract.

DEOBSTRUENT Clearing obstruction from the natural ducts of the body.

DEPURATIVE Removing wastes from body, purifying blood.

DETERGENT   A cleansing action.

DIAPHORETIC   Promoting sweating.   Commonly used as an aid for relief of the common cold.

DIURETIC   Promoting flow of urine.

EMMENAGOGUE   Promoting menstruation.

EMOLLIENT   Softening and soothing skin when applied externally.

EXPECTORANT   Loosening phlegm in the mucous membrane of the bronchial and nasal passages, thus facilitating its expulsion.

HEMOSTATIC   Checking internal bleeding.

HEPATIC   Affecting the liver.

LAXATIVE   A gentle cathartic that helps to promote bowel movements.

MUCILAGINOUS   A soothing quality for inflamed parts.

NERVINE   Calming nervous irritation from excitement, strain, or fatigue.

PECTORAL   Relieving ailments of the chest and lungs.

REFRIGERANT   Generally cooling in effect, also reduces fevers.

SEDATIVE   Calming the nerves.

STIMULANT   Increasing or quickening various functions of the body, such as digestion and appetite.   It does this quickly, whereas a tonic stimulates general health over a period of time.

STOMACHIC   Strengthing and toning the stomach and stimulating the appetite.

TONIC   Invigorating or strengthening the system.

VASODILATOR   Widening blood vessels.

VERMIFUGE   Destroying and helping to expel intestinal worms.

VULNERARY   Application for external wounds.

REFERENCES

Clymer, R. Swinburne, M.D.: *Nature's Healing Agents.* (Philadelphia: Dorrance & Co., 1963).

Heinerman, John: *Medical Doctors' Guide to Herbs.* (Provo, Utah: Bi-World Publishers, Inc., 1977.)

Kloss, Jethro: *Back to Eden.* (New York: Beneficial Books, 1971.)

Lehane, Brendan: *The Power of Plants.* (Maidenhead, England: McGraw-Hill, 1977.)

Lewis, Walter: *Medical Botany.* (New York: John Wiley & Sons, 1977.)

Lucas, Richard: *Nature's Medicines.* (N. Hollywood, Calif.: Wilshire Book Co., 1977.)

Lust, Benedict, M.D.: *About Herbs.* (Wellingborough Northants, England: Weatherby Woolnough, 1961.)

Lust, John: *The Herb Book.* (New York: Bantam Books, 1974.)

Meyer, Joseph: *The Herbalist.* (Glenwood, Ill.: Meyerbooks, 1976.)

Null, Gary: *Herbs for the Seventies.* (New York: Robert Speller & Sons, 1972.)

Rodale Herb Book. (Emmaus, Pa.: Rodale Press, 1976.)

Sherborne House Book of Herbs. (Sherborne, Gloucestershire, England: Coombe Springs Press.)

Thomson, William, M.D.: *Herbs That Heal.* (New York: Charles Scribner's Sons, 1976.)

Wren, R.W.: *Potter's New Cyclopaedia.* (New York: Harper & Row, 1972.)

Foods, Beverages, and Supplementary Foods

Many factors influence eating patterns and therefore affect nutrition. For example, taste preferences, states of health, and various social and cultural customs all determine what foods a person eats. Poor nutrition may be the result of consuming too little, too much, or the wrong kinds of food, because of any number of reasons.

The foods and beverages we consume should provide our bodies with the nutrients necessary for good health. Protein builds and maintains body cells, and carbohydrates, fats, and some protein provide calories for energy. Vitamins and minerals help regulate the many chemical reactions within the body. For individual recommended dietary allowances of nutrients, see the "Nutrient Allowance Chart" on pages 247 to 248.

Fresh, raw fruits and vegetables are generally more nutritious than prepared ones, although many kinds of foods are more palatable when cooked. Studies indicate that considerable losses of nutrients, especially the B complex, vitamin C, and the bioflavonoid complex, occur during storage and cooking. It is essential to select, store, and prepare foods wisely in order to obtain these nutrients. Precautions should also be taken to avoid foodborne illnesses caused by the growth of harmful bacteria. Some basic rules for storing and preparing foods in order to retain their nutrient content and to prevent food poisoning are as follows:

Cook meats, especially pork and poultry, thoroughly in order to kill harmful bacteria.

Guard against the growth of harmful bacteria by immediately refrigerating leftovers or foods cooked for later use. Do not allow them to cool to room temperature first.

Keep perishable foods—especially chopped and processed meats, custards, pastries, and dairy products—in the refrigerator to avoid bacterial contamination.

Destroy cans that bulge or canned contents that bubble out when the can is opened, in order to avoid food poisoning.

Ensure thorough cooking of frozen foods by allowing them to thaw completely before cooking, unless otherwise stated on frozen food packages.

Avoid soaking fruits, vegetables, or meats in water to protect against the loss of water-soluble vitamins.

Store fresh foods as soon as possible to minimize nutrient loss.

Supplementary foods may be useful for further increasing the nutritional value of meals. Supplementary foods must also be stored and prepared properly in order to prevent nutrient loss.

In the following section, food groups, beverages, and supplementary foods are discussed alphabetically in terms of their nutrient content and special features. This information is intended for use with the "Table of Food Composition" on pages 199 to 234 and the "Nutrient Allowance Chart" on pages 247 to 248.

Any reference to a body disorder or disease in connection with a food or beverage is not meant to be prescriptive, but merely represents research findings.

FOODS

EGGS

Eggs are an excellent source of complete protein; they contain all essential amino acids. (One large egg contains 7 or 8 grams of first-class protein.) Also found in eggs are vitamins A, B_2, D, and E; niacin; copper; iron; phosphorus; and unsaturated fats. The egg yolk contains the richest known source of choline, found in lecithin and necessary for keeping the cholesterol within the egg emulsified. The egg yolk also contains biotin, one of the B-complex vitamins.

Eggs should be kept refrigerated at all times (at 45° to 55°F) because temperature variations will cause the whites to become thin. A soiled egg should be wiped clean with a dry cloth rather than washed, to preserve the natural protective film on the porous eggshell. This film prevents odors, flavors, molds, and bacteria from entering the egg. Eggs retain their freshness and quality better if stored large end up in their original carton.

Raw eggs should not be consumed in great quantity because the whites contain a protein called avidin, which may be harmful to the body if consumed over a long period of time, since it interferes with the use of biotin. However, avidin is inactivated by heat.

FIBER

Fiber is the part of food that is not digested by the human body, such as the skin of an apple and the husk of a wheat kernel. The normal functioning of the intestinal tract depends upon the presence of adequate fiber. A low-fiber diet has been associated with heart disease, cancer of the colon and rectum, diverticulosis, varicose veins, phlebitis, and obesity.

FISH

Fish are excellent sources of high-grade protein, polyunsaturated fatty acids, and minerals, especially iodine and potassium.

Fish are categorized as freshwater fish, saltwater fish, and shellfish. These types differ slightly in nutritive value. Freshwater fish provide magnesium, phosphorus, iron, and copper. Saltwater fish and shellfish are rich in iodine, fluorine, and cobalt. The unsaturated fat content of fish and shellfish varies with the species and season of year. Fatty fish, such as halibut, mackerel, and salmon, are good sources of vitamins A and D. Herring, oysters, and sardines contain vanadium and zinc. Shellfish are low in fatty acids but are relatively high in cholesterol.

Fish and shellfish may be purchased fresh, frozen, canned, salted, dried, or smoked. Because of the possibility of bacterial infection, fresh fish and shellfish should not remain at room temperature for more than two hours. They should be well wrapped, stored in the coldest part of the refrigerator, and used within two days.

Fish and shellfish are best cooked at low temperature (300° to 325°F) and should not be overcooked in order to preserve flavor, juices, and nutrients.

FRUITS

Fresh fruits are good sources of vitamins and minerals, especially vitamins A and C, carbohydrates in the form of cellulose and natural sugars, and water. They are good substitutes of such high-carbohydrate foods as candy, cookies, and cakes, which contain few nutrients.

Yellow fruits, such as apricots, cantaloupe, and persimmons, are good sources of carotene, which is converted to vitamin A. Aside from acerola cherries and rose hips, the best natural sources of vitamin C are the citrus fruits, such as oranges, grapefruit, lemons, and tangerines; other sources of vitamin C are cantaloupe, strawberries, and tomatoes.

Apples and bananas contain valuable bulk fiber in the form of indigestible cellulose, which is needed for regular bowel movement. Bananas are high in magnesium and may be useful for treatment of diarrhea, colitis, ulcers, and certain cases of protein allergies. Bananas and pears are the highest in natural sugars.

Fruits may be fresh, frozen, dried, or canned, but nutrient values will decrease if fruits are not properly stored or if they are refrigerated for extended periods of time. Fresh fruits offer the richest source of vitamins and minerals as well as appetite appeal in color, flavor, and texture. Fresh fruits purchased in season will be higher in nutrient quality and more economical in price than frozen, dried, or canned fruits. It is preferable to obtain ripe rather than green fruits, since ripe fruits contain simple sugars that are very easily assimilated by the digestive system. Fruits that are not fully ripe should be allowed to ripen at room temperature and then should be stored in a cool, dark place or in the refrigerator.

Fresh fruits should always be washed prior to eating so that any possible chemical residue is removed, and should be eaten whole or peeled thinly so that nutrients found in the skin are conserved. If fruits are to be cooked, they should be cooked quickly.

Frozen fruits compare favorably in nutrient content with fresh fruits, but some loss of nutritional value may occur in the processes of drying and canning, if done improperly. Dried fruits, rich in thiamine and iron, should be softened and cooked in the same water and then stored in a cool, dry place. Home-canned fruits should be stored in a dark place to preserve their vitamin C content. Water-packed and light-syrup fruits are preferable to those packed in heavy syrups that contain large amounts of sugar.

FRUIT JUICES

Fresh fruit juices usually have a pleasing flavor and are easily digested. Although the nutritive value of the whole fruit is somewhat higher, juice is an excellent source of vitamins and minerals.

Juice should be extracted from chilled fruit immediately prior to serving. It should not be allowed to stand for a long period of time after extraction, because vitamin C will be lost. Juices should be refrigerated in covered containers to ensure that vitamin C will not be lost through oxidation.

GRAINS

Grains are often referred to as cereals; they are the seeds of various grasses such as wheat, rye, oats, rice, and barley. Often called the "staff of life," they provide the bulk of the world's food supply. Common foods made from these grains are flours, breads, breakfast cereals, and macaroni.

Breads and Cereals

The main constituent of breads is flour. Flour is the product resulting from the milling process, which involves grinding and sifting of cleaned grains. The type of flour or grain from which it originates often determines the color, texture, flavor, and nutritive value of the bread. Cereals can be made from a variety of grains, such as corn, barley, oats, wheat, etc.

Whole-grain flour is the result of the first milling process. Whole-grain flour contains the germ of the grain, which possesses the most nutrients, and must be refrigerated to prevent rancidity. Whole-grain breads should be stored at room temperature or frozen until used. Refrigerated bread loses moisture and thus becomes stale faster than bread that is frozen or that which is kept at room temperature.

All-purpose flour is a blend of different wheat grains. Bleached flour has been whitened to create a more uniform flour. Self-rising flour contains added salt and leavening in proper proportions. *Enriched flour* has the nutrients thiamine, riboflavin, and niacin of the vitamin B complex, and sometimes iron, returned to it. This enrichment process also applies to other "enriched" products, such as breakfast cereals and macaroni.

Rice

Whole brown rice contains a generous supply of B vitamins, plus calcium, phosphorus, and iron. *Wild rice* contains twice as much protein, four times as much phosphorus, eight times as much thiamine, and twenty times as much riboflavin as white rice. *White rice*, dehulled polished rice, has no significant amount of B vitamins but may also be enriched, as are flour and cereals. *Converted rice* has undergone a process similar to milling and it has a somewhat higher vitamin content than white rice.

TOTAL NUTRIENTS IN THE KERNEL OF WHEAT[1]

Germ is 2½% of Kernel

Of the whole kernel
the germ contains:

64% Thiamine
26% Riboflavin
21% Pyridoxine
8% Protein
7% Pantothenic Acid
2% Niacin

Bran is 14% of Kernel

Of the whole kernel
the bran contains:

73% Pyridoxine
50% Pantothenic Acid
42% Riboflavin
33% Thiamine
19% Protein

Endosperm is 83% of Kernel

Of the whole kernel
the endosperm contains:

70-75% Protein
43% Pantothenic Acid
32% Riboflavin
12% Niacin
6% Pyridoxine
3% Thiamine

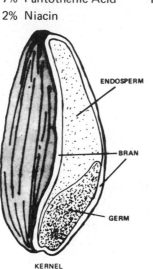

ENDOSPERM

BRAN

GERM

KERNEL
(magnification)

Other Nutrients Found in the Whole Wheat
Grain are:

Calcium	Chlorine
Iron	Sodium
Phosphorus	Silicon
Magnesium	Boron
Potassium	Barium
Manganese	Silver
Copper	Inositol
Sulphur	Folic Acid
Iodine	Choline
Fluorine	Vitamin E

And other trace materials

Whole Grains

The structure of a whole grain may be separated into three different parts (see illustration). The *germ* is the heart of the grain, which sprouts when the seed is planted. It is especially rich in the B vitamins, vitamin E, protein, unsaturated fat, minerals (especially iron), and carbohydrates. The *endosperm* constitutes the largest part of the grain. It is composed chiefly of carbohydrates in the form of starch, with some incomplete protein and traces of vitamins and minerals. The *bran* portion of the grain is the covering. It is composed chiefly of the carbohydrate cellulose, with traces of B vitamins, minerals (especially iron), and incomplete proteins.

While the entire grain is edible, the bran and germ are often removed during milling in order to reduce the

chance of rancidity and to improve the storage quality of the grain. At the same time, important nutrients such as the B vitamins, vitamin E, and iron are lost. In order to enrich flour, bread, and cereal products, thiamine, riboflavin, and iron are added during processing.

LEGUMES

Legumes are plants that have edible seeds within a pod. They include peas, beans, lentils, and peanuts. Legumes are a rich source of incomplete protein, iron, thiamine, riboflavin, and niacin. When sprouted, they provide an excellent source of vitamin C.

Legumes are a hearty and versatile food. Because of their high but incomplete protein content, legumes can be used as a meat substitute when used with other complementary protein foods.

Dried legumes should be stored in tightly covered containers in a cool, dry place. They should be cooked

[1]*The Art of Nutritious Cooking* (Bismarck, N.Dak.: Nutrition Search, 1974), p. 15.

in liquid to soften their cellulose fiber and to restore flavor and moisture that is lost in the drying process. If one adds baking soda when cooking legumes to speed up the softening of the cellulose, the thiamine content of the legumes will be destroyed.

Soybeans

Generous supplies of soybean products may serve as the major protein source in a meatless diet. However, the balance of essential amino acids in soybeans is not the same as that in meats; therefore more grams of this protein are required to supply the essential amino acids adequately. In addition, soybeans contain vitamins and minerals in a natural relationship that is similar to the human body's needs.

Soy flour, oil, and milk are used in a variety of home-cooked and commerical products. Soy flour has a creamy yellow color and a slightly nutty taste. It is a rich source of protein, the vitamin B complex, calcium, phosphorus, potassium, magnesium, and iron. Soybean oil contains large amounts of linoleic acid, an unsaturated fatty acid essential to the human body. Soybean oil is stable against oxidation and flavor deterioration because of its lecithin and vitamin E content. Soy milk is often recommended for persons who are allergic to cow's milk. Soy milk is low in fat, carbohydrates, calcium, phosphorus, and riboflavin but rich in iron, thiamine, and niacin.

Some forms of soy protein are made into commercial imitation-meat items. Pressed soybean cakes, the product resulting from grinding the soybean residue after the soybeans have been processed for oil, can be added to a variety of cooked dishes. Sprouted soybeans contain increased amounts of vitamin C.

MEATS

"Meat" commonly refers to the flesh of animals; it is the most important source of first-class protein in the modern diet. In addition to protein, beef, lamb, and pork are good sources of the B-complex vitamins (especially thiamine and riboflavin), phosphorus, iron, sulfur, potassium, and copper. Poultry, also a good source of protein, contains the B-complex vitamins (especially niacin), iron, and phosphorus.

The quality of beef, lamb, and pork is designated by the cut—Prime, Choice, or Good—when purchased over the counter. The meat's flavor, tenderness, and ease of cooking vary with the grade and do not affect its nutritional value. In general, lean cuts with less fat are preferable. Prime and Choice cuts of meat are often not the highest in protein content because the animals were "fattened" before slaughter and the lean contains marbling, or fat granules, to increase tenderness. Good grades, therefore, may be more lean and contain more protein per pound. Luncheon meats, frankfurters, and sausages are usually high in fats.

Variety, or organ, meats are usually richer in vitamins and minerals than muscle meats. Variety meats include the liver, tongue, kidneys, heart, brains, and sweetbreads (glands of calves or lambs). Liver is a very rich source of complete protein and B vitamins, especially riboflavin, niacin, and B_{12}. It is also a good source of vitamins A, C, and D; iron; phosphorus; and copper. Because of the high iron and vitamin B_{12} content, liver can aid the body in combating iron-deficiency anemia and pernicious anemia.

Both raw and cooked meat should be refrigerated at a temperature of 30° to 32°F. In order to be at their best flavor and nutritive value, meats should be used within two or three days after purchase. Ground meats and variety meats should be used within 24 hours to prevent spoilage. Meat should not be soaked in water because this leads to loss of water-soluble nutrients. Nearly all meats freeze well and maintain their quality if wrapped and stored properly, although meat that is frozen for more than six months may show freezer burn (drying) and changes in texture. Meats should be frozen quickly and kept at temperatures of −10°F or lower to retard deterioration.

It is preferable that meats be cooked without adding fats or water; broiling and baking at moderate temperatures are recommended. Juices obtained during cooking contain valuable nutrients and should be served with the meat. Pork, or any raw product containing pork, should be cooked thoroughly to kill any trichinosis organisms that may be present. The temperature at the center of a pork roast should be at least 160° to 185°F.

Poultry that is inspected for quality is graded A, B, or C, A being the top quality. White poultry meat is especially rich in niacin and is easier to digest than dark meat, since it contains less fat and connective tissue. Dark meat, however, is superior to white meat as a source of thiamine and riboflavin.

Chilled raw poultry may be kept one or two days in

the coldest part of the refrigerator. Stuffing from cooked poultry should be removed and stored separately in a covered container. The body cavity or skin of chickens and turkeys may contain a bacteria that causes food poisoning. In order to prevent a large bacterial growth due to moisture, one should store these birds with loose wrapping so that the surface of the bird will be slightly dry. It is also recommended that poultry be frozen without stuffing and stuffed immediately prior to cooking. Poultry should be thawed completely to enable thorough cooking. Poultry should be cooked thoroughly; the temperature at the center should be about 190°F.

MILK AND MILK PRODUCTS

Milk and milk products are excellent sources of calcium, complete protein, and riboflavin. Milk also contains phosphorus, thiamine, and vitamins B_6 and B_{12}, but it contains little iron or vitamin C. A glass of milk contains about 300 milligrams of calcium; three glasses of milk daily supply the needed amount of calcium for adults; children and adolescents need four or five glasses per day.

Milk is available in several forms. Most milk is pasteurized to kill bacteria and thereby to prevent the spread of milkborne diseases. The pasteurization process involves heating the milk to a high temperature and cooling it rapidly. Homogenized milk is that which has its fat content finely dispersed throughout, and because of this, it is more easily digested than nonhomogenized milk.

Whole milk usually contains about 3.5 percent fat. Skim milk is whole milk from which the fat is removed. Two percent milk contains two percent fat, which gives it more body and flavor than skim milk. Fortified milk has one or more nutrients, commonly vitamins A and D, added. Nonfat dry milk and fluid skim milk, unless fortified, contain no significant amounts of vitamin A or D because these fat-soluble vitamins are removed with the fat; but they are rich in protein, calcium, and vitamin B_2.

People who are allergic to milk may substitute buttermilk, goat's milk, yogurt, and possibly soy milk, although soy milk lacks much of the value of cow's milk because it is low in calcium and phosphorus.

Buttermilk may be obtained from the residue of the butter-making process, or it may be cultured. Most commercial buttermilk is made by the latter process, in which a harmless bacteria is added to skim milk or churned buttermilk.

Evaporated milk is whole milk with one-half of its water content removed. Condensed milk has water removed and sugar added. Dried milk results from the removal of 95 to 98 percent water from whole milk; nonfat dry milk is skim milk with the water removed.

Butter

Butter is made from milk products, contains vitamins A and D, and is high in fat content. Butter should be kept in the refrigerator and left in its original wrapper until ready for use, to retain its flavor and consistency.

Cheese

Cheese is made by separating most of the curd, or milk solids, from the whey or water part of the milk. Its texture and flavor vary with ripening (aging). Most cheeses contain protein, milk, fat, calcium, phosphorus, vitamin A, and riboflavin. The best way to store cheese is by leaving it in its original wrapper in the refrigerator. If the wrapper is torn, protect the surface from drying out by covering exposed surface with waxed paper, foil, or plastic. Cheeses with a strong odor should be kept in a container with a tight cover.

Yogurt

Milk that has been fermented by a mixture of bacteria and yeasts forms a custardlike product called yogurt. The milk is defatted and soured with *Lactobacillus acidophilus* and other bacteria that are necessary for health of the intestine. Yogurt aids digestion and controls the action of the intestine in favorably stimulating the kidneys.

Yogurt contains the B-complex vitamins and has a higher percentage of vitamins A and D than does the milk it was made from; it is also high in protein.

The beneficial bacteria in yogurt make it a natural antibiotic. Yogurt has been found to be beneficial in treating high cholesterol level, arthritis, constipation, diarrhea, gallstones, halitosis, hepatitis, kidney disorders, and skin diseases.

Yogurt made at home is preferable to commercial yogurt because many of the preservatives added to yogurt found in grocery stores tend to nullify its therapeutic effects.

NUTS

Nuts are the dry fruits or seeds of some kinds of plants, usually of trees. Some readily available nuts are pecans, filberts, Brazil nuts, walnuts, almonds, and cashews. The soft inside part of the nut is the meat, or kernel, and the outer covering is the shell. Nuts are a concentrated food source of proteins, unsaturated fats, the B-complex vitamins, vitamin E, calcium, iron, potassium, magnesium, phosphorus, and copper.

Nuts may be eaten fresh, roasted, boiled, or in the form of flour or butter. Nuts may interfere with digestion unless they are chewed well or chopped into fine particles. When nuts are purchased in the shell, attention should be paid to the firmness of the seal, since partially cracked nuts soon become dry and rancid. Nuts that are shelled should be stored preferably in the refrigerator, in airtight containers, to preserve their freshness and to prevent oxidation and rancidity of their fat content.

OILS

The term "oil" generally refers to fats in a liquid state. Vegetable oils, such as corn, cottonseed, safflower, soybean, olive, and sunflower, are widely used in cooking. These oils are important in the diet because of their content of unsaturated fatty acids, especially linoleic acid, which is necessary for growth and maintenance of the cells.

Oils may be removed from seeds, such as the safflower, or from beans, such as the soybean, by heat extraction or by pressing. Oils removed by pressing are referred to as "cold-pressed" and retain their vitamin A and E content better than those extracted by heat.

Margarine is a popular butter substitute made from solidified vegetable oils. Margarine contains 87 percent fat along with some salt and flavoring compounds to make it resemble butter in taste. Margarine is fortified with vitamin A, which makes it nutritionally comparable to butter, although margarine is sometimes preferred to butter because it has a higher unsaturated fatty acid content while butter has a higher saturated fatty acid content.

Oils, margarine, and all other fats should be kept refrigerated. They should also be well covered to prevent the absorption of odors from other foods.

SEASONINGS, HERBS, SPICES, AND EXTRACTS

Seasonings, herbs, spices, and extracts are usually derived from foods. They normally have little nutritive value because they are consumed in minute amounts. However, they give variety to the flavor of foods, stimulate the appetite, and encourage the flow of digestive juices. Seasonings, herbs, spices, and extracts are usually derived from the bark, roots, fruits, berries, or leaves of plants, shrubs, or trees.

Salt, or sodium chloride, is the most commonly used seasoning as well as an essential body mineral. Most people, however, consume many times too much salt, the body needs only a small amount, about two or three grams per day. An excess of table salt may cause mineral imbalances in the body because the sodium in it upsets the potassium and calcium levels in the body. Salt may be plain or iodized; salt used in the home should be iodized salt.

Salt substitutes are often used by people who must restrict their intake of sodium. Unrefined salt from evaporated seawater contains many trace minerals, is an especially good source of iodine, and may be found in a refined form.

Pepper ranks next to salt as a common seasoning. Pepper is available in two forms, black and white. Both forms are obtained from the dried berries of the same tropical vine, but they differ in the manner of processing.

Herbs and spices lose their true bouquet and flavor after six months of shelf life. They should be stored in tightly covered containers away from heat and light so that they will not become dry and stale.

Liquid extracts, including vanilla, almond, and fruit extracts (such as lemon and orange), should be stored in a cool, dry place so as not to develop off-flavors or aromas. They must be tightly capped to prevent evaporation.

SEEDS

Seeds are the ripened ovules of plants. The most important nutritive elements of seeds are the B-complex vitamins; vitamins A, D, and E; unsaturated fats; proteins; phosphorus; calcium; and a trace of fluorine.

Edible seeds such as pumpkin seeds, sesame seeds, and sunflower seeds are rich in protein; the B complex; vitamins A, D, and E; phosphorus; calcium; iron; fluorine; iodine; potassium; magnesium; zinc; and unsaturated fatty acids. Sesame seeds are high in calcium content. Sunflower seeds contain up to 50 percent protein.

Seeds have a variety of uses and may be eaten raw, dried, roasted, or cooked. Pumpkin, sesame, and sunflower seeds are popular snack foods, and others, such as caraway, dill, poppy, and anise, are used as seasonings. Seeds can be especially nutritious additions to soups, salads, casseroles, and baked goods. Sunflower-seed oil may be extracted for use in cooking and baking.

Unhulled seeds have a long shelf life, provided they are kept in a cool, dry place in a tightly covered container. Hulled seeds should be refrigerated immediately and used promptly because oxidation of their fat content may make them rancid.

SWEETENERS

Sugars and other concentrated sweets furnish quick energy to the body in readily digestible form. Cane and beet sugars, jellies, jams, candy, syrup, molasses, and honey are concentrated sources of sugar. Fruits are a natural source of sugar and furnish bulk in the diet.

Sugar is a major carbohydrate source but is completely devoid of protein, vitamins, and minerals and is not considered nutritious. Refined white sugar, in granulated or powdered form, and brown sugar are made from either sugar cane or sugar beet. White sugar contains no vitamins or minerals. The B vitamins needed for its assimilation must be obtained from other sources, either foods or supplements. Sugar leads to an imbalance in the calcium-phosphorus relationship. Sugar may also be a contributing factor in the development of overweight,

diabetes, arthritis, tooth decay, pyorrhea, asthma, mental illness, nervous disorders, and low blood sugar. Natural sources of sugar, such as fruits, usually contain adequate supplies of vitamins essential for digestion and metabolism. Brown sugar has a slightly higher nutritive value than white sugar.

Artificial Sweeteners

Certain sugar-substitute sweetening agents may be employed by diabetics or persons who must reduce their caloric intake. Saccharine and sorbitol are sugar substitutes that have little energy, or caloric, value.

Carob

Carob is a natural sweetener rich in B vitamins and minerals with a flavor similar to that of chocolate. It is often used as a substitute for chocolate or cocoa, especially by people who are allergic to chocolate or who wish to avoid the caffeine it contains. Carob also contains a fair amount of protein, sugar, and some calcium and phosphorus. It is available in tablet, powder, syrup, and wafer forms.

Chocolate and Cocoa

Chocolate, cocoa, and foods flavored with these substances from the cocoa bean are usually prepared with large amounts of sugar that add carbohydrates to the diet while adding no significant amounts of vitamins and minerals. Chocolate and cocoa contain two stimulants, caffeine and theobromine, which speed up the heartbeat and stimulate the central nervous system. Chocolate also contains oxalic acid, an excess of which could interfere with calcium absorption. Cocoa is lower in fat than chocolate and therefore will keep for longer periods of time. It is slightly higher in nutritive value than chocolate.

Honey

Honey is one of Nature's finest energy-giving foods, consisting of carbohydrates in the most easily digestible form. Honey varies in texture, flavor, and color, depending upon place of origin and the flowers from which the nectar was gathered. Because honey is almost twice as sweet as cane or beet sugar, smaller amounts of it are needed for sweetening purposes. Honey contains large amounts of carbohydrates in the form of sugars, small amounts of minerals, and traces of the B-complex vitamins and vitamins C, D, and E.

Molasses

Molasses is a thick, sticky syrup, light to dark brown in color, with a strong, distinctive flavor. Blackstrap molasses is the residue left after the last possible extraction of sugar from the cane or beet (see "Blackstrap Molasses," p. 194). Ordinary molasses is a good mineral and vitamin source, rich in iron, calcium, copper, magnesium, phosphorus, pantothenic acid, inositol, vitamin E, and the B vitamins.

VEGETABLES

Vegetables are composed primarily of carbohydrates and water and contain very little protein. Vegetables also provide vitamins, minerals, and bulk to the diet and contribute appetite appeal through color, texture, and flavor. In general, light-green vegetables provide vitamins, minerals, and a large amount of the carbohydrate cellulose, necessary to provide bulk in the diet. Yellow and dark-green vegetables are excellent sources of vitamin A. Vegetable leaves are usually rich in calcium, iron, magnesium, vitamin C, and many of the B vitamins. The greener the leaf, the richer it will be in nutrients. Potatoes are relatively high in protein and are excellent sources of vitamin A, vitamin C, niacin, thiamine, and riboflavin as well as iron and calcium. A medium-size potato contains about 90 calories.

Vegetables are commonly available in fresh, frozen, canned, or dried forms. Fresh raw vegetables generally contain more vitamins and minerals than the processed products, although quick-freezing causes almost no nutrient loss. Properly canned vegetables usually contain as many vitamins and minerals as home-cooked fresh vegetables, but dried vegetables show a considerably greater loss of nutrients.

Before being eaten or cooked, fresh vegetables should be thoroughly washed so that chemical sprays and dirt are removed. The vegetable skins should be left on or pared as thinly as possible, so that the vitamins and minerals are preserved. Cooking time should be kept to a minimum when vegetables are boiled in water so that

nutrients are conserved and flavor is retained. Baked vegetables will have a higher concentration of nutrients than boiled vegetables.

VEGETABLE JUICES

Fresh vegetable juices are an excellent source of minerals and vitamins. Juices from dark-green and yellow vegetables are especially high in vitamin A. People who want a change from raw or cooked vegetables may find juices appealing and easy to digest. Vegetable juices may also be the preferred form for persons suffering from disorders of the digestive system.

BEVERAGES

Beverages such as alcohol, coffee, cola, and tea add little nutritive value to the diet, except for water. However, milk drinks and fruit and vegetable juices contribute fair amounts of protein, fat, vitamins, and minerals to the diet.

ALCOHOLIC BEVERAGES

Alcoholic beverages may be those produced by fermentation only, such as ale, beer and most wines, and those that are distilled, such as whiskey. Alcoholic beverages supply little to the diet except calories. (See "Alcoholism," p. 109.)

CARBONATED BEVERAGES

Carbonated beverages are high in sugar content and have no nutritional value whatsoever. In order to hold the sugar in suspension and keep it from crystallizing, all soft drinks contain acid, usually orthophosphoric or citric, which eats away tooth enamel and can impair the appetite and the stomach. Certain soft drinks, especially cola, contain large amounts of caffeine, which stimulates the metabolism and leads to depletion of valuable nutrients in the body.

COFFEE

Coffee is produced from the coffee bean. It contains no nutrients but does contain caffeine. Coffee quickens the respiration process, strengthens the pulse, raises the blood pressure, stimulates the kidneys, excites the functions of the brain, and temporarily relieves fatigue or depression. If consumed in excess, coffee can cause increased nervous symptoms, aggravate heart and artery disorders, and irritate the lining of the stomach. It may also create inositol and biotin deficiencies, prevent iron from being properly utilized, and cause other vitamins to be pumped through and out of the body before they can be properly absorbed.

Coffee substitutes are powdered vegetable preparations that are used as coffee alternatives. They usually have barley or chicory-root bases and contain no caffeine.

TEA

Tea is similar to coffee in that it contains caffeine; it contains tannin, or tannic acid, and essential oils as well. The caffeine is the stimulating element; the tannin gives it its color and body; the oils give it flavor and aroma. Tannin in its concentrated form has had harmful effects on the mucous membrane of the mouth and the digestive tract, but it is generally believed that tannin does not occur in significant enough amounts in tea to be harmful. Tea actually has little nutritive value with the exception of its fluoride content. Herbal teas are preferred to commercial teas because of their therapeutic value, depending upon the herbs used in brewing the tea.

SUPPLEMENTARY FOODS

Supplementary foods may be useful for individuals who wish to increase the nutritional value of their meals. Supplements may be in the form of tablets, liquids, powders, syrups, capsules, granules, or bars; various forms may have differing nutrient characteristics. *Any*

information concerning ailments is not meant to be prescriptive, but merely represents research findings.

ALFALFA

Alfalfa is a leguminous plant that is particularly rich in vitamin K and calcium and contains significant amounts of nearly every other vitamin and mineral. The seeds, sprouts, and leaves of the plant are edible but are also available in the form of tablets, powder, or tea.

BLACKSTRAP MOLASSES

Blackstrap molasses is a truly rich source of minerals and vitamins. As the last possible extraction of the cane in refining sugar, it is the richest in nutrients of the sugar-related products. It contains more calcium than milk, more iron than many eggs, and more potassium than any food, and it is an excellent source of B vitamins. It is also rich in copper, magnesium, phosphorus, pantothenic acid, inositol, and vitamin E. One tablespoon of blackstrap molasses contains 3 milligrams of iron and over 100 milligrams of calcium. It is also a good source of natural sugar. Recommended daily dosage is one tablespoon dissolved in one cup lukewarm water or milk, one-half that amount is recommended for children. Molasses may be used as a sugar substitute in cereals and may be eaten instead of jam or jelly. Varicose veins, arthritis, ulcers, dermatitis, hair damage, eczema, psoriasis, angina pectoris, constipation, colitis, anemia, and nervous conditions may respond to supplementing the diet with this mineral-rich molasses.

BONE MEAL

Bone meal is a flourlike substance consisting of the finely ground bones of cattle. As a good supplemental source of calcium, bone meal is especially recommended for anyone whose milk intake must be limited. It also contains phosphorus and the trace minerals copper, manganese, nickel, and fluorine, which are essential for the complete nutrition of teeth and bones. Bone meal can usually be given safely in any dose. The recommended intake of bone meal is three tablets or an equivalent amount per day.

BREWER'S YEAST

Brewer's yeast is a nonleavening yeast that can be added to all foods to increase their nutritional value. Brewer's yeast is one of the best sources of B vitamins and minerals. It contains 16 amino acids, 14 minerals, and 17 vitamins. Brewer's yeast is high in phosphorus in relation to calcium; therefore, 8 ounces of skim milk or four tablespoons of dry powdered milk should be taken with every tablespoon of yeast. The recommended supplemental allowance of brewer's yeast is one tablespoon daily.

Wheat germ and brewer's yeast taken daily may be helpful in preventing heart trouble. Brewer's yeast may protect against toxicity of large does of vitamin D. It is used to prevent constipation and is a good source of enzyme-producing agents.

Brewer's yeast is one of the best sources of RNA, a nucleic acid that is important in keeping the body immune to the degenerative diseases, including dry and wrinkled skin and low resistance to diseases as age advances.

Brewer's yeast is available in powder, flake, and tablet forms.

DESICCATED LIVER

Desiccated liver is concentrated beef liver, in powder or tablet form, which has been dried in a vacuum at a low temperature so that most of the original nutrient value of liver is conserved. Desiccated-liver tablets, rich in vitamin A, vitamin C, vitamin D, iron, calcium, phosphorus, and copper, are recommended to supplement the diet if liver is not eaten once or twice a week. Desiccated liver may be combined with soups, baked goods, and other foods.

LECITHIN

Lecithin is a natural constituent of every cell of the human body and helps to emulsify cholesterol in the body. Lecithin is available both naturally in egg yolk, soybeans, and corn and as a supplement in capsule, liquid, and granule forms. Lecithin is high in phosphorus and unites with iron, iodine, and calcium to give power and vigor to the brain and aid in the digestion and absorption of fats. Lecithin also consists of ordinary fat, unsaturated fatty acids, and choline.

Lecithin may break up cholesterol and allow it to pass through arterial walls, helping to prevent atherosclerosis. It has also been found to increase immunity against virus infections and to prevent the formation of gallstones. Even distribution of body weight is also aided by lecithin. Lecithin plays an important part in maintaining a healthy nervous system and is found naturally in the myelin sheath, a fatty protective covering for the nerves. Lecithin also helps to cleanse the liver and purify the kidneys.

The National Research Council has not yet established a Recommended Dietary Allowance for lecithin, although it has been suggested that it should be taken daily. There are no known toxic levels for lecithin.

ROSE HIPS AND ACEROLA CHERRIES

Rose hips are the urn-shaped seeds at the base of rose blossoms. They are excellent sources of vitamin A, the B complex, vitamin E, vitamin K, and the bioflavonoids. They can be used either fresh or dried and can be made into tea, jam, syrup, or soup. Another small fruit, the acerola cherry, is a rich natural source of vitamin C and is frequently used together with rose hips to make organic vitamin C supplements. Rose hips and acerola cherries are available as a supplement in the forms of powder, syrup, tablets, and capsules.

SEAWEED

Seaweed is a vegetable from the ocean which is rich in minerals. Sea plants have an advantage over land crops because they grow in seawater, in which the minerals are constantly being renewed. Seaweed is rich in all necessary minerals. There are several varieties of seaweed, including kelp, nori, and Irish moss, all of which are salty in flavor. Kelp is one of the best natural sources of iodine; it is also rich in B-complex vitamins; vitamins D, E, and K; calcium; and magnesium. It is often used as a salt substitute and is available in dried, powdered, and tablet forms. Dulse is dark red in color and is rich in iodine. It can be used fresh in salads, but it should be soaked several times in water first. Seaweed is beneficial in maintaining the health of the mucous membranes and in treating arthritis, constipation, nervous disorders, rheumatism, colds, and skin irritations.

WHEAT GERM

Wheat germ is the heart of the kernel of wheat. It is an excellent source of protein (24 grams per one-half cup), B-complex vitamins, vitamin E, and iron. It also contains copper, magnesium, manganese, calcium, and phosphorus. It is high in phosphorus in relation to calcium, so 8 ounces of skim milk or 4 tablespoons of dry milk powder should be taken with every tablespoon of wheat germ. Wheat germ contains a vegetable oil and therefore should be tightly covered and refrigerated. Wheat-germ oil is extracted from wheat germ; it is a supplemental food high in unsaturated fatty acids and is one of the richest known sources of vitamin E.

SOME RICH SOURCES OF NUTRIENTS

CARBOHYDRATES
Whole grains
Sugar, syrup, and honey
Fruits
Vegetables

FATS
Butter and margarine
Vegetable oils
Fats in meats
Whole milk and milk products
Nuts and seeds

PROTEIN
Meats, fish, and poultry
Soybean products
Eggs
Milk and milk products
Whole grains

WATER
Beverages
Fruits
Vegetables

VITAMIN A
Liver
Eggs
Yellow fruits and vegetables
Dark-green fruits and vegetables

Whole milk and milk products
Fish-liver oil*

VITAMIN B$_1$
Brewer's yeast
Whole grains
Blackstrap molasses
Brown rice
Organ meats
Meats, fish, and poultry
Egg yolks
Legumes
Nuts

VITAMIN B$_2$
Brewer's yeast
Whole grains
Blackstrap molasses
Organ meats
Egg yolks
Legumes
Nuts

VITAMIN B$_6$
Meats
Whole grains
Organ meats
Brewer's yeast
Blackstrap molasses
Wheat germ
Legumes

Green leafy vegetables
Desiccated liver*

VITAMIN B$_{12}$
Organ meats
Fish and pork
Eggs
Cheese
Milk and milk products

VITAMIN B$_{13}$
Root vegetables
Liquid whey

BIOTIN
Egg yolks
Liver
Unpolished rice
Brewer's yeast
Whole grains
Sardines
Legumes

CHOLINE
Egg yolks
Organ meats
Brewer's yeast
Wheat germ
Soybeans
Fish
Legumes
Lecithin*

FOLIC ACID
Dark-green leafy vegetables
Organ meats
Brewer's yeast
Root vegetables
Whole grains
Oysters
Salmon
Milk

INOSITOL
Whole grains
Citrus fruits
Brewer's yeast
Molasses
Meat
Milk
Nuts
Vegetables
Lecithin*

LAETRILE
Whole kernels of apricots, apples, cherries, peaches, and plums

NIACIN
Lean meats
Poultry and fish
Brewer's yeast
Peanuts

*Denotes the supplemental form.

Milk and milk products
Rice bran
Desiccated liver*

PARA-AMINOBENZOIC ACID

Organ meats
Wheat germ
Yogurt
Molasses
Green leafy vegetables

PANGAMIC ACID

Brewer's yeast
Rare steaks
Brown rice
Sunflower, pumpkin, and sesame seeds

PANTOTHENIC ACID

Organ meats
Brewer's yeast
Egg yolks
Legumes
Whole grains
Wheat germ
Salmon

VITAMIN C

Citrus fruits
Rose hips
Acerola cherries
Alfalfa seeds, sprouted
Cantaloupe
Strawberries
Broccoli
Tomatoes
Green peppers

VITAMIN D

Salmon
Sardines
Herring
Vitamin D–fortified milk and milk products
Egg yolks
Organ meats

Fish-liver oils*
Bone meal*

VITAMIN E

Cold-pressed oils
Eggs
Wheat germ
Organ meats
Molasses
Sweet potatoes
Leafy vegetables
Desiccated liver*

VITAMIN F

Vegetable oils
Butter
Sunflower seeds

VITAMIN K

Green leafy vegetables
Egg yolks
Safflower oil
Blackstrap molasses
Cauliflower
Soybeans

BIOFLAVONOIDS

Citrus fruits
Fruits
Black currants
Buckwheat

CALCIUM

Milk and milk products
Green leafy vegetables
Shellfish
Molasses
Bone meal*
Dolomite*

CHLORINE

Table salt
Seafood
Meats
Ripe olives
Rye flour

Dulse*

CHROMIUM

Corn oil
Clams
Whole-grain cereals
Brewer's yeast

COBALT

Organ meats
Oysters
Clams
Poultry
Milk
Green leafy vegetables
Fruits

COPPER

Organ meats
Seafood
Nuts
Legumes
Molasses
Raisins
Bone meal*

FLUORIDE

Tea
Seafood
Fluoridated water
Bone meal*

IRON

Organ meats and meats
Eggs
Fish and poultry
Blackstrap molasses
Cherry juice
Green leafy vegetables
Dried fruits
Desiccated liver*

MAGNESIUM

Seafood
Whole grains

Dark-green vegetables
Molasses
Nuts
Bone meal*

MANGANESE

Whole grains
Green leafy vegetables
Legumes
Nuts
Pineapples
Egg yolks

MOLYBDENUM

Legumes
Whole-grain cereals
Milk
Liver
Dark-green vegetables

PHOSPHORUS

Fish, meats, and poultry
Eggs
Legumes
Milk and milk products
Nuts
Whole-grain cereals
Bone meal*

POTASSIUM

Lean meats
Whole grains
Vegetables
Dried fruits
Legumes
Sunflower seeds

SELENIUM

Tuna
Herring
Brewer's yeast
Wheat germ and bran
Broccoli
Whole grains

*Denotes the supplemental form.

SODIUM
Seafood
Table salt
Baking power and baking
soda
Celery

Processed foods
Milk products
Kelp*

SULFUR
Fish

Eggs
Meats
Cabbage
Brussel sprouts

VANADIUM
Fish

ZINC
Sunflower seeds
Seafood
Organ meats
Mushrooms
Brewer's yeast
Soybeans

SECTION VII

Table of Food Composition

The foods in this table have been divided according to food groups and similar types of foods that do not belong to any one group. The chart runs alphabetically according to food groups, with the items in each group also being alphabetized. The first group analyzed is Beverages; the second is Breads, Flours, Cereals, Grains, and Grain Products, and so on. If you are unable to locate a particular food in a group, this does not necessarily mean that it has not been included. Check the Index in the back of the book, and look for the name indicated by an asterik.

Food values have been calculated so as to permit easy computation. All figures are, of necessity, averages of different food samples. *The blank spaces on the chart do not indicate an absence of a particular nutrient, but rather that meaningful analysis of the food for that nutrient is lacking.* Only the zero confirms the absence of a nutrient.

There are three major factors that influence the nutrient content of foods—first, the inherent characteristics of the plant or animal; second, environmental conditions affecting the plant or animal; and third, the method of handling, processing, and cooking the plant or animal material. The content of trace minerals such as selenium, copper, and zinc depends on the soil in which they are grown and where they are grown, and will therefore vary significantly in foods from area to area.

Vitamin E values have been given in milligrams. To approximate the value in IUs, multiply milligrams by 1.5. For example, if 3 milligrams of vitamin E are present, multiply 3 by 1.5, which makes 4.5 IU of vitamin E.

See page 234 for the abbreviations and symbols used in the chart.

CONTENTS: TABLE OF FOOD COMPOSITION

Beverages	200
Breads, Flours, Cereals, Grains, and Grain Products	200
Dairy Products	204
Desserts and Sweets	206
Fish, Seafood, and Seaweed	210
Fruits and Fruit Juices	212
Meat and Poultry	216
Nuts, Nut Products, and Seeds	220
Oils, Fats, and Shortening	222
Salad Dressings and Sauces	222
Soups	222
Spices and Herbs	224
Vegetables, Legumes, Sprouts, and Vegetable Juices	226

Food Item	Measure	Weight g	Calories	Carbohydrate g	Protein g	Fiber g	Saturated fat g	Unsaturated fat g	Total fat g	Cholesterol mg	Vitamin A IU	Vitamin B₁ mg	Vitamin B₂ mg	Vitamin B₆ mg
BEVERAGES														
Alcoholic														
Beer, 4.5% alcohol	1 cup	240	101	9.1	.72				0			.01	.07	.2
Daiquiri	3.5 oz	100	122	5.2	.1							.014	.001	
Gin, rum, vodka, whiskey, 86 proof	1 oz	28	70	t	0				0		0	0	0	
Martini	3.5 oz	100	140	.3	.1						4	t	t	
Tom Collins	10 oz	300	180	9	.3						0	.03	t	
Wines														
Sweet, 18.8% alcohol	1 cup	240	329	18.4	.24				0			.02	.05	.1
Dry, 12.2% alcohol	1 cup	240	204	9.6	.24				0			t	.02	.1
Common														
Club soda	1 cup	240	0	0	0	0			0		0	0	0	
Coffee, clear	1 cup	240	5	.8	.3	0			.1		0	.02	.02	t
Cola drinks	1 cup	240	94	19	0				0		0	0	0	
Fruit-flavored drinks	1 cup	240	110	29	0	0			0		0	0	0	
Diet drinks	1 cup	240	t		0	0			0		0	0	0	
Ginger ale	1 cup	240	74	19	0	0			0		0	0	0	
Root beer	1 cup	240	98	25	0	0			0		0	0	0	
Tea, clear	1 cup	240	4	.9	.1	t			t		0	0	.04	
BREADS, FLOURS, CEREALS, GRAINS, AND GRAIN PRODUCTS														
Barley														
Pearled, pot or Scotch, dry	1 cup	200	696	154	19.2	2.14	.48	1.52	2.2		0	.42	.14	
Pearled, light, dry	1 cup	200	698	158	16.4	.7	t	2	2		0	.24	.1	.448
Bran, wheat, raw	1 cup	57	121	35.4	9	5.2	.42	1.76	2.6		0	.41	.2	.468
Bran flakes, 40%, fortified	1 cup	35	106	28.2	3.6	1			.6		1650	.41	.49	.134
Bulgur (parboiled wheat), dry	1 cup	170	602	129	19	3	.34	1.48	2.5		0	.48	.24	.38
Breads														
Biscuit, enr.	2″ diam	28	103	12.8	2.1	.1	1	3	4.8		t	.06	.06	
Cornbread, whl grd	2″ sq	45	93	13.1	3.3	.2	.81	2.25	3.2	30	68	.06	.09	
Cracked wheat, enr	1 slice	23	60	12	2	.1	.1	.4	.6		t	.03	.02	.02
Cracked wheat, enr, toasted	1 slice	19	60	11.8	2	.1	.1	.4	.6		t	.02	.02	
English muffin, enr[1]	1 avg	130	27	4				1			t	.23	.136	
French or Vienna, enr	1 slice	20	58	11.1	1.8	t	.14	.45	.64		t	.06	.04	.01
Italian, enr	1 slice	20	55	11.3	1.8	t	t	.17	.3			.06	.05	
Pita, whole wheat, sesame	1 avg	42.5	140	24	6				2		t	.2	.068	
Pumpernickel	1 slice	32	79	17	2.9	.4			.4			.07	.04	.05
Raisin, enr	1 slice	23	60	12.3	1.5	.2	.18	.46	.64		t	.01	.02	
Rye, American	1 slice	23	56	12	2.1	.1			.3			.04	.02	.02
White, enr	1 slice	23	62	11.6	2	t	.16	.53	.79		t	.06	.05	.009
White, enr, toasted	1 slice	20	62	11.6	2	t	.1	.5	.7		t	.05	.05	
Whole wheat	1 slice	23	56	11	2.4	.4	.11	.42	.7		t	.06	.02	.04
Whole wheat, toasted	1 slice	19	55	11	2.4	.4	.1	.4	.7		t	.04	.02	
Breadcrumbs, enr, dry	1 cup	100	392	73.4	12.6	.3	1	3	4.6		t	.22	.3	
Buns (hamburger, hot dog), enr	1 avg	40	119	21.2	3.3		.5	1.6	2.2		t	.11	.07	
Cornflakes, fortified	1 cup	25	97	21	2				.1		1180	.29	.35	.016
Corn-grits (hominy), degermed, enr, ckd	1 cup	245	125	27	2.9	.2	.03	.17	.25		150[2]	.1	.07	t
Corn meal, whl grd, dry	1 cup	118	427	88	10.6	1.2	.46	3	4		566[2]	.35	.09	.29
Corn meal, degermed, enr, ckd	1 cup	238	119	25.5	2.4	.2	.05	.33	.5		142[2]	.14	.1	
Cornstarch	1 tbsp	8	29	7	t	t	t	.04	.05		0	0	.006	t
Crackers														
Graham, plain	1 lg	14.2	55	10.4	1.1	.22	.3	.9	1.3		0	.01	.03	
RyKrisp, Ralston	2 avg	12.6	42	9.6	1.6	.3			.15			.04	.03	
Soda	1 avg	2.8	12.5	2	.26	.008	.075	.225	.37		0	t	.001	
Soup or oyster	10	7.5	33	5.3	.7				1		0	t	t	
Whole wheat, Ak-Mak	4 pieces	28	117	18.9	4.64				2.33		14	.06	.04	
Zwieback	1 piece	7	31	5.4	.9	.02	.2	.4	.6		3	.004	.005	

[1] Thomas'.

[2] Based on yellow corn; the white variety has only a trace.

[3] No added salt. Added salt specified by manufacturer is 264 mg/cup cornmeal; 708 mg/cup cream of wheat; 353 mg/cup farina; 523 mg/cup oatmeal; 519 mg/cup wheat-meal cereal.

Vitamin B₁₂ mcg	Biotin mcg	Folic Acid mg	Niacin mg	Pantothenic Acid mg	Vitamin C mg	Vitamin E mg	Sodium mg	Phosphorus mg	Potassium mg	Calcium mg	Iron mg	Magnesium mg	Copper mg	Manganese mg	Selenium mg	Zinc mg
0	t		1.44	.19			17	72	60	12	t		.3		.46	.07
	t				8			3		4	.1					
			0		0		t	0	1	0	0					
	t							1		5	.1					
	t				21			6		6	t					
0			.48	.07			10		184	16		24		.72		
0		.002	.24	.07			12	24	221	22	.96	12	.3	.72	12	.24
			0		0		59	t								
0			.9	.008	0		2.3	5	83	4.6	.23	21.8	.05	.22	.3	.05
			0		0		2									.05
			0		0		18									
			0		0											.02
			0		0		18		.1							
			0		0		18									.02
			.1		1		1.6	4	58	5	.2	8	1.13	1.66	.1	.04
0		.04	7.4		0			580	592	68	5.4	71.4				
0			6.2	1	0		6	378	320	32	4	71.4	.8	3.36		
0		.147	12	1.65	0		5.13	727	639	67.8	8.49	279	.9		35.9	5.59
0		.04	4.1	.31	12		207	125	137	19	12.4		.213			1.26
0		7.7	7.8	1.12	0			575	389	49	6.3					
			.5		t		175	49	33	34	.4					
			.3		t		283	95	71	54	.5					
0		.01	.3	.14	t		122	29	31	20	.3	8				
			.3		t		120	29	30	20	.2	8				
			2		t					20	1.08		.1			
0		.002	.5	.08	t		116	17	18	9	.4	4				
			.5	.1	t		117	15	15	3	.4					.01
			2.4		t					40	1.8					
0			.4	.16			182	73	145	27	.8	23				.365
			.2		t		84	20	54	16	.3	6				
0		.006	.3	.1			128	34	33	17	.4	10	.06	.3		.4
t	.2	.009	.6	.1	t	.23	117	22	24	20	.6	5	.05	.07	6.44	.2
			.6		t		117	22	24	19	.5	5	.03			
0	.46	.013	.6	.174	t	.3	121	52	63	23	.5	18	.06		15.5	.5
			.6		t		119	52	62	22	.5	18				
			3.5		t		736	141	152	122	3.6		.2			.38
			.9		t		202	34	38	30	.8	14				.21
0		.003	2.9	.048	9		251	9	30	1–7	.6	3	.043	.012	.6	.08
0			1				502	25	27	2	.7	7				
0	t	.019	2.2	.65			1	263	293	20	2.1	125	.156			2.1
0			1.2			.354	t[3]	33	38	2	1	16				.3
			.002		0		.32	2.4		.32	0		.04	.16	.004	
			.2		0		95	21	55	6	.2	5.68	.03			
			.15				111	49		7	.5		.042			
0			.03		0	.1	31	2.5	3.4	.6	.04	.81	.001			
			.1		0		83	7	9	2	.1					
	3.29	.012	1.05	.18	1.6	.33		.01		21.3	.45	41	.08			.9
			.1				18.2	5.04	11		.95	.04				

Food Item	Measure	Weight g	Calories	Carbohy-drate g	Protein g	Fiber g	Satu-rated fat g	Unsatu-rated fat g	Total fat g	Choles-terol mg	Vitamin A IU	Vitamin B₁ mg	Vitamin B₂ mg	Vitamin B₆ mg
Cream of wheat, ckd	1 cup	200	133	28.2	4.5	.1			4		0	.11	.07	
Farina, enr, ckd	1 cup	245	103	21.3	3.2	.2	.074	.25	.49		0	.1	.07	
Flour														
Buckwheat, dark, sftd	1 cup	100	333	72	11.7	1.6	.47	1.76	2.5		0	.58	.15	.578
Buckwheat, light, sftd	1 cup	100	347	79.5	6.4	.5	.24	.83	1.2		0	.08	.04	
Carob (St. John's bread)	1 tbsp	8	14	6.5	.4	.64			.1					
Corn	1 cup	117	431	89.9	9.1		.35	2.34	3		400	.23	.07	
Gluten, wheat	1 cup	140	529	66.1	58	.6			2.7		0			
Pastry, wheat, sftd	1 cup	100	364	79.4	7.5	.2			.8		0	.03	.03	.045
Peanut, defatted	1 cup	60	223	18.9	28.7	1.62	1.2	4	5.5			.45	.13	
Potato	1 cup	110	386	87.9	8.8	1.76			.88		t	.46	.15	.008
Rice, granulated	1 cup	125	479	107	7.5	.2			.4		0	.52	.14	.2
Rye, dark, sftd	1 cup	128	419	87.2	20.9	3.07	.42	1	3.3			.78	.28	.384
Rye, light, sftd	1 cup	80	286	62.3	7.5	.3			.8			.12	.05	.07
Soy, full-fat, stirred	1 cup	72	303	21.9	26.4	1.7	2.5	10.6	14.2		79	.61	.22	.48
Soy, low-fat, stirred	1 cup	100	356	36.6	43.4	2.5	1.02	4.88	6.7		80	.83	.36	.68
Soy, defatted, stirred	1 cup	138	450	52.6	64.9	3.2	1.17	23	2.76		55	1.5	.47	1
Wheat, all purpose, sftd	1 cup	110	400	83.7	11.6	.3			1.1		0	.07	.06	.066
Wheat, all purpose, enr, sftd	1 cup	110	400	83.7	11.6	.3			1.1		0	.48	.28	.066
Wheat, whole, stirred	1 cup	120	400	85.2	16	2.8	t	2	2.4		0	.66	.14	.41
Granola[4]	1 cup	85	390	57	9				15			.09	.034	
Macaroni, enr, ckd	1 cup	140	151	32.2	4.8	.1			1		0	.2	.11	.029
Millet, whl grain, dry	1 cup	228	746	166	22.6	7.3	1.96	4.1	6.8		0	1.66	.87	
Muffins														
Plain, enr	1 avg	40	118	16.9	3.1	.1	1	3	4		40	.07	.09	
Bran, enr	1 avg	40	104	17.2	3.1	.72	1.2	2.4	3.9		90	.06	.1	
Corn meal, whl grd	1 med	45	130	19.1	3.2	.2	2.3	2.2	4.6		140	.08	.08	
Whole wheat	1 avg	40	103	20.9	4	.6			1.1		t	.14	.05	
Noodles, egg, enr, ckd	1 cup	160	200	37.3	6.6	.2	1	1	2.4	50	112	.22	.13	.04
Oat flakes, fortified	1 cup	37	147	26.7	6.67	.5			2.1			.5	.57	.67
Oatmeal (rolled oats), ckd	1 cup	240	132	23.3	4.8	.5	.4	1.76	2.4		0	.19	.05	.024
Pancakes														
Plain, enr	4″ diam	27	62	9.2	1.9	.1	.5	1.3	1.9		30	.05	.06	
Buckwheat, from mix	4″ diam	27	54	6.4	1.8	.2	.8	1.5	2.5		60	.03	.04	
Whole wheat[5]	4″ diam	45	74	8.8	3.4				3.2		80	.09	.07	
Pasta, whole wheat, dry[6]	4 oz	113	400	78	20				1		200	.6	.85	
Pizza, cheese, 14″ diam	⅛	65	153	18.4	7.8	.2	2	3	5.4		410	.04	.13	
Popcorn, plain	1 cup	14	54	10.7	1.8	.3	t	.6	.7			.055	.02	.03
Pretzel, twisted	1 avg	16	62	12.1	1.6	.05			.7		0	.003	.008	.003
Rice														
Brown, raw	1 cup	196	704	152	14.8	1.6			3.6		0	.68	.08	1
Brown, ckd w/salt	1 cup	150	178	38.2	3.8	.45	.31	.94	1.2		0	.14	.03	
Instant, enr, ckd w/salt	1 cup	165	180	39.9	3.6	.1			t		0	.21		
Parboiled, enr, ckd w/salt	1 cup	175	186	40.8	3.7	.2	.1	.24	.4		0	.19	.02	
White, ckd w/salt	1 cup	205	223	49.6	4.1	.2	.1	.24	.4		0	.04	.02	
White, enr, dry	1 cup	195	708	157	13.1	.4	.4	.9	1.5		0	.86	.06	.3
White, enr, ckd w/salt	1 cup	205	223	49.6	4.1	.2	.1	.24	.4		0	.23	.02	
Wild, raw	1 cup	160	565	121	22.6	.12			1.1		0	.72	1.01	
Rice, puffed, fortified w/o salt, sugar	1 cup	15	60	13.4	.9	.1			.1		0	.07	.01	.01
Rice polish or bran	1 cup	105	278	60.6	12.7	2.4	2.44	9.34	12.8		0	1.93	.19	
Rolls														
Danish, enr	1 avg	42	179	19.4	3.1	t	3.25	6.5	10		130	.03	.06	
Dinner, enr	1 avg	38	113	20.1	3.1	.1	.54	1.49	2.2		t	.11	.07	
Hard, enr	1 avg	50	156	29.8	4.9	.1	.28	.77	1.6		t	.13	.12	
Whole wheat	1 avg	35	90	18.3	3.5	.6			1		t	.12	.05	
Shredded wheat, biscuit	1 avg	25	89	20	2.5	.5	.09	.38	.5		0	.06	.03	.06
Spaghetti, enr, ckd	1 cup	140	155	32.2	4.8	.2			.6		0	.2	.11	
Tapioca, dry	1 cup	152	535	131	.9	.15			.3		0	0	.15	
Tortilla, yellow corn	6″ diam	30	63	13.5	1.5	.3			.6		6	.04	.015	.022

[4]Nature Valley; made with oats, brown sugar, honey, and sesame seeds.
[5]25% soya powder; prepared with egg, milk, and oil.
[6]Erewhon; made with 96% durum flour and 4% vegetable flour.

Vitamin B₁₂ mcg	Biotin mcg	Folic Acid mg	Niacin mg	Pantothenic Acid mg	Vitamin C mg	Vitamin E mg	Sodium mg	Phosphorus mg	Potassium mg	Calcium mg	Iron mg	Magnesium mg	Copper mg	Manganese mg	Selenium mg	Zinc mg
			.85		0		3.7³	110		13	1.4	8				
0			1.3		0		2³	29	22	10	2–12	8	.25			.2
0			2.9	1.5	0		1	347	656	33	5		.7	2.09		
			.4		0		1	88	320	11	1	48				
								6		28	.33					
			1.6		0		1	92		7	2.1					
					0		3	196	84	56						
0			.7	.32	0		2	73	95	17	.5	26				.3
			16.7		0		5	432	712	62	2.1	216				
0			3.74		19		37.4	196	1747	36.3	18.9					
0			7.2		0			120		11	6.8	35				
0			3.5	1.7	0		1	686	1101	69	5.8	147	.54			
0		.069	.5	.58	0		1	148	125	18	.9	58	.3			
0	49	.311	1.5	1.22	0		1	402	1195	143	6	178				
0			2.6	2.08	0		1	634	1859	263	9.1	289				
0			3.6	3.06	0		1	904	2512	366	15.3	428				
0	1.1	.024	1	.51	0	1.87	2	96	105	18	.9	28	.21		21.7	.77
0	1.1	.024	3.9	.51	0	1.87	2	96	105	18	3.2	28	.21		21.7	.77
0	6	.065	5.2	1.32	0	3.12	4	446	444	49	4	136	.6		77.4	2.88
			t					80		20	1.08	32	.08			.6
0			1.5		0		1³	70	85	11	1.2	25	.028			.7
			5.24		0	4		709	980	45.6	15.5	369				
			.6		t		176	60	50	42	.6	11				
			1.6		t		179	162	172	57	1.5					
			.5		t		223	97	59	50	.6	48				
			1.2		t		226	112	117	42	1	45				
t			1.9		0		3³	94	70	16	1.4		.27			
2		.13	3.2			.09	420	133	133	53	3.1	53.7	.274	1.81		
0			.2	.236	0		.8³	137	146	22	1.4	50	.07			1.18
			.4		t		115	38	33	27	.4	6.59	.02			.37
			.2		t		125	91	66	59	.4	13.2				
			.4		t					50	.54					
			8		10.8			400		20	5.4					
			.7		5		456	127	85	144	.7					.79
0			.3		0		t	39	33.6	2	.4		.04			.574
t			.1	.09	0	t	269	21	21	4	.2		.024			.173
0	18	.032	9.2	2.1	0	3	16	432	420	64	3.2	172	.4	3.2	77.2	3.6
			2.1		0		423	110	105	18	.8	45				.9
			1.7		0		450	31	t	5	1.3					.33
			2.1		0		627	100	75	33	1.4		.47			.526
			.8		0		767	57	57	21	.4	12	.04			.8
0	5.86	.02	6.8	1.26	0	.7	10	183	179	47	5.7	13	.2	2.1	65.1	2.5
			2.1		0		767	57	57	21	1.8	12	.04			.8
0			9.9	1.63	0		11	542	352	30	6.7	144				
0		.003	.7	.049	0		t	14	15	3	.3		.051		.403	.18
		.039	29.6		0		t	1161	750	72	16.9					
			.3		t		156	46	48	21	.4	8				35
			.8		t		192	32	36	28	.7	14				.46
			1.4		t		313	46	49	24	1.2	8				.4
			1.1		t		197	98	102	37	.8	40				
0		.011	1.1	.155	0		1	97	87	11	.9	33			1.1	.62
0			1.5		0		1³	70	85	11	1.3	27				
		.012	0		0		5	27	27	15	.6	3	.14	1.04		
0			.3	.016	0			42		60	.9	32				

Food Item	Measure	Weight g	Calories	Carbohydrate g	Protein g	Fiber g	Saturated fat g	Unsaturated fat g	Total fat g	Cholesterol mg	Vitamin A IU	Vitamin B_1 mg	Vitamin B_2 mg	Vitamin B_6 mg
Waffles, plain, enr	5½" diam	75	209	28.1	7	.1	2	5	7.4		248	.13	.19	
Wheat germ														
Raw	1 cup	100	363	46.7	26.6	2.5	1.88	8.18	10.9	0	2	.68	.92	
Toasted[7]	1 cup	96	368	48	29	1.7	1.59	8	11.2		110	1.76	.8	1.1
Wheat flakes, fortified	1 cup	30	106	24.2	3.1	.5	.11	.47	.72		1410	.35	.42	.088
Wheat, puffed, fortified w/o sugar, salt	1 cup	15	54	11.8	2.3	.2			.2		0	.08	.03	.02
Wheatmeal cereal														
Dry	1 cup	125	423	90.4	16.9	.75	.325	.94	2.75		0	.64	.16	.489
Cooked	1 cup	245	110	23	4.4				.7		0	.15	.05	
DAIRY PRODUCTS														
Cheese														
American, pasteurized, processed	1 oz	28	107	.5	6.5	0	5.58	2.82	8.86	27	340	.006	.11	.02
Blue	1 oz	28	103	.66	6	0	5.3	2.44	8.15	21	204	.008	.108	.047
Brick	1 oz	28	103	.79	6.59	0	5.32	2.66	8.4	27	307	.004	.1	.018
Brie	1 oz	28	95	.13	5.88	0			7.85	28	189	.02	.147	.067
Camembert, domestic	1 oz	28	84	.5	5.6	0	4.33	2.19	6.9	20	262	.01	.21	.064
Cheddar, American	1 oz	28	112	.36	7	0	5.98	2.93	9.4	30	300	.008	.106	.021
Cheddar, American, grated, not packed	1 cup	113	455	1.45	28	0	23.8	11.7	37.4	119	1197	.03	.424	.084
Cheese spread, American, pasteurized, processed	1 oz	28	81	2.3	4.5	0	3.78	1.94	6	16	223	.003	.122	.033
Colby	1 oz	28	112	.73	6.74	0	5.73	2.9	9.1	27	293	.004	.106	.022
Cottage, creamed, not packed	1 cup	210	217	5.6	26.2	0	5.99	3	9.47	31	342	.044	.342	.141
Cottage, 2% fat, not packed	1 cup	226	203	8.2	31	0	2.76	1.37	4.36	19	158	.054	.418	.172
Cottage, dry, not packed	1 cup	145	123	2.68	25	0	.396	.182	.61	10	44	.036	.206	.119
Cream	1 oz	28	105	.6	2.2	0	5.88	3.64	10.6	31	430	.006	.06	.013
Edam	1 oz	28	101	.4	7.7	0	4.98	2.49	7.8	25	260	.01	.11	.022
Gjetost	1 oz	28	132	12.09	2.74	0	5.43	2.5	8.37					
Gouda	1 oz	28	101	.63	7.07	0	4.99	2.39	7.78	32	183	.009	.095	.023
Gruyere	1 oz	28	115	15	8.45	0	5.36	3.34	9.17	31	346	.017	.079	.023
Limberger	1 oz	28	93	.14	5.68	0	4.75	2.58	7.72	26	363	.023	.143	.024
Monterey	1 oz	28	106	.19	6.94	0			8.58		269		.11	
Mozzarella	1 oz	28	80	.63	5.51	0	3.73	2.08	6.12	22	225	.004	.069	.018
Mozzarella, part skim, low moisture	1 oz	28	79	.89	7.79	0	3.08	1.52	4.85	15	178	.006	.097	.022
Muenster	1 oz	28	104	.32	6.64	0	5.42	2.66	8.52	27	318	.004	.091	.016
Parmesan, hard	1 oz	28	110	.8	10	0	4.65	2.29	7.3	19	300	.011	.094	.026
Parmesan, grated	1 tbsp	5	23	.19	2.08	0	.95	.47	1.5	4	35	.002	.019	.005
Port du Salut	1 oz	28	100	.16	6.74	0	4.73	2.86	8	35	378		.068	.015
Provolone	1 oz	28	100	.61	7.25	0	4.84	2.32	7.55	20	231	.005	.091	.021
Ricotta, whl milk	1 cup	246	428	7.48	27.7	0	20.4	9.87	31.9	124	1205	.032	.40	.11
Ricotta, part skim	1 cup	246	340	12.6	28	0	12.1	6	19.5	9	1063	.052	.455	.049
Roquefort	1 oz	28	105	.57	6.1	0	5.46	2.77	8.69	26	297	.011	.166	.035
Swiss	1 oz	28	107	.96	8.06	0	5.04	2.34	7.78	26	240	.006	.103	.024
Swiss, pasteurized, processed	1 oz	28	95	.6	7.01	0	4.55	2.18	7.09	24	229	.004	.078	.01
Cheese souffle, cheddar	1 cup	95	207	5.9	9.4		8.57	6.67	16.2	159	760	.05	.23	
Cream														
Half and half	1 cup	242	315	10.4	7.16	0	17.3	9.07	27.8	89	1050	.085	.361	.094
Half and half	1 tbsp	15	20	.64	.44	0	1.07	.56	1.72	6	65	.005	.022	.006
Coffee or table	1 tbsp	15	29	.55	.4	0	1.8	.96	2.9	10	108	.005	.022	.005
Sour, cultured	1 cup	230	493	9.8	7.27	0	30	15.7	48.7	102	1817	.081	.343	.037
Whipping, lt	1 cup	239	699	7.07	5.19	0	46.2	23.8	73.9	265	2694	.057	.299	.067
Whipping, hvy	1 cup	238	821	6.64	4.88	0	54.8	28.7	88.1	326	3499	.052	.262	.062
Eggs														
Raw, ext lge	1	64	94	.5	7.4	0	2.18	2.67	7.24	351	680	.06	.17	.077
Raw, lge	1	57	82	.5	6.5	0	1.94	2.37	6.44	312	590	.05	.15	.068
Raw, med	1	50	72	.4	5.7	0	1.75	2.08	5.65	274	520	.05	.13	.06
Raw, sm	1	40	65	.4	5.2	0	1.36	1.66	4.5	219	470	.04	.12	.048

[7]Used mainly as a ready-to-eat cereal.

Vitamin B₁₂ mcg	Biotin mcg	Folic Acid mg	Niacin mg	Pantothenic Acid mg	Vitamin C mg	Vitamin E mg	Sodium mg	Phosphorus mg	Potassium mg	Calcium mg	Iron mg	Magnesium mg	Copper mg	Manganese mg	Selenium mg	Zinc mg
			1	.5	t		356	130	109	85	1.3	19				
		.328	4.2	2.2	0	15	3	1118	827	72	9.4	336	1.3		83.3	14.3
0		.42	4.8	1.15	10		2	1080	912	48	8					14.8
0			3.5		11		310	83	81	12	1.3		.132		3.3	.691
0			1.2		0		1	48	51	4	.6		.052			.312
			5.9				3	498	463	56	4.6	128	.32		30	4.5
			1.5		0		t³	127	118	17	1.2					
.197		.002	.02	.137	0	.28	406	216	46	174	.11	6	.017	.004	2.52	.85
.345		.01	.288	.490	0		396	110	73	150	.09	7	.011	.003		.75
.28		.006	.033	.081	0		159	127	38	191	.1	7	.007	.003		.74
.468		.018	.108	.196	0		178	53	43	52	.14					
.367	1	.018	.2	.387	0		239	98	53	110	.1	6	.022	.011		.68
.234	1	.005	.023	.117	0		176	145	28	211	.19	8	.031	.003		.88
.935		.021	.09	.467	0		701	579	111	815	.77	31				3.51
.113		.002	.037	.194	0		381	202	67	158	.09	8	.009	.005		.73
.234			.026	.06	0		171	129	36	194	.22	7	.012	.003		.87
1.31		.026	.265	.447	t		850	277	177	126	.29	11	.04	.007	11.3	.78
1.61		.03	.325	.547	t		918	340	217	155	.36	14				.95
1.2	3	.021	.225	.236	0		19	151	47	46	.33	6				.68
.12		.004	t	.077	0		70	23	21	17	.1	2	.011	.001		.15
.435		.005	.023	.08	0		274	136	53	225	.12	8	.008	.003		1.06
		.001	.23		0		170	126		113						
		.006	.018	.096	0		232	155	34	198	.07	8				1.11
.454		.003	.03	.159	0		95	172	23	287	.3	12				
.295		.016	.045	.334	0		227	111	36	141	.2	6				.6
					0		152	126	23	212	.2	8	.009	.003		.85
.185		.002	.024	.018	0		106	105	19	147	.05	5				.63
.262		.003	.034	.026	0		150	149	27	207	.07	7	.008	.003		.89
.418		.003	.029	.054	0		178	133	38	203	.12	8	.009	.002		.8
.002			.077	.128	0		205	197	42	320	.23	13	.101	.006		.78
		t	.016	.026	0		93	40	5	69	.05	3	.018			.16
.425		.005	.017	.06	0		151	102		184						
.415		.003	.044	.135	0		248	141	39	214	.15	8	.007	.003		.92
.831			.256		0		207	389	257	509	.94	28	.085	.024		2.85
.716			.192		0		307	449	308	669	1.08	36				3.3
.182	.8	.014	.208	.491	0		513	111	26	188	.16	8	.01	.009		.59
.475		.002	.026	.122	0	.098	74	171	31	272	.3	10	.036	.005	2.83	1.11
.348			.011	.074	0		388	216	61	219	.17	8				1.02
			.2		t		346	185	115	191	1					
.796		.006	.189	.699	2.08		98	230	314	254	.17	25				1.23
.049		t	.012	.043	.13		6	14	19	16	.01	2				.08
.033		t	.009	.041	.11		6	12	18	14	.01	1	.033		.075	.04
.690		.025	.154	.828	1.98		123	195	331	268	.14	26				.62
.466	.119	.009	.1	.619	1.46	1.4	82	146	231	166	.07	17				.6
.428	.071	.009	.093	.607	1.38	3	89	149	179	154	.07	17				.55
.99	13	.041	.039	1.11	0	.64	70	118	74	31	1.3	7.68	.13	.032	14.8	.922
.88	11	.036	.035	.986	0	.57	61	103	65	27	1.2	6	.1	.029	13.2	.84
.773	10	.032	.031	.864	0	.5	54	90	57	24	1	5	.09	.025	11.6	.72
.618	8	.026	t	.69	0	.4	49	82	52	22	.9	4	.05	.02	9.24	.576

Food Item	Measure	Weight g	Calories	Carbohydrate g	Protein g	Fiber g	Saturated fat g	Unsaturated fat g	Total fat g	Cholesterol mg	Vitamin A IU	Vitamin B₁ mg	Vitamin B₂ mg	Vitamin B₆ mg
Raw, white	1 lg	33	17	.3	3.6	0	0	0		0	0	.002	.094	.001
Raw, yolk	1 lg	17	59	.1	2.79	0	1.72	3	5.7	312	580	.043	.074	.053
Fried[8]	1 lg	46	99	.53	5.37	0	2.41	1	6.4	312	640	.033	.126	.05
Hard cooked	1 lg	57	82	.5	6.5	0	1.9	3.36	5.8	312	590	.04	.14	.065
Omelet or scrambled[9]	1 egg	64	111	1.5	7.2	0	2.82	3.31	7.08	314	690	.05	.18	.058
Poached	1 lg	50	82	.5	6.5	0	1.67	2.94	5.8	312	590	.04	.13	.051
Dried, whole	2 tbsp	10	60	.48	4.58	0	1.26	2.22	4.18	210	600	.03	.118	.04
Eggnog[10]	1 cup	254	342	34.4	9.68	0	11.3	6.53	19	149	894	.086	.483	.127
Ice cream, hard	1 cup	133	269	31.7	4.8	0	8.92	4.67	14.3	59	543	.052	.329	.061
Ice milk, hard	1 cup	131	184	29	5.16	0	3.51	1.84	5.63	18	214	.076	.347	.085
Milk														
Buttermilk	1 cup	244	99	11.7	8.1	0	1.34	.7	2.16	9	81	.083	.337	.083
Chocolate, whole	1 cup	250	208	25.9	7.92	.3	5.26	2.79	8.48	30	500[11]	.092	.405	.1
Condensed, sweetened	1 cup	306	982	166	24.8	0	16.8	8.46	26.6	104	1004	.275	1.27	.156
Dried, whole	1 cup	128	635	49.2	33.7	0	21.4	11	34.2	124	1180	.362	1.54	.387
Dried, whole, instant	1 cup	68	527	40.1	27.7				28.9	65	1190	.3	1.53	
Dried, nonfat	1 cup	120	435	62.4	43.4	0	.6	.28	.92	24	43[12]	.498	1.86	.433
Dried, nonfat, instant	1 cup	68	244	35.5	23.9	0	.32	.15	.49	12	18.4[12]	.281	1.19	.235
Evaporated, whole, unsw	1 cup	252	338	25.3	17.2	0	11.6	6.5	19.1	74	612	.118	.796	.126
Evaporated, skim, unsw	1 cup	256	198	28.9	19.3	0	.31	.174	.52	10	1000	.114	.788	.14
Goat, whole	1 cup	244	168	10.9	8.69	0	6.5	3.07	10.1	28	451	.117	.337	.112
Human	1 oz	30.8	21	2.12	.32	0	.62	.66	1.35	4	74	.004	.011	.003
Low-fat	1 cup	244	121	11.7	8.12	0	2.92	1.52	4.68	18	500[11]	.095	.403	.105
Malted[13]	1 cup	265	236	26.6	10.8	.13	5.96	3.46	9.94	37	376	.204	.538	.18
Skim	1 cup	245	86	11.8	8.35	0	.287	.132	.44	4	500[11]	.088	.343	.098
Whole	1 cup	244	159	11.4	8.5	0	5.07	2.65	8.15	33	350	.093	.395	.102
Sherbet	1 cup	193	270	58.7	2.16	t	2.38	1.24	3.82	14	185	.033	.089	.025
Whey, sweet, dry	1 tbsp	7.5	26	5.56	.96	0	.05	.02	.08	t	3	.039	.165	.044
Yogurt														
Whole milk, plain	8 oz	227	139	10.6	7.88	0	4.76	2.24	7.38	29	279	.066	.322	.073
Low-fat, plain, 12 g protein[14,15]	8 oz	227	144	16	11.9	0	2.27	1.07	3.52	14	150	.1	.486	.11
Skim, plain, 13 g protein[15]	8 oz	227	127	17.4	13	0	.264	.124	.41	4	16	.109	.531	.12
Low-fat, fruit, 9 g protein[14,15,16]	8 oz	227	225	42.3	9.04	.27	1.68	.79	2.61	10	111	.077	.368	.084
Low-fat, fruit, 11 g protein[14,15,16]	8 oz	227	239	42.2	11	.27	2.06	.97	3.2	12	136	.093	.449	.102
DESSERTS AND SWEETS														
Apple or brown Betty[17]	1 cup	215	325	63.9	3.4	1.4	2.15	2.2	7.5		220	.13	.09	
Apple butter	1 tbsp	17.6	33	8.2	.1	.2			.1		0	t	t	
Boston cream pie, ⅛ cake	1 piece	103	311	51.4	5.2	0	3	5	9.7		220	.03	.11	
Brownies, enr, 2 × 2 × ¾"	1 piece	30	146	15.3	2	.2	1.5	6	9.4	25.5	60	.05	.03	
Cake														
Angel food, 1/10 cake	1 piece	45	121	27.1	3.2	0			.1		0	.004	.06	
Chocolate, devils food, no icing, 2 × 3 × 2"	1 piece	45	165	23.4	2.2	.1			7.7		68	.009	.045	

[8]Made with ½ tsp fat and dash of salt.

[9]Made with 1½ tbsp milk, ½ tsp fat, and dash of salt.

[10]Made with 8 oz whole milk, one egg, and 3 tsp sugar.

[11]Value if vitamin A is added.

[12]Value based on data without added vitamin A. If vitamin A is added, each cup of reconstituted milk contains 500 IU.

[13]Made with 8 oz whole milk, 3 heaping tsp malt powder.

[14]Fat content may vary with resultant variation in vitamin A and fat constituents.

[15]Contains nonfat milk solids.

[16]Carbohydrate and calorie content may vary because of amount of sugar or honey added, and/or the level and solids content of added flavoring material.

[17]Made with enriched bread.

Vitamin B$_{12}$ mcg	Biotin mcg	Folic Acid mg	Niacin mg	Pantothenic Acid mg	Vitamin C mg	Vitamin E mg	Sodium mg	Phosphorus mg	Potassium mg	Calcium mg	Iron mg	Magnesium mg	Copper mg	Manganese mg	Selenium mg	Zinc mg
.021	2	.005	.029	.08	0		48	5	46	3	.01	2.97	.025	.013	1.88	.01
.647	9	.026	.012	.753	0	.51	9	97	17	24	.95	2.72	.045	.015	2.96	.58
.581		.022	.026	.763	0		144	80	58	26	.92	5	.023			.64
.749		.027	.034	.985	0		61	103	65	27	1.2	6.84				.821
.638		.022	.042	.819	0		164	121	93	51	1.1	8	.032			.7
.616		.024	.026	.86	0		61	103	65	27	1.2	6	.015			.72
.001			.024	.638	0		52	68	48	22	.78	4	.018			.54
1.14		.002	.267	1.06	3.8		138	278	420	330	.51	47				1.17
.625		.003	.134	.654	.7	.399	116	134	257	176	.12	18	.2			1.4
.875		.003	.118	.662	.76		105	129	265	176	.18	19				.55
.537	5		.142	.674	2.4	.118	257	219	371	285		27	.047			1.03
.835		.012	.313	.738	2.28		149	251	417	280	.6	33				1.02
1.36	9	.034	.643	2.3	7.96		389	775	1136	868	.58	77	.66			2.88
4.16	17	.047	.827	2.91	11.1		475	993	1702	1168	.6	108	.4			4.28
			.7		6		425	743	1397	954	.5					
4.84	19	.06	1.14	4.28	8.1		642	1162	2153	1508	.38	132				4.9
2.72		.034	.606	2.2	3.79		373	670	1160	837	.21	80				3
.41	7	.02	.488	1.61	4.74	.75	266	510	764	658	.48	60	.075		3.02	1.94
.61		.022	.444	1.88	2.16		294	496	846	738	.74	68				2.3
.159	5	.001	.676	.756	3.15		122	270	499	326	.12	34	.095	.019		.73
.014	t	.002	.055	.069	1.54	.069	5	4	16	10	.01	1	.015	t		.05
.888		.012	.21	.78	2.32		122	232	377	297	.12	33				.95
1.04		.022	1.28	.766	2.31		215	307	529	347	.29	52				1.14
.926	5	.013	.216	.806	2.4	t	126	247	406	302	.1	28	.1		11	.98
.871	5	.012	.205	.766	2.29	.293	120	228	351	291	.12	33	.5	.005	3.17	.93
.158		.014	.131	.062	3.86		88	74	198	103	.31	15				1.33
.177		.001	.094	.419	.11		80	70	155	59	.07	13				.15
.844		.017	.17	.883	1.2		105	215	351	274	.11	26				1.34
1.28		.025	.259	1.34	1.82		159	326	531	415	.18	40				2.02
1.39		.028	.281	1.46	1.98		174	355	579	452	.2	43				2.2
.967		.019	.195	1.01	1.36		121	247	402	314	.14	30				1.5
1.18		.024	.238	1.24	1.68		147	301	491	383	.16	37				1.86
		.9		2			329	47	215	39	1.3	14	.774			
		t		t			t	6	44	2	.1		.065			
		.2		t			192	104	92	69	.5					
		.2		t			75	44	57	12	.6					
		.1		0			127	10	40	4	.1	6.76				
		.1	.1	t			132	62	63	33	.4		.144			

Food Item	Measure	Weight g	Calories	Carbohydrate g	Protein g	Fiber g	Saturated fat g	Unsaturated fat g	Total fat g	Cholesterol mg	Vitamin A IU	Vitamin B_1 mg	Vitamin B_2 mg	Vitamin B_6 mg
Gingerbread, enr, 3 × 3 × 2″	1 piece	117	371	60.8	4.4	t			12.5		110	.14	.13	
Pound, old-fashioned, 3 × 3 × $\frac{1}{2}$″	1 piece	30	142	14.1	1.7	t			8.8		84	.009	.03	
Pound, low-fat, 3 × 3 × $\frac{1}{2}$″	1 piece	30	123	16.4	1.9	t			5.6		87	.01	.03	
Sponge, $\frac{1}{10}$ cake	1 piece	50	149	27	3.8	0	1	1	2.85	123	225	.03	.07	
White, no icing	1 piece	50	188	27	2.3	1	2	5	8		15	.005	.04	.025
Cake icing														
Chocolate	1 cup	275	1034	185	8.8	t	21	15	38.2		580	.06	.28	
White, boiled	1 cup	94	297	75.5	1.3	0			0		0	t	.03	
Candied citron	1 oz	28	89	22.7	.1	.39			.1					
Candy														
Caramel, plain or chocolate	1 piece	5	20	3.88	.2	.01	.357	.179	.536		t	.002	.009	
Chocolate milk bar, plain	1 oz	28	147	16.1	2.2	.112	5	3	9.2		80	.02	.1	
Chocolate fudge	1″ cube	21	84	15.8	.6	.04	1.5	.752	3		t	t	.02	
Mint patty, chocolate-covered	$1\frac{3}{8}$″ diam	11	45	8.9	.2	t			1.2		t	t	.01	
Peanut brittle	1 oz	25	119	23	1.6	.125	.5	1.75	2.6		0	.05	.01	
Chocolate														
Bitter or baking	1 oz	28	143	8.2	3	.7	8	6	15		20	.01	.07	
Bittersweet	1 oz	28	135	13.3	2.2	.5			11.3		10	.01	.05	
Semisweet	1 oz	28	144	16.2	1.2	.28	5.6	3.79	10.1		10	t	.02	
Chocolate syrup	1 tbsp	18.7	46	11.7	.45	.1	t	t	.49		t	.005	.015	
Cookies														
Chocolate chip, enr, $2\frac{1}{3}$″ diam	1	10	51	6	.55	t	1	2	3		10	.01	.01	
Fig bar	1	14	50	10.5	.55	.238	.14	.42	.775		15	.005	.01	
Gingersnap, 2″ diam	1	7	29.4	5.59	.39	t			.62		5	.003	.004	
Macaroon	1 med	14	67	9.3	.7	.3	2.24	.84	3.2		0	.006	.02	
Oatmeal w/raisin, 3″ diam	1	14	63	10.3	.9	.1			2.2		7	.015	.011	
Vanilla wafer	1	3.67	17	2.73	.2	t			.6		4.67	.067	.027	
Custard, baked	1 cup	265	305	29.4	14.3	0	7	6	14.6	278	930	.11	.5	
Doughnut														
Cake, plain	1 avg	32	125	16.4	1.5	t	1	4	6		26	.05	.05	
Raised, plain	1 avg	30	124	11.3	1.9	.1	1.8	5.69	8		18	.05	.05	
Eclair, custard, chocolate icing	1 avg	100	239	23.2	6.2	0	4	8	13.6		340	.04	.16	
Honey	1 tbsp	21	64	17.3	.1	0			0		0	.002	.014	.004
Jams, preserves	1 tbsp	20	54	14	.1	.1			t		t	t	.01	.005
Jellies	1 tbsp	18	49	12.7	t	0			t		t	t	.01	
Molasses														
Blackstrap	1 tbsp	20	43	11	0							.02	.04	.054
Light	1 tbsp	20	50	13	0							.01	.01	
Pie														
Apple, $\frac{1}{6}$ of 9″ pie	1 piece	160	410	61	3.4	.6	4.74	11.8	17.8	156	48	.03	.03	
Meringue, lemon, $\frac{1}{6}$ of pie	1 piece	140	357	52.8	5.2	t	4.67	8.33	14.3	130	238	.05	.11	
Pecan, $\frac{1}{6}$ of pie	1 piece	160	668	82	8.2	.8	5.36	28	36.6		256	.25	.11	
Pumpkin, $\frac{1}{6}$ of pie	1 piece	150	317	36.7	6	.8	5.77	9.23	16.8	91	3700	.04	.15	
Piecrust, baked, enr, 9″	1	135	675	59.1	8.2	.3	12	30	45.2		0	.27	.19	
Pudding														
Bread w/raisins, enr	1 cup	265	496	75.3	14.8	.2	7.95	5.3	16.2	170	800	.16	.5	
Chocolate, cornstarch	1 cup	260	385	66.8	8.1	.2	7	4	12.2	30	390	.05	.36	
Rice w/raisins	1 cup	265	387	70.8	9.5	.133	5.3	2.65	8.2	29	290	.08	.37	
Tapioca cream	1 cup	165	221	28.2	8.3	0	4	3	8.4		480	.07	.3	
Sugar														
Beet or cane, granulated	1 cup	200	770	199	0	0			0		0	0	0	
Beet or cane, granulated	1 tbsp	12	46	11.9	0	0			0		0	0	0	
Brown, packed	1 cup	220	821	212	0	0			0		0	.02	.07	
Powdered	1 cup	120	462	119	0	0			0		0	0	0	
Raw, brown	1 tbsp	14	14	12.7	.06				.07		t	.003	.016	
Syrup														
Maple	1 tbsp	20	50	12.8	0	0			0		0			
Corn	1 tbsp	20	57	14.8	0	0			0		0	0	.002	

Vitamin B$_{12}$ mcg	Biotin mcg	Folic Acid mg	Niacin mg	Pantothenic Acid mg	Vitamin C mg	Vitamin E mg	Sodium mg	Phosphorus mg	Potassium mg	Calcium mg	Iron mg	Magnesium mg	Copper mg	Manganese mg	Selenium mg	Zinc mg
			1.1		0		277	76	531	80	2.7					
			.1		0		33	24	18	6	.2					
			.1		t		53	31	23	12	.2		.027			
		.003	.1		t		84	56	44	15	.6					
			.1	.15	t	4.21	162	46	38	32	.1					1
			.6		1		168	305	536	165	3.3					
			t		0		134	2	17	2	t					
							82	7	34	24	.2					
			.018		t		11.4	6.25	9.64	7.5	.071					
		.002	.1		t	.308	27	65	109	65	.3	16.2	.137			.129
			t		t		40	18	31	16	.2					.192
			t		t		20	6	10	6	.1		.004			.038
			1		0		9	27	43	10	.7					
			.4		0	3.12	1	109	235	22	1.9	81.8	.748			
			.3		0		1	81	174	16	1.4					
			.1		t		1	43	92	9	.7					
			.1		0		10	17	53	3	.3	11.8	.08			.15
		.001	.1		t		34.8	10	11.8	3.5	.2					.096
			.05		t		35.3	8.5	27.8	11	.15					
			.03		t		40	3.3	32.3	5.1	.16					
			.1		0		5	12	65	4	.1					
			.1		t		23	14	52	3	.4		.015			.183
			t		0	.009	9.33	2.33	2.67	1.33	t	.588	.027			.011
			.3		1		209	310	387	297	1.1					
		.003	.4	.12	t	.81	160	61	29	13	.4	7	.035			2
		.007	.4		0		70	23	24	11	.5	6				
			.1		t		82	112	122	80	.7					
		.001	.1	.04	t		1	1	11	1	.1	.6	.008	.006		016
		.002	t	t	0		2	2	18	4	.2	1	.062			.006
			t		1		3	1	14	4	.3	.72	.016			
1.8		.002	.4	.1			19	17	585	137	3.2	51.6	.284			
			t				3	9	183	33	.9	9.2	.2		5.2	
		.006	.6	.176	2	.32	482	35	128	1	.5		.096			.143
			.3		4		395	69	70	20	.7					
			.5		t		354	165	197	75	4.5					
			.8	.778	t		321	104	240	76	.8					
			2.4		0	1.17	825	67	67	19	2.3					.715
			1.3		3		533	302	570	289	2.9		.212			
			.3		1	1.79	146	255	445	250	1.3					
		.013	.5		t		188	249	469	260	1.1		.08			.82
		.003	.2		2		257	180	223	173	.7		.066			
			0		0		2	0	6	0	.2		.04			.1
			0		0		t	0	t	0	t		.002			.006
			.4		0		66	42	757	187	7.5		.77			
			0		0		1	0	4	0	.1		.024			
			.04		.3			6		7	.6		.059			
					0		3	3	26	33	.2		.09			
			t		.1			3		9	.8		.072		2.8	

FISH, SEAFOOD, AND SEAWEED[18]

Food Item	Measure	Weight g	Calories	Carbohydrate g	Protein g	Fiber g	Saturated fat g	Unsaturated fat g	Total fat g	Cholesterol mg	Vitamin A IU	Vitamin B₁ mg	Vitamin B₂ mg	Vitamin B₆ mg
Abalone	1 lb	453	445	15.4	84.8	0			2.3			.83	.62	
Agar-agar		100		74.6	2.3	0			.1		0	0	0	
Anchovy, canned	3 fillets	12	21	t	2.3	0	.2	.45	.767					.014
Bass	1 lb	453	472	0	85.7	0	2.04	5.8	9.5			.46	.13	
Bluefish	1 lb	453	531	0	93	0			15			.52	.43	
Carp	1 lb	453	522	0	81.6	0	3.44	13.1	19.1		770	.04	.18	
Catfish	1 lb	453	467	0	79.8	0	3.9	9.29	14.1			.18	.13	
Caviar, sturgeon, granular	1 rd tsp	10	26	3.3	2.7				1.5	30				
Clams														
Fresh	4 lg or 9 sm	100	82	1.3	14				1.9	120		.1	.19	.08
Canned	1 cup	200	104	5.6	15.8				1.4	240		.02	.22	.166
Cod	1 lb	453	354	0	79.8	0	.544	1.54	3.31	227	0	.27	.33	1.02
Crab														
Steamed	1 lb	453	422	2.3	78.5				8.6	453	9830	.72	.38	1.36
Canned, drained, packed	1 cup	160	162	1.8	27.8				4	161		.13	.13	.48
Dulse		100				.7			3					
Eel	1 lb	453	1057	0	72.1	0	19	30	83	227	7300	1	1.66	1.04
Flounder, sole, or sandabs	1 lb	453	358	0	75.8	0	1.26	2.54	5.44	227		.24	.23	.77
Frog's legs	4 lg	100	73	0	16.4	0			.3	40	0	.14	.25	.12
Haddock	1 lb	453	358	0	83	0	.498	1.22	2.99	272		.19	.29	.80
Halibut	1 lb	453	454	0	94.8	0	.91	2.72	4.98	227	2000	.29	.3	1.95
Herring														
Fresh	1 lb	453	798	0	78.5	0	8.7	16.2	28.1	386	520	.1	.68	1.68
Canned	1 cup	200	416	0	39.8	0			.8				.36	.32
Hijiki		100		42.8	5.6	13			.8		150	.01	.2	
Kelp	1 tbsp	14.2		5.53	1.03	.97			.157				.046	
Kombu		100		54.9	7.3	3			1.1		430	.08	.32	
Lobster	1 lb	453	413	2.3	76.7	0			8.6	900	t	1.84	.23	
Mackerel														
Fresh	1 lb	453	866	0	86.2	0	11	27.5	44.4	431	2040	.66	1.49	2.99
Canned, drained	1 cup	210	384	0	40.4	0			12.4	199	920	.12	.44	.54
Nori		100		44.3	35.6	4.7			.7		11,000	.25	1.24	
Oysters														
Fresh	1 lb	453	299	15.4	38.1				8.2	227	1410	.64	.82	.23
Canned	1 cup	240	158	8.2	20.2		1.97	2.02	4.3	108	740	.34	.43	.089
Perch														
Ocean	1 lb	453	431	0	86.2	0	1.86	7.57	11.3		136	.41	.36	1.04
Yellow	1 lb	453	413	0	88.5	0			4.1	317	136	.27	.77	1.04
Pike, walleye	1 lb	453	422	0	87.5	0	.725	2.08	5.4			1.13	.73	.52
Pollock, fillet	1 lb	453	431	0	92.5	0	.544	2.49	4.1			.23	.46	.56
Salmon														
Fresh	1 lb	453	984	0	102	0	22	23	60.8	272	1359	.45	.36	3.18
Pink, canned	1 cup	220	310	0	45.1	0	4	2	13	77	150	.07	.4	.66
Sockeye, canned	1 cup	220	376	0	44.7	0	1.65	9.94	14.7	77	510	.09	.35	.66
Sardines, canned in oil, drained	1 oz	28	58		6.8				3.1	20	60	.01	.06	.05
Scallops	1 lb	453	367	15	69.4				.9	159		.18	.29	
Shad	1 lb	453	771	0	84.4	0			45.4			.68	1.09	
Shrimp														
Fresh	1 lb	453	413	6.8	82.1				3.6	680	40.5	.09	.14	.45
Canned, drained	1 cup	128	148	.9	31				1.4	192	66.8	.01	.04	.077
Smelt	1 lb	453	445	0	84.4	0			9.5			.04	.56	
Snails	3.5 oz	100	90	2	16.1				1.4					

[18]Values are for raw flesh only unless stated otherwise. One lb fish steaks = 4 svgs. One lb fish fillets = 5 svgs.

[19]The flesh of some oysters is high in vitamin C, containing from 22 to 38 mg/100 gr.

[20]Based on frozen scallops, possibly brined.

Vitamin B₁₂ mcg	Biotin mcg	Folic Acid mg	Niacin mg	Pantothenic Acid mg	Vitamin C mg	Vitamin E mg	Sodium mg	Phosphorus mg	Potassium mg	Calcium mg	Iron mg	Magnesium mg	Copper mg	Manganese mg	Selenium mg	Zinc mg
								866		168	10.9					
								8		400	5					
			0		0			25		20						
			9.6	2.32			308	871	1160							
			8.8				336	1102		104	2.7					
t			6.7	.68	5		227	1148	1297	227	4.1	68				
.01			7.7	2.12			272		1497		1.8		.77			
							220	36	18	28	1.2					
.098	2	.003	1.5	.3			36	183	235	12	3.4	63			55	1.5
			2					274	280	110	8.2					
3.6	.91	.005	10	.544	9		318	880	1733	45	1.8	127	2.27	.045	186	
45.4	22.7	.018	12.7	2.72	9			794		195	3.6	154	5.89			19.5
16	8	t	8.6	.959			1600	291	176	72	1.3	61	1.66		81.6	
								22		567	6.3					
4.5			6.2	.68	6.43		353	916	1119	82	3.2	81.5	.136	.14		
5.4			7.6	3.86			354	885	1551	54	3.6	136	.815	.091	152	3.2
			1.2	.37			55	147	308	18	1.5					
5.9	1.36	.005	13.6	.59	0	2.72	277	894	1379	104	3.2	109	1.04	.091		
4.5	9.06	.009	37.8	1.25	t		245	957	2037	59	3.2		1.04	.045		3.2
40.5			16.4	4.4	2.27	9.06	535	1161	1436	258	5	118	1.36	.091		
16				1.4				594		294	3.6					
			4		0			56		1400	29					
				.784			429	34.3	753	156	.014	104	t			
			1.8		11		2500	150		800	10					
2.3	22.7	.002	6.6	6.8	t		1359	830	1178	132	2.7	77.9	9.97	.18	471	8.2
40	9.06	.005	37.1	3.86	t	7.25	652	1084	1622	23	4.5	127	.725	.091		
			12	.94				574		388	4.4					
			10		10		600	510		260	12					
81.6	4.53	.018	11.3	1.13		t[19]	331	649	549	426	24.9	145	5.44	.906	222	338
			6				175	343	290	226	13.2					
4.5			11.3	1.63	13.6		286	960	1769	208	4.53					
4.5			7.9	1.63			308	816	1043	90.6	2.7					
			10.5			.906	231	971	1447	90.6	1.8	136	1.13	.091		
4.5			7.1	1.36			218		1588							
18.1	4.53	.009	32.6	5.9	41		217	844	1771	358	4.1	131	.906	.045		
15.2		.001	17.6	1.07			851	629	794	431	1.8	65	.154	.15		
15		.001	16.1	1			1148	757	757	570	2.6	63.8	.11			
2.8	5.6	t	1.5	.238	t		233	141	167	124	.8		.011			
5.4	1.36	.002	5.8	.6			1155[20]	943	1796[20]	118	8.2		.544		349	
			38.1	2.76			245	1179	1497	91	2.3					
4.1			14.5	1.27	t		635	753	998	286	7.3	190	1.95		906	
		.003	2.3	.269	t		80	337	156	147	4			218		
			6.1					1234			1.8				557	
										170	3.5	250	.4	1.6		

Food Item	Measure	Weight g	Calories	Carbohydrate g	Protein g	Fiber g	Saturated fat g	Unsaturated fat g	Total fat g	Cholesterol mg	Vitamin A IU	Vitamin B₁ mg	Vitamin B₂ mg	Vitamin B₆ mg
Snapper	1 lb	453	422	0	89.8	0	1.09	2.9	5.44			.78	.11	
Swordfish	1 lb	453	535	0	87.1	0			18.1		7170	.24	.23	
Trout, rainbow	1 lb	453	885	0	97.5	0	11	13	51.7	249	t	.34	.92	3.13
Tuna														
Canned in oil, drained	1 cup	160	315	0	46.1	0	4.8	6.4	13.1	104	130	.08	.19	.39
Canned in water	1 cup	200	254	0	56	0			1.6	126			.2	.85
Wakame		100		51.4	12.7	3.6			1.5		140	.11	.14	
Whitefish	1 lb	453	703	0	85.7	0	3.9	15.7	37.2		10,250	.64	.54	
FRUITS AND FRUIT JUICES														
Acerola (Barbados cherry)														
Raw	10 fruits	100	23	5.6	.3	.4			.2			.02	.05	.009
Juice	1 cup	242	56	11.6	1	.73			.7			.05	.15	.01
Apple														
Raw	1 med	180	96	24	.3	1.8			1		150	.05	.03	.05
Dried	1 cup	85	234	61	.9	2.6			1.4			.05	.1	.115
Juice, unsw	1 cup	248	117	29.5	.2	.26			t			.02	.05	.075
Applesauce, unsw	1 cup	244	100	26.4	.5	1.3			.5		100	.05	.02	.07
Apricot														
Raw	3 avg	114	55	13.7	1.1	.7			.2		2890	.03	.04	.077
Canned, hvy syrup	1 cup	258	222	56.8	1.5	1			.3		4490	.05	.05	.139
Dried	1 cup	130	338	86.5	6.5	3.9			.7		14,170	.01	.21	.22
Nectar	1 cup	251	143	36.6	.8	.5			.3		2380	.03	.03	
Avocado, raw, pitted	1 avg	200	334	12.6	4.2	3.2			32.8		580	.22	.4	.84
Banana, raw	1 avg	150	127	33.3	1.6	.8			.3		270	.08	.09	.76
Blackberries														
Raw	1 cup	144	84	18.6	1.7	5.9			1.3		290	.04	.06	.07
Canned, hvy syrup	1 cup	256	233	56.8	2	6.5			1.5		330	.03	.05	.06
Juice, unsw	1 cup	245	91	19.1	.7	t			1.5			.05	.07	
Blueberries														
Raw	1 cup	145	90	22.2	1	2.2			.7		150	.04	.09	1
Canned, hvy syrup	1 cup	240	242	62.4	1	2.16			.4		96	.02	.02	
Frozen, sweetened, unthawed	1 cup	230	242	61	1.4	2			.7		70	.09	.12	.124
Boysenberries, frozen, unsw	1 cup	126	60	14.4	1.5	3.38			.4		210	.03	.16	.071
Cantaloupe, raw	¼ avg	100	30	7.5	.7	.3			.1		3400	.04	.03	.086
Casaba melon, raw	1/10 avg	245	38	9.1	1.7	1.2			t		40	.06	.04	
Cherries														
Sour, raw, pitted	1 cup	155	90	22.2	1.9	.4			.5		1550	.08	.09	.095
Sour, canned, hvy syrup	1 cup	270	119	29.6	2.2	.2			.5		150	.05	.05	.118
Sweet, raw	1 cup	130	82	20.4	1.5	.52			.4		130	.06	.07	.041
Sweet, canned, hvy syrup	1 cup	279	208	52.6	2.3	.2			.5		150	.05	.05	.084
Crabapple, raw	3.5 oz	100	68	17.8	.4	.6			.3		40	.03	.02	
Cranberry, raw	1 cup	100	46	10.8	.4	1.4			.7		40	.03	.02	.035
Cranberry sauce														
Home-prepared[23]	1 cup	277	493	126	.6	1.94			.8		60	.03	.03	
Canned	1 cup	277	404	104	.3	.55			.6		60	.03	.03	.06
Currants														
Black, raw	3.5 oz	100	54	13.1	1.7	2.4			.1		230	.05	.05	.066
Red or white, raw	1 cup	133	67	16	1.87	4.5			.267		160	.05	.07	.049
Dates, pitted	10 med	100	274	72.9	2.2	2.3			.5		50	.09	.1	.153
Elderberries, raw	3.5 oz	100	72	16.4	2.6	7			.5		600	.07	.06	.23
Figs														
Raw	2 lg	100	80	20.3	1.2	1.2			.3		80	.06	.05	.113
Canned, hvy syrup	1 cup	259	218	56.5	1.3	1.7			.5		80	.08	.08	

[21]Applies to dietary low-sodium pack. Regular water pack with salt added is 1733 mg/cup.
[22]Range may be from 2400–5300 mg.
[23]Made with 1 lb cranberries and 2 cups sugar.

Vitamin B$_{12}$ mcg	Biotin mcg	Folic Acid mg	Niacin mg	Pantothenic Acid mg	Vitamin C mg	Vitamin E mg	Sodium mg	Phosphorus mg	Potassium mg	Calcium mg	Iron mg	Magnesium mg	Copper mg	Manganese mg	Selenium mg	Zinc mg
							304	971	1465	73	3.6	127				
4.5			36.4	.85				885		86	4.1					
22.7			38	8.85	t		177		2129	86	4.53		1.5		.136	
1.6	.8	.024	19	.32				374		13	3			.192		1.76
4.4	1	.03	26.3	.64			82[21]	380	558	32	3.2			.24		
			1		15		2500	260		1300	13					
			13.6		t		236	1225	1356		1.8		.861			
0			.3		.1066		7	9	68	10	.2					
0			1	.49	3872[22]		7	22		24	1.2					
0	1.8	.014	.2	.19	7	1.33	2	17	182	12	.5	14.4	.16	.126	.9	.09
0			.4		9		4	44	484	26	1.4	18.7	.2			
0	1.2	.002	.2	.05	2		2	22	250	15	1.5	10	.5			
0		.003	.1	.2	2		5	12	190	10	1.2	12.2	.85		.488	.24
0		.003	.6	.26	11		1	25	301	18	.5	13.7	.12	.2		
0			1	.237	10		3	39	604	28	.8	17	.13	.2		
0		.018	4.3	.98	16		34	140	1273	87	7.2	80.6	.455	.36		
0			.5		8		t	30	379	23	.5					
0		.102	3.2	2.14	28		8	·84	1208	20	1.2	90	.8	4		.7
0	6	.042	1	.39	15	.6	2	39	550	12	1	49	.24	.96	1.5	.3
0	.6	.018	.6	.345	31		1	27	245	46	1.3	43	.23	.9		
0			.5	.195	18		3	31	279	54	1.5					
0			.7	.2	25		2	29	417	29	2.2	51.5				
0		.009	.7	.231	20		1	19	117	22	1.5	8.7	.22	.4		
			.4		14		2	20	132	22	1.4	9.6				
0			.9	.278	18		2	25	152	14	.9	9.2				
0			1.3	.269	16		1	30	193	32	2	22.5				
0	3	.03	.6	.25	33	.14	12	16	251	14	.4	17	.05	.04		.06
			.8		18		17	22	351	20	.6					
0	.6	.012	.6	.213	16		3	29	296	34	.6	21	.18	.045		
0			.5	.28	7		2	32	323	37	.7		.16			
0	.52	.01	.5	.339	12		2	22	223	26	.5	18	.156	.039		
0			.5		8		3	33	323	39	.8	25.2	.168			
			.1		8		1	13	110	6	.3					
0		.002	.1	.219	11		2	10	82	14	.5	8	.11	.3		
			.3		6		3	14	105	19	.6	5.5				.017
0			.1		6		3	11	83	17	.6	5.5				.017
0	2.4		.3	.398	200		3	40	372	60	1.1	10	.13			
0	3.46		.3	.085	54.7		2.68	30.7	343	42.7	1.3	21	.17	.78		
0		.021	2.2	.78	0		1	63	648	59	3	58	.22	.15		
0	2	.017	.5	.14	36			28	300	38	1.6					
0		.01	.4	.3	2		2	22	194	35	.6	20	.07	.128		
0			.5	.179	3		5	34	386	34	1					

Food Item	Measure	Weight g	Calories	Carbohydrate g	Protein g	Fiber g	Saturated fat g	Unsaturated fat g	Total fat g	Cholesterol mg	Vitamin A IU	Vitamin B₁ mg	Vitamin B₂ mg	Vitamin B₆ mg
Dried	5 med	100	274	69.1	4.3	5.6			1.3		80	.1	.1	.175
Fruit cocktail, canned, hvy syrup	1 cup	255	194	50.2	1	1			.3		360	.05	.03	.3
Gooseberries														
Raw	1 cup	150	59	14.6	1.2	2.9			.3		440	.22	.045	.018
Canned, hvy syrup	1 cup	200	180	46	1	2.4			.2		380			
Granadilla (passion fruit), raw	3.5 oz	100	90	21.2	2.2				.7		700	t		.13
Grapefruit														
Raw	½ med	100	41	10.8	.5	.2			.1		10	.04	.02	.034
Canned in syrup	1 cup	254	178	45.2	1.5	.5			.3		30	.08	.05	.05
Juice, unsw	1 cup	250	98	23	1.2	t			.2		200	.1	.05	.027
Grapes														
American (slip skin), raw	1 cup	153	106	24	2	.9			1.5		150	.08	.05	.12
European (adherent skin), raw	1 cup	160	107	27.7	1	.8			.5		160	.08	.05	.13
Thompson seedless, canned, hvy syrup	1 cup	256	197	51.2	1.3	.4			.3		180	.1	.03	
Juice, unsw	1 cup	253	167	42	.5	t			t			.1	.05	.1
Guava, raw	1 med	100	62	15	.8	5.6			.6		280	.05	.05	
Honeydew melon, raw	2" wide	150	49	11.5	1.2	.9			.5		60	.06	.05	.084
Kumquat, raw	1 med	20	12	3.2	.2	.74			t		110	.01	.02	
Lemon														
Raw, peeled	1 med	110	20	6	.8	.4			.2		10	.03	.01	.08
Juice, unsw	1 tbsp	15.2	4	1.2	.1	t			t		t	t	t	.007
Peel, grated	1 tbsp	6		1	.1				t		t	t	t	
Lemonade, frozen concentrate, diluted	1 cup	248	107	28.3	.1	t			t		10	.01	.02	.012
Lime														
Raw	1 sm	80	19	6.4	.5	.5			.1		10	.02	.01	
Juice, unsw	1 tbsp	15.4	4	1.4	t	t			t		t	t	t	
Loganberries, raw	1 cup	144	89	21.5	1.4	4			.9		290	.04	.06	
Loquats, raw	10 fruits	160	59	15.3	.5	.8			.2		830			
Lychees														
Raw	10 fruits	150	58	14.8	.8	.45			.3				.05	
Dried	3.5 oz	100	277	70.7	3.8	1.4			1.2					
Mango, raw	1 fruit	300	152	38.8	1.6	2.7			.9		11,090	.12	.12	
Nectarine, raw	1 avg	150	88	23.6	.8	.6			t		2280			
Olives														
Green	2 med	13	15	.2	.2	.2			1.6		40	.004	.01	.003
Ripe	2 lg	20	37	.6	.2	.3			4		14	t	t	.003
Greek (salt-cured)	3 med	20	67	1.7	.4	.8			7.1					
Orange														
Raw	1 avg	180	64	16	1.3	.9			.3		260	.13	.05	.108
Juice, unsw	1 cup	248	112	25.8	1.7	.3			.5		500	.22	.07	1
Juice, frozen concentrate, diluted, unsw	1 cup	249	122	28.9	1.7	t			.2		540	.23	.03	.07
Papaya														
Raw	½ med	150	58	15	.9	1.8			.15		2625	.06	.06	
Juice, canned	1 cup	250	120	30.2	1				0		5000	.04	.02	
Peach														
Raw	1 med	115	38	9.7	.6	.69			.1		1330	.02	.05	.026
Canned, hvy syrup	1 cup	256	200	51.5	1	1			.3		1100	.03	.05	.06
Dried	1 cup	160	419	109	5	5			1.1		6240	.02	.3	.16
Pear														
Raw	1 avg	200	122	30.6	1.4	2.8			.8		40	.04	.08	.034
Canned, hvy syrup	1 cup	255	194	50	.5	1.5			.5		10	.03	.05	.038
Dried	1 cup	180	482	121	5.6	6.2			3.2		130	.02	.32	

Vitamin B$_{12}$ mcg	Biotin mcg	Folic Acid mg	Niacin mg	Panto-thenic Acid mg	Vitamin C mg	Vitamin E mg	Sodium mg	Phospho-rus mg	Potas-sium mg	Calcium mg	Iron mg	Magne-sium mg	Copper mg	Manga-nese mg	Sele-nium mg	Zinc mg
0		.03	.7	.435	0		34	77	640	126	3	71	.28	.35		
0			1	.92	5		13	31	411	23	1	17	.075			
0	.7		.45	.429	50		2	23	233	27	.8	13.5	.12	.06		
					20		2	18	196	22	.6					
			1.5		30		28	64	348	13	1.6	29				
0	3	.011	.2	.283	38	.26	1	16	135	16	.4	12	.04	.01		
0			.5	.3	76		3	36	343	33	.8	27	.1			
0	1.7	.052	.5	.32	95	.1	2	38	405	22	.5	30	.05			.075
0	3	.011	.5	.112	6		5	18	242	24	.6	19.5	.135	.124		
0	3.2	.011	.5	.119	6		5	32	278	19	.6	9.6	.15	.13		
			.5		5		10	33	269	20	.8					
0	.9	.005	.5	.175	t		5	30	293	28	.8	32.5	.22		10	
0			1.2	.15	242		4	42	289	23	.9	13				
0			.9	.31	35		18	24	377	21	.6	6.7	.09	.027		
					7		1	4	44	12	.1					
0		.012	.1	.19	39		1	12	102	19		9	.15	.04		
0		t	t	.015	7		t	2	21	1	t	1.2	.012	.001		.002
			t		8		t	1	10	8	t					
0		.012	.2	.027	17		1	3	40	2	.1	2.5				.025
0		.003	.1	.217	25		1	12	69	22	.4					
0			t	.047	5		t	2	16	1	t	.81	.005	.001		
			.6		35		1	24	245	50	1.7	36	.21			
					1			44	429	25	.5					
					38		3	38	153	7	.4					
							3	181	1100	33	1.7					
0			2.5	.48	81	3	16	30	437	23	.9	54	.36	.078		1.41
0		.007		.025	18		8	33	406	6	.7	19.5	.12	.057		
0		t	.065	.002	0		312	2	7	8	.2	2.86	.06	.007		.007
0				.003			150	3	5	21	.3					.06
							658	6								
0	1.8	.083	.5	.45	66	.43	1	20	263	54	.5	19.8	.11	.045	2.5	26
0	.8	.136	1	.47	124		2	42	496	27	.5	49	.2		14.9	.09
0		.136	.9	.41	120		2	42	503	25	.2	25	.025			.09
0			.45	.327	84		4.5	24	351	30	.45	11.4	.015	.013		
		.008	.2		111			24		44	.8					
0	2	.004	1	.177	7		1	19	202	9	.5	11.5	.09	.11	.46	.2
0	.5	.001	1.5	.15	8		5	31	333	10		15	.15	.1	.512	.25
0			8.5		29		26	187	1520	77		76.7	.48	1.07		
0	.2	.028	.2	.14	8		4	22	260	16	.6	14	.3	12	1.2	
0			.3	.055	3		3	18	214	13	.5	13	.1		.51	
			1.1		13		13	86	1031	63	2.3	55.8				

Food Item	Measure	Weight g	Calories	Carbohydrate g	Protein g	Fiber g	Saturated fat g	Unsaturated fat g	Total fat g	Cholesterol mg	Vitamin A IU	Vitamin B₁ mg	Vitamin B₂ mg	Vitamin B₆ mg
Persimmon														
Japanese, raw	1 med	100	77	19.7	.7	1.6			.4		2710	.03	.02	
Native, raw	1 med	100	127	33.5	.8	1.5			.4					
Pineapple														
Diced, raw	1 cup	155	81	21.2	.6	.5			.3		110	.14	.05	.132
Canned, hvy syrup	1 cup	255	189	49.5	.8	.7			.3		130	.2	.05	.185
Juice, unsw	1 cup	250	138	33.8	1	.2			.3		130	.13	.05	.24
Plantain (baking banana), raw	1 lg	365	313	82	2.9	1.4			1.1		²⁴	.16	.11	
Plums														
Damson, raw	2 med	100	66	17.8	.5	.4			t		300	.08	.03	.052
Prune type, raw	3 med	100	75	19.7	.8	.4			.2		300	.03	.03	.052
Purple, canned, hvy syrup	1 cup	272	214	55.8	1	.8			.3		3130	.05	.05	
Pomegranate, raw	1 lg	275	97	25.3	.8	.5			.5		t	.05	.05	
Pricklypear, raw		100	42	10.9	.5	1.6			.1		60	.01	.03	
Prunes														
Dehydrated, nugget type	1 cup	100	344	91.3	3.3	2.2			.5		2170	.12	.22	.5
Dried, softenized	1 cup	185	411	108	3.4	1.96			1		2580	.14	.27	.44
Cked, unsw	1 cup	250	253	66.7	2.1	2			.6		1590	.07	.15	
Juice, unsw	1 cup	256	197	48.6	1	t			.3			.03	.03	
Quince, raw	3.5 oz	100	57	15.3	.4	1.7			.1		40	.02	.03	
Raisins, packed	1 cup	165	477	128	4.1	1.4			.3		30	.18	.13	.396
Raspberries														
Black, raw	1 cup	134	98	21	2	7.65			1.9		t	.04	.12	.08
Red, raw	1 cup	123	70	16.7	1.5	4			.6		100	.04	.11	.072
Frozen, sweetened, un-thawed	1 cup	250	245	61.5	1.8	5.5			.5		180	.05	.15	.095
Juice, unsw	1 cup	120	49	12.8	t	t			0		120	.02		.04
Rhubarb, diced, raw	1 cup	122	20	4.5	.7	.7			.1		120	.04	.09	.036
Strawberries														
Raw	1 cup	150	56	12.6	1	2			.8		90	.04	.1	.082
Frozen, sweetened, un-thawed	1 cup	255	278	70.9	1.3	2			.5		80	.05	.15	.112
Tangelo, raw	1 med	170	39	9.2	.5				.1					
Tangerine, raw	1 med	116	39	10	.7	.5			.2		360	.05	.02	.08
Watermelon														
Slice	6″ × 1½″	600	156	38.4	3	1.8			1.2		3540	.18	.18	
Balls or cubes	1 cup	100	26	6.4	.5	.3			.2		590	.03	.03	.068
Meat and Poultry²⁵														
Beef²⁶														
Chuck roast	1 lb	454	905	0	78.8	0	36	34	75	270	130	.34	.7	1.27
Club steak	1 lb	454	1443	0	58.9	0	63.4	60.7	132	261	260	.25	.52	1.27
Corned, boneless	1 lb	454	1329	0	71.7	0	54	52	113			.14	.68	.56
Dried, chipped	3 oz	85	173	0	29.1	0	2.55	2.55	5.4			.06	.272	
Flank steak	1 lb	454	653	0	98	0	12.4	11.9	25.9	261	50	.42	.87	1.27
Ground beef, lean	1 lb	454	812	0	93.9	0	22	21	45.4	295	90	.4	.83	1.97
Ground beef, regular	1 lb	454	1216	0	81.2	0	48	44	96.2	307	160	.35	.72	1.5
Heart	1 lb	454	490	3.2	77.6	0	5	7.72	16.3	680	90	2.42	3.98	1.13
Kidney	1 lb	454	130	.9	15.4	0			6.7	1700	690	.36	2.55	1.95
Liver	1 lb	454	140	5.3	19.9	0	6.8	5	17.3	1360	43,900²⁷	.25	3.26	3.8

²⁴Value varies with color; white varieties have 10 IU/100 gms, deep yellow varieties up to 1200 IU/100 gms.

²⁵Values are for raw meat only, unless stated otherwise. If meats are cooked at low temperatures, proteins are not altered. However, high temperatures and overcooking can harm some of the essential amino acids and decrease their health-promoting value. With the possible exception of folic acid, the B vitamins are not depleted at low temperatures except at the surface of the meat. Above the boiling point, the B vitamins are destroyed in proportion to the temperature. The B vitamins and minerals dissolve in water and can be lost if meats are soaked or boiled and the cooking water is not used. Juices that seep from frozen meats during thawing and those that drip into the broiling pan can be used in gravy or added to soup stock.

²⁶Beef steak contains .63 mg vitamin E/100 gms; beef has approx. 13.6 mcg biotin/lb; lean beef contains 19 mg zinc/lb.

²⁷Values vary widely in all kinds of liver, ranging from 450 IU/lb.

Vitamin B₁₂ mcg	Biotin mcg	Folic Acid mg	Niacin mg	Panto-thenic Acid mg	Vitamin C mg	Vitamin E mg	Sodium mg	Phospho-rus mg	Potas-sium mg	Calcium mg	Iron mg	Magne-sium mg	Copper mg	Manga-nese mg	Sele-nium mg	Zinc mg
			.1		11		6	26	174	6	.3	8				
					66		1	26	310	27	2.5					
0		.017	.3	.24	26		2	12	226	26	.8	20	.09	1.57	.93	
0		.002	.5	.25	18		3	13	245	28	.8	20	.25		2.04	
0		.003	.5	.25	23		3	23	373	38	.8	30	.15			
0		.058	1.6	.86	37		13	79	1012	18	1.8					
0	t	.006	.5	.186	6		2	17	299	18	.5	9	.1	.1		
0	t	.002	.5	.186	4		1	18	170	12	.5	9	.15	.1		
			1		5		3	26	367	23	2.3					
0			.5	1.64	6		5	12	399	5	.5					
			.4		22		2	28	166	20	.3					
0		.005	2.1	.35	4		11	107	940	90	4.4	32	.16		.18	
0		.007	2.6	.85	5		13	127	1117	82	6.3	74	.52			
			1.5		2		9	79	695	51	3.8	50	.42			.79
			1		5		5	51	602	36	10.5	25.6	.05			.025
			.2		15		4	17	197	11	.7	6	.13	.04		
0	7	.007	.8	.074	2		45	167	1259	102	5.8	57.7	.41	.47		.3
0	2.5	.007	1.2	.324	24		1	29	267	40	1.2	40.5	.24	.68		
0	2.28	.006	1.1	.288	31		1	27	207	27	1.1	24	.22	.61		
0			1.5	.317	53		3	43	250	33	1.5	27.5				
0					18			14		29	1	21				
0		.009	.4	.102	11		2	22	306	117	1	19	.02			.44
0	1.6	.024	.9	.51	88		2	32	246	32	1.5	18	.11	.09		.12
0			1.3	.337	.35	.48	3	43	286	36	1.8	23				
					26											
0		.021	.1	.24	27		2	15	108	34	.3	11	.08	.04		
			1.2		42		6	60	600	42	3	48	.24			
0	4	.008	.2	.3	7		1	10	100	7	.5	8	.04	.02		
5.4		.032	18.9	1.81	0		276	731	1261	49	11.8	80	.45			
5.4		.032	14.1	1.81			206	539	942	34	8.7	81				
3.9			7.7		0		5897	567	272	41	10.9					9
1.56			3.2		0		3660	343	170	17	4.3					
5.4		.032	23.5	1.81	0		343	912	1568	59	14.5	100	.09			
8.2		.032	22.5	2.81	0			871		54	14.1	95				15
6.4		.032	19.5	2.13	0			708	1070	45	12.2	77	.27		94	
50	36	.014	34.1	11.3	9		390	885	875	23	18.1	82	1.32			
141	40.9	.363	6.4	17.5	15		176	219	225	11	7.4	50	1.14	.36	640	
363	454	.99	13.6	35	31	6.36	136	352	281	8	6.5	59	12.7	1.23	206	17

Food Item	Measure	Weight g	Calories	Carbohydrate g	Protein g	Fiber g	Saturated fat g	Unsaturated fat g	Total fat g	Cholesterol mg	Vitamin A IU	Vitamin B₁ mg	Vitamin B₂ mg	Vitamin B₆ mg
Porterhouse steak	1 lb	454	1603	0	60.8	0	71	68	148	261	300	.26	.55	1.27
Rib roast	1 lb	454	1673	0	61.8	0	74.9	71.8	156	261	310	.27	.55	1.27
Round steak	1 lb	454	863	0	88.5	0	26	25	53.9	261	110	.38	.79	1.27
Rump roast	1 lb	454	1167	0	67	0	47	46	97.4	261	190	.29	.6	1.27
Sirloin steak	1 lb	454	1316	0	71	0	52	50	112	261	220	.3	.63	1.27
T-bone steak	1 lb	454	1596	0	59	0	70	89	168	261	300	.25	.53	1.27
Tongue	1 lb	454	714	1.4	56.5	0			52		0	.42	.99	.43
Brains, all kinds	1 lb	454	567	3.6	47.2	0			39	320	0	1.05	1.18	.68
Chicken[28]														
Back	1 lb	454	385	0	40.4	0	11.1	24	39	368	760	.13	.55	2.27
Breast	1 lb	454	394	0	74.5	0	5.3	11	18	239	270	.18	.57	3.1
Canned	1 cup	205	406	0	44.5	0	8	12	24		470	.08	.25	.6
Drumstick	1 lb	454	313	0	51.2	0	8.67	18.8	30.7	239	340	.18	.87	1.47
Gizzard	1 lb	453	513	3.2	91.2	0			12.2	658		.12	.89	
Heart	10 med	100	157	1.6	20.5	0			7	170	30	.12	.91	.363
Liver	1 lb	454	585	13.2	89.4	0	7.54	9.44	20.4	2517	54,890[27]	.86	11.3	3.4
Neck	1 lb	454	329	0	33.7	0			20.5	368	660	.1	.53	1.47
Thigh	1 lb	454	435	0	61.6	0	9.49	20.6	33.5	368	620	.2	1.13	1.47
Wing	1 lb	454	325	0	41.1	0	15.3	32.9	52.7	368	530	.09	.32	3.1
Chili con carne w/beans	1 cup	255	339	31	19	1.5	7.5	7.5	15.6		150	.08	.18	
Corned beef hash w/potato	1 cup	220	398	23.5	19.4	1.25	11	11	24.9		t	.02	.2	.165
Duck, ready to cook	1 lb	454	1213	0	59.5	0	31	80	130	318		.29	.71	
Frankfurter	1 lb	454	1402	8.2	56.7	0	51	72	131	295		.71	.9	.64
Goose, ready to cook	1 lb	454	1172	0	54.3	0	41	88	153			.25	.63	2.72
Lamb[29]														
Leg	1 lb	454	845	0	67.7	0	35	24	61.7	265		.59	.82	1.05
Chops	1 lb	454	1146	0	63.7	0	54.3	37.8	97	270		.57	.79	1.05
Liver	1 lb	454	617	13.2	95.3	0	6.9	6.63	19.6	1361	229,070[27]	1.81	14.9	1.36
Shoulder	1 lb	454	1082	0	59	0	52	36	92	270		.53	.73	1.05
Liver pate	1 tbsp	13	60	.6	1.5	0			5.7			.01	.04	
Pheasant, ready to cook	1 lb	454	596	0	95.9	0	16	31	52					
Pork[30]														
Bacon, sliced	1 lb	454	3016	4.5	38.1	0	101	179	314	999	0	1.64	.52	.57
Bacon, Canadian	1 lb	454	980	1.4	90.7	0	23	33	65.3		0	3.75	1.01	
Boston butt	1 lb	454	1220	0	65.9	0	37	53	104	232	0	3.2	.77	1.3
Chops	1 lb	454	1065	0	61	0	32	45	89	260	0	2.97	.71	1.3
Feet, pickled	1 lb	454	903	0	75.8	0	24	34	67.1					
Ham, cured	1 lb	454	1535	1.2	66.7	0	50	70	138	318	0	3.36	.817	1.25
Ham, deviled	1 cup	225	790	0	31.3	0	30	39	72.7		0	.32	.23	
Ham, minced	1 lb	454	1034	20	62.1	0	28	38	76.7		0	1.68	1	
Picnic	1 lb	454	1083	0	59	0	33	47	92.2	232	0	2.87	.69	1.3
Spareribs	1 lb	454	976	0	39.2	0	32	46	89.7	232	0	1.91	.46	2.18
Potted meat, all kinds	1 cup	225	558	0	39.4	0			43.2			.07	.5	
Rabbit, ready to cook	1 lb	454	581	0	75	0	11	13	29	295	136	.29	.2	1.58
Sausage														
Blood	1 lb	454	1787	1.4	64	0			167					.17
Bologna	1 lb	454	1379	5	54.9	0	54	69	133			.72	.98	.45
Braunschweiger	1 lb	454	1447	10.4	67.1	0	45	63	124		29,620	.78	6.55	
Brown and serve	1 lb	454	1783	12.2	61.2	0			163					
Cervelat	1 lb	454	2046	7.7	112	0	50	50.4	123		0	1.22	1.04	.64
Country-style	1 lb	454	1565	0	68.5	0	51	72	141			1	.87	
Headcheese	1 lb	454	1216	4.5	70.3	0	36	51	99.8		0	.18	.45	
Knockwurst	1 lb	454	1261	10	64	0	45.5	70.5	123			.77	.95	
Liverwurst	1 lb	454	1393	8.2	73.5	0			116		28,800	.91	5.9	.86

[28]Whole chicken per lb contains 15 gms total fat, 5 gms sat. fat, and 9 gms uns. fat. Chicken contains .25 mg vitamin E/100 gms and approx. 4.54 mcg biotin/lb.
[29]Lamb contains 13.6 mg zinc/lb in lean meat only, no fat. Lamb contains approx. 13.6 mcg biotin/lb.
[30]Lean meat only, no fat.

Vitamin B12 mcg	Biotin mcg	Folic Acid mg	Niacin mg	Pantothenic Acid mg	Vitamin C mg	Vitamin E mg	Sodium mg	Phosphorus mg	Potassium mg	Calcium mg	Iron mg	Magnesium mg	Copper mg	Manganese mg	Selenium mg	Zinc mg
5.4		.032	14.6	1.81			213	559	973	33	9	71	.54			
5.4		.032	14.8	1.81			216	630	989	38	9.2	71				
5.4		.032	21.3	1.81			310	890	1416	53	13.1	97	.318		165	
5.4		.032	16.1	1.81			235	616	1072	39	10	71				
5.4		.032	17.1	1.81			249	652	1138	42	10.5	71	.182			
5.4		.032	14.2	1.81			207	543	946	32	8.8	100	.545			
13.6	13.6		17.2	6.89	0		252	627	679	28	7.2	41	.32			
18.1	31.8	.055	20.1	11.8	82		567	1415	993	45	10.9	54.5	.95			
		.014	10.5	3.6	11.4		377	453	1630	29	4.2	168	1	.091		8.17
2		.027	28.3	3.63	11.4		377	767	1630	39	4.3	82	.636	.091	48	3.18
1.58			9	1.7	8			506	283	43	3.1		.22			
1.8		.05	11.7	4.54	11.4		377	506	1630	35	4.4	168	1	.091	55	8.17
			20.3				295	476	1089	45	13.2	59	.363	.499		13
4	8	.003	5.2	2.56	6		79	142	158	23	1.7	14	.23			2.9
113		1.65	49	27.2	79		318	1070	780	54	35.8	91	.27	1.18		11
1.8		.05	6.5	4.54	11.4		377	396	1630	24	4.1	168	1	.091		12.3
1.8		.05	19.3	4.54	11.4		377	633	1630	41	5.4	168	1	.091		8.17
2		.027	9.1	3.63	11.4		377	451	1630	22	3.3	82	.636	.091		7.26
			3.3				1354	321	594	82	4.3					4.1
			4.6				1188	147	440	29	4.4					
			24.8		36		386	655	1294	37	6		1.86	.136		
5.9		.018	12.2	1.95			4990	603	998	32	8.6		.36			9.1
			22.1				386	583	1907	33	5.3		1.5	.227		
8.2		.018	19	2		3.6	237	593	1083	39	5.1	61	.27			
8.2		.018	18.5	2		3.5	223	567	1019	35	4.7	55	.73		78	
472	454	.99	76.5	32.7	152		236	1583	916	45	49.4	64	25	1.04		
8.2		.018	17 1	2		3.6	206	516	942	35	3.9	50				
			.3													
3.2	31.8		8.3	1.5		1.82	3084	490	590	59	5.4	54	.726			
			21.2		0		8578	816	1778	54	13.6	91				
2	18.2	.036	17.1	2.23		3.18	231	735	1054	38	9.8					14.5[30]
2	18.2	.036	15.9	2.23	0	3.2	214	690	978	36	9.3	68	1.41		98.5	10[30]
2	22.7	.036	18.2	2.05	0		3415	763	1067	41	10.4	62	.136	.27		12.7[30]
			3.6					207			18	4.7				
			15.4					404		36	9.5					
2	18.2	.036	15.4	2.23		3.18	207	664	944	34	9	67				12.7[30]
4.54	22.7	.036	10.2	2.95	9.08	2.7	137	432	627	22	5.9	86.3		.27		
			2.7										.158			
			45.9	2.8		4.5	154	1261	1379	72	4.7					
		.023	12				5897	581	1043	32	8.2		.091			8.2
			37					1111		45	26.8					12.7
								971		50	12.7					
			24.9					1334		64	12.2					
			14					762		41	10.4					
		.009	4					785		41	10.4					
			11.8					699		36	9.5					
63.1		.136	25.9	12.6				1080		41	24.5					

Food Item	Measure	Weight g	Calories	Carbohydrate g	Protein g	Fiber g	Saturated fat g	Unsaturated fat g	Total fat g	Cholesterol mg	Vitamin A IU	Vitamin B1 mg	Vitamin B2 mg	Vitamin B6 mg
Polish-style	1 lb	454	1379	5.4	71.2	0	41	64.4	117		0	1.54	.86	
Pork, link or bulk	1 lb	454	2259	t	42.6	0	83	118	230		0	1.95	.76	.75
Salami	1 lb	454	2041	5.4	108	0	53.5	89.5	151			1.68	1.13	.56
Thuringer	1 lb	454	1393	7.3	84.4	0			111			.51	1.17	
Vienna, canned	7 saus	113	271	.3	15.8	0			22.4			.09	.15	.083
Turkey														
Dark meat, ckd	1 lb	454	921	0	136	0	10.9	24.1	37.6	458	t	.18	1.04	
Light meat, ckd	1 lb	454	798	0	149	0	5.1	11.3	17.7	349	t	.23	.64	
Canned	1 cup	205	414	0	42.8	0	8	16	25.6		270	.04	.29	
Veal (calf)[31]														
Breast	1 lb	454	828	0	65.6	0	29.3	28	61	254		.48	.87	1.22
Chuck	1 lb	454	628	0	70.4	0	17	17	36	320		.52	.94	1.22
Cutlet	1 lb	454	681	0	72.3	0	19.7	18.8	41	254		.53	.96	1.22
Liver	1 lb	454	635	18.6	87.1	0			21.3	1361	102,060[27]	.9	12.3	3.04
Rib roast	1 lb	454	723	0	65.7	0	23.5	22.6	49	254		.48	.87	1.22
Rump roast	1 lb	454	573	0	68	0	14.9	14.2	31	254		.5	.9	1.22
Sweetbreads (pancreas)	1 lb	454	426	0	80.7	0			9.1	1135		.37	.76	
Venison (deer)	1 lb	454	572	0	95	0	11	5	18			1.03	2.19	

NUTS, NUT PRODUCTS, AND SEEDS[32]

Food Item	Measure	Weight g	Calories	Carbohydrate g	Protein g	Fiber g	Saturated fat g	Unsaturated fat g	Total fat g	Cholesterol mg	Vitamin A IU	Vitamin B1 mg	Vitamin B2 mg	Vitamin B6 mg
Almonds														
Raw	1 cup	142	849	27.7	26.4	3.85	6.2	67	77		0	.34	1.31	.142
Roasted and salted	1 cup	157	984	30.6	29.2	3.85	7.3	78.8	90.6		0	.08	1.44	.149
Almond meal	1 oz	28	116	8.2	11.2	.64	.4	4.5	5.2		0	.09	.48	
Brazil nuts, raw	1 cup	140	916	15.3	20	4.2	18.7	69.3	93.7		t	1.34	.17	.238
Cashews, roasted	1 cup	140	785	41	24.1	1.96	10.9	49.3	64		140	.6	.35	
Chestnuts														
Fresh	1 cup	160	310	67.4	4.6	1.66	.44	2.04	2.7		0	.35	.35	.527
Dried	1 cup	100	377	78.6	6.7	2.5			4.1			.34	.39	
Coconut														
Fresh, shredded, not packed	1 cup	80	277	7.5	2.8	2.7	24.3	2	28.2		0	.04	.02	.035
Dried, shredded, sweetened	1 cup	62	344	33	2.24	2.55			24.2		0	.025	.019	
Milk[33]	1 cup	240	605	12.5	7.7		51.4	4.2	59.8		0	.07	t	
Water (liquid from coconuts)	1 cup	240	53	11.3	.7	t			.5		0	t	t	.045
Hazelnuts (filberts), raw	1 cup	135	856	22.5	17	1.05	4.2	59	84.2		144	.62	.738	.735
Hickory nuts, raw	15 sm	15	101	2	2.1	.3	.9	8.8	10.1			.08		
Lychee nuts, dried	6 avg	15	45	10.5	.5	.48			.1					
Macadamia nuts, roasted	6 avg	15	109	1.5	1.4	.375	1.64	8.9	11.7		0	.032	.018	
Peanuts, roasted	1 cup	144	838	29.7	37.7	3.89	15.4	50.5	70.1		t	.46	.19	.576
Peanut butter	1 tbsp	15	86	3.2	3.9	.33	1.5	6.1	8.1		0	.018	.02	.05
Pecans, halves, raw	1 cup	108	742	15.8	9.9	2.3	5.4	63.8	76.9		140	.93	.14	.183
Pine nuts, raw	1 oz	28	180	5.8	3.7	.31	1.7	11.7	14.3		10	.36	.07	
Pistachio nuts, shelled	30 avg	15	88	2.8	2.9	.3	1.1	6.5	8		34.4	.1		
Pumpkin and squash seeds, dried, hulled	1 cup	140	774	21	40.6	2.66	11.8	51	65.4		100	.34	.27	
Sesame seeds, dried, hulled	1 cup	150	873	26.4	27.3	3.6	11.2	64	80			.27	.2	.126
Sunflower seeds, dried, hulled	1 cup	145	812	28.9	34.8	5.5	8.2	56.9	68.6		70	2.84	.33	1.8
Walnuts														
Black, chopped, raw	1 cup	125	785	18.5	25.6	2.13	4.5	61.6	74.1		380	.28	.14	
English, halves, raw	1 cup	100	651	15.8	14.8	2.1	4.5	49.5	64		30	.33	.13	.73

[31]Veal contains 12.7 mg zinc/lb lean meat only, no fat.

[32]All nuts and seeds are unsalted, unless stated otherwise. For salted nuts, the sodium content is approx. 280 mg/cup.

[33]Liquid from mixture of coconut meat and water.

Vitamin B12 mcg	Biotin mcg	Folic Acid mg	Niacin mg	Pantothenic Acid mg	Vitamin C mg	Vitamin E mg	Sodium mg	Phosphorus mg	Potassium mg	Calcium mg	Iron mg	Magnesium mg	Copper mg	Manganese mg	Selenium mg	Zinc mg
2.4		.064	14.1	3.09			3357	798		41	10.9	41				15
6.4			10.4					417	635	23	6.4					
			24					1284		64	16.3					
			19.2					971		50	12.7					
			2.9					173		9	2.4					
		.032	19.1	5			449	962	1805	36	10.4		.545	.136		14.1
		.023	50.3	2.68			372	962	1864	36	5.4		.454	.136		7.26
			9.6							21	2.9					
5.7	22.7	.023	22	3.23			230	652	1050	39	9.7					
5.7	22.7	.023	23.6	3.23			246	722	1126	40	10.5					
5.7	22.7	.023	24.2	3.23			253	734	1157	41	10.9	73	1.14			
272			51.8	36.3	161		331	1510	1275	36	39.9	73	36			17
5.7	22.7	.023	22	3.23	0		230	664	1051	38	9.8	52	1.14		.136	
5.7	22.7	.023	22.8	3.23			238	699	1090	38	10					
63.6	63		11.7				281	1521	1130	41	4.54	68	.27			
			28.6		0		318	1129	1525	45	22.7	150				
0	25	.136	5	.668	t	21.3	6	716	1098	332	6.7	386	1.18	2.7	2.8	
0			5.5	.393	0		311	791	1214	369	7.4					4.02
			1.8		0		2	259	397	120	2.4					
0		.006	2.2	.323	14	9.1	1	970	1001	260	4.8	351	2.14	3.9	144	7.1
0		.095	2.5	1.82			21	522	650	53	5.3	374				6.1
0	2.1		1	.756	9.6	.8	10	141	726	43	2.7	65.6	.67	5.9		
			.8		0		4	170	875	57	3.3					
0		.031	.4	.16	2	.8	18	76	205	10	1.4	37	.368	1.05		
0			.248		2.5		11	696	219	9.94	1.24	46	.33			
			1.9		5			240		38	3.8					
0			.2	.12	5		60	31	353	48	.7	67				
0		.097	1.2	1.54	t	28	3	455	950	282	4.6	313	1.72	5.67	2.7	4
					0					4	.4	24	.214			
					5				165	4	.3					
			.2		0			36		8	.3					
0	49	.153	24.6	3		9.36	7	586	1009	104	3.2	252	.62	2.17		
0	5.8	.013	2.4		0		18	59	123	11	.3	26	.085			
0		.026	1	1.7	2	1.5	t	312	651	79	2.6	142	1.14	1.54	3.24	
			1.3		t			171		3	1.5					
		.009	.21		0			75	145	19.6	1.09	23.7	.168			
		.144	3.4					1602		71	15.7					
0			8.1		0			888		165	3.6	270	2.39			
0			7.8	2				1214	1334	174	10.3	57	2.57			
			.9				4	713	575	t	7.5	238	1.74			2.82
0	37	.066	.9	.9	2	1.5	2	380	450	99	3.1	131	1.39	1.8		2.26

Food Item	Measure	Weight g	Calories	Carbohydrate g	Protein g	Fiber g	Saturated fat g	Unsaturated fat g	Total fat g	Cholesterol mg	Vitamin A IU	Vitamin B₁ mg	Vitamin B₂ mg	Vitamin B₆ mg
OILS, FATS, AND SHORTENING														
Bacon fat	1 tbsp	14	126		0	t			14					
Butter	1 tbsp	14.2	102	.1	.1	0	6.3	4.1	11.5	35	470	t	.001	t
Butter	1 cup	227	1625	.9	1.4	0	101	66.2	184	570	7500	t	.02	.006
Chicken fat	1 tbsp	14	126	0	0				14					
Lard	1 tbsp	13	117	0	0	0	4.9	7.3	13	12	0	0	0	.003
Margarine														
Regular	1 tbsp	14.2	102	.1	.1	0	2.1	9	11.5	0[34]	470	t	t	
Whipped	1 tbsp	9.4	68	t	.1	0	1.4	6	7.6	0[34]	310	t	t	
Oils														
Cod-liver	1 tbsp	14	126	0	0	0			14	119	11,900		0	
Corn	1 tbsp	14	126	0	0	0	1.4	11	14	t	t	t	t	
Cottonseed	1 tbsp	14	126	0	0	0	3.4	9.7	14	0	0	0	0	
Olive	1 tbsp	14	124	t	t	0	1.5	11.2	14	t	0	0	0	
Peanut	1 tbsp	14	124	t	t	0	2.4	10.2	14	t	0	0	0	
Safflower	1 tbsp	14	124	0	0	0	1.1	11.8	14	t	t	t	t	
Soybean	1 tbsp	14	124	t	t	0	2	9.8	14	t	0	0	0	
Sesame	1 tbsp	14	120	t	t	0	1.9	10.9	14	t	0	0	0	
Sunflower	1 tbsp	14	124	t	t	0	1.8	12	14	t	0	0	0	
Wheat germ	1 tbsp	14	124	t	t	0	2.34	8.8	14	t	0	0	0	
Vegetable shortening	1 tbsp	12.5	111	0	0	0	3.1	9	12.5			0	0	
SALAD DRESSINGS AND SAUCES														
Barbecue sauce	1 tbsp	15	14	1.25	.238	.09	.106	.875	1.08		56	.002	.002	
Catsup, tomato	1 tbsp	15	16	3.8	.3	.075			.1		210	.01	.01	.016
Chili sauce	1 tbsp	17	16	4	.5	.126			.1		210	.02	.01	
Hollandaise sauce	1 tbsp	12.5	45	.1	.55				4.6		257	.007	.011	
Horseradish, prepared	1 tbsp	15	6	1.4	.2	.108			t					.022
Mayonnaise	1 tbsp	14	101	.3	.2	t	2	8	11.2	10	40	t	.01	
Miso, takka		100	249	42.8	9	2			5.2		0	.1	.15	
Mustard	1 tbsp	15	15	.9	.9	.3			.9					
Salad dressings														
Blue or Roquefort cheese, regular	1 tbsp	15	76	1.1	.7	t	1.6	5.5	7.8		30	t	.02	
Blue or Roquefort cheese, low calorie	1 tbsp	16	12	.7	.5	.01	.5	.3	.9		30	t	.01	
Caesar	1 tbsp	15	73	.6	.3				8					
French, regular	1 tbsp	16	66	2.8	.1	.04	1.1	4.5	6.2					
French, low calorie	1 tbsp	16	15	2.5	.1	.04	.1	.5	.7					
Green goddess	1 tbsp	15	72	.8	.1				7.4					
Italian	1 tbsp	15	83	1	t	t	1.6	6.6	9		t	t	t	
Russian	1 tbsp	15	74	1.6	.2	.045	1.4	5.5	7.6		100	.01	.01	
Thousand Island, regular	1 tbsp	16	80	2.5	.1	.04	1.4	5.7	8		50	t	t	
Thousand Island, low calorie	1 tbsp	15	27	2.3	.1	.04	.4	1.4	2.1		50	t	t	
Soy sauce	1 tbsp	18	12	1.7	1	0			.2		0	t	.05	
Tartar sauce	1 tbsp	14	31	.9	.1	.042			3.1	7	30	t	t	
Umeboshi		100	17	3.4	.3	.3			.8		0	.06	.09	
Vinegar	1 tbsp	15	2	.9	t	0			0					t
White sauce, medium	1 tbsp	16	27	1.5	.65	t	1	.71	2.05	2.06	82	.005	.025	
Worcestershire sauce	1 tbsp	15	12	2.7	.3				0					
SOUPS[35]														
Asparagus, cream of	1 cup	240	65	10.1	2.4	.8			1.7		310	.05	.1	
Bean and pork	1 cup	250	168	21.8	8	1.8	1.3	3.9	5.8		650	.13	.08	
Beef														
Consomme or bouillon	1 cup	240	31	2.6	5	.14			0		t	t	.02	
Noodle	1 cup	245	140	14.2	7.8	.15	.8	1.6	2.6		120	.1	.12	

[34]Value for all vegetable fat; ⅔ animal fat and ⅓ vegetable fat has 7 mg/tbsp.

[35]All soups are diluted with water.

Vitamin B$_{12}$ mcg	Biotin mcg	Folic Acid mg	Niacin mg	Panto-thenic Acid mg	Vitamin C mg	Vitamin E mg	Sodium mg	Phospho-rus mg	Potas-sium mg	Calcium mg	Iron mg	Magne-sium mg	Copper mg	Manga-nese mg	Sele-nium mg	Zinc mg
t					0	.35	140	2	3	3	0	.28	.004	.006		.01
t					0	5.2	2240	36	52	45	0	4.5	.067	.09		.2
0		0			0	.14	.039	.39	.026	.129	.013		.004			.03
		t	t		0	1.25	140	2	3	3	0		.006			.03
		t	t		0	.89	93	2	2	2	0		.004			.03
			0			3.6	.014									
		t			t	11	t	0	0	t	t					.025
		0			0	10.9	0	0	0	0	0					.025
		0			0	.714	.001	0	t	.07	.01		.01			.025
		0			0	1.8	t	0	0	t	0		.001			.025
		t			t	10.5	t	0	0	t	t					.025
		0			0	7.9	t	0	0	t	0		.056			.025
		0			0	2.3	t	0	0	t	0					.025
		0			0	1.3	t	0	0	t	0					
		0			0	21.5	t	0	0	t	0					
		0			0	0	0	0	0	0	0					
		.001	.05		.8		127	3	27	3.3	.125					.005
0		.001	.2		2		156	8	54	3	.1		.089			.039
			.2		2		201	3	56	2	.1					
			t		t			19.5		6	.225					
0							14	5	44	9	.1	5	.021			.16
		t	t		0		84	4	5	3	.1	.28	.034			.022
			1.5		0			250		150	60					
							195	21	21	18	.3	7.2	.06			.032
		t			t		164	11	6	12	t					.038
		t			t		177	8	5	10	t					
							236									
						1.3	219	2	13	2	.1	1.4				.012
						.2	126	2	13	2	.1					
						1.54	140									
		t				1.8	314	1	2	2	t		.105			.017
			.1		1	1.34	130	6	24	3	.1					.065
		t			t	1.5	112	3	18	2	.1					.021
		t			t	.33	105	3	17	2	.1					
		.005	.1		0		1319	19	66	15	.9					
		t			t		99	4	11	3	.1					
			.6		0		9400	26		6.1	2					
0							t	1	15	1	.1	.2	.014		13.3	.015
			.05		.125		59	15	21.7	18	.05					
								9		15	.9					
		.047	.7				984	38	120	26	.7					
			1		3		1008	128	395	63	2.3					
		.01	1.2				782	31	130	t	.5		1.85			
			2.2		2		1872	98	157	15	1.7		.09			3

Food Item.	Measure	Weight g	Calories	Carbohy-drate g	Protein g	Fiber g	Satu-rated fat g	Unsatu-rated fat g	Total fat g	Choles-terol mg	Vitamin A IU	Vitamin B₁ mg	Vitamin B₂ mg	Vitamin B₆ mg
Celery, cream of	1 cup	240	86	8.9	1.7	.84	.9	3.7	5		190	.02	.05	
Chicken														
Consomme or bouillon	1 cup	240	22	1.9	3.4	t			t					
Cream of	1 cup	240	94	7.9	2.9	.3	.9	4.3	5.8		410	.02	.05	
Gumbo	1 cup	240	55	7.4	3.1	.1			1.4		220	.02	.05	
Noodle	1 cup	240	62	7.9	3.4	.25			1.9		50	.02	.02	
w/rice	1 cup	240	48	5.8	3.1	.12			1.2		140	t	.02	
Chili beef	1 cup	250	168	23.4	7.9	1.1			4.7		851	.09	.08	
Clam chowder														
Manhattan	1 cup	245	81	12.3	2.2	.4			2.5		880	.02	.02	
New England	1 cup	240	130	10.5	4.3	.25			7.7		48	.05	.1	
Minestone	1 cup	245	105	14.2	4.9	.9			3.4		2350	.07	.05	
Mushroom, cream of	1 cup	240	134	10.1	2.4	.12	1.3	7.3	9.6		70	.02	.12	
Onion	1 cup	240	65	5.3	5.3	.5			2.4		t	t	.02	
Oyster stew	1 cup	240	120	8	5.88	.1			8		240	.07	.19	
Pea, split	1 cup	245	145	20.6	8.6	.5	1	1.8	3.2		440	.25	.15	
Potato, cream of	1 cup	260	115	12	3.6	.45	3	2	5.7		442	.05	.07	
Tomato	1 cup	245	88	15.7	2	.7	.4	1.7	2.5		1000	.05	.05	
Turkey noodle	1 cup	240	79	8.4	4.3	.12	.8	1.8	2.9		190	.05	.05	
Vegetable														
Beef	1 cup	245	78	9.6	5.1	.65			2.2		2700	.05	.05	
Vegetarian	1 cup	245	78	13.2	2.2	.9			2		2940	.05	.05	
SPICES AND HERBS														
Allspice, grd	1 tsp	1.9	5	1.37	.12	.41	.05	.05	.17	0	10	.002	.001	
Anise seed	1 tsp	2.1	7	1.05	.37	.31		.28	.33	0				
Basil, grd	1 tsp	1.4	4	.85	.2	.25			.06	0	131	.002	.004	
Bay leaf, crumbled	1 tsp	.6	2	.45	.05	16	.01	.02	.05	0	37	t	.003	
Caraway seed	1 tsp	2.1	7	1.05	.42	.27	.01	.22	.31	0	8	.008	.008	
Cardamom, grd	1 tsp	2	6	1.37	.21	.23	.01	.03	.13	0		.004	.004	
Celery seed	1 tsp	2	8	.83	.36	.24	.04	.39	.5	0	1			
Chervil, dried	1 tsp	.6	1	.3	.14	.07			.02	0				.007
Chili powder	1 tsp	2.6	8	1.42	.32	.58			.44	0	908	.009	.021	
Cinnamon, grd	1 tsp	2.3	6	1.84	.09	.56	.01	.02	.07	0	6	.002	.003	
Cloves, grd	1 tsp	2.1	7	1.29	.13	.2	.09		.42	0	11	.002	.006	
Coriander leaf, dried	1 tsp	.6	2	.31	.13	.06			.03	0		.008	.009	
Coriander seed	1 tsp	1.8	5	.99	.22	.52	.02	.27	.32	0		.004	.005	
Cumin seed	1 tsp	2.1	8	.93	.37	.22			.47	0	27	.013	.007	
Curry powder	1 tsp	2	6	1.16	.25	.33			.28	0	20	.005	.006	
Dill seed	1 tsp	2.1	6	1.16	.34	.44	.02	.22	.31	0	1	.009	.006	
Dill weed, dried	1 tsp	1	3	.56	.2	.12			t	0		.004	.003	.015
Fennel seed	1 tsp	2	7	1.05	.32	.31	.01	.23	.3	0	3	.008	.007	
Fenugreek seed	1 tsp	3.7	12	2.16	.85	.37			.24	0		.012	.014	
Garlic powder	1 tsp	2.8	9	2.04	.47	.05			.02	0		.013	.004	
Ginger, grd	1 tsp	1.8	6	1.27	.16	.11	.03	.04	.11	0	3	.001	.003	
Mace, grd	1 tsp	1.7	8	.86	.11	.08	.16	.26	.55	0	14	.005	.008	
Marjoram, dried	1 tsp	.6	2	.36	.08	.11			.04	0	48	.002	.002	
Mustard seed, yellow	1 tsp	3.3	15	1.15	.82	.22	.05	.83	.95	0	2	.018	.013	
Nutmeg, grd	1 tsp	2.2	12	1.08	.13	.09	.57	.08	.8	0	2	.008	.001	
Onion powder	1 tsp	2.1	7	1.69	.21	.12			.02	0		.009	.001	
Oregano, grd	1 tsp	1.5	5	.97	.17	.22	.04	.09	.15	0	104	.005		
Paprika	1 tsp	2.1	6	1.17	.31	.44	.04	.2	.27	0	1273	.014	.037	
Parsley, dried	1 tsp	.3	1	.15	.07	.03			.01	0	70	.001	.004	.003
Pepper														
Black	1 tsp	2.1	5	1.36	.23	.28	.03	.03	.07	0	4	.002	.005	
Red or cayenne	1 tsp	1.8	6	1.02	.22	.45	.06	.2	.31	0	749	.006	.017	

*Present, but approximate value in milligrams unavailable.

Vitamin B12 mcg	Biotin mcg	Folic Acid mg	Niacin mg	Pantothenic Acid mg	Vitamin C mg	Vitamin E mg	Sodium mg	Phosphorus mg	Potassium mg	Calcium mg	Iron mg	Magnesium mg	Copper mg	Manganese mg	Selenium mg	Zinc mg
			t	1.1	t		955	36	108	48	.5					
							722	72		12	1.2		.02			
			.5		t		970	34	79	24	.5					
			1.2		5		950	24	108	19	.5		.27			
			.7		t		979	36	55	10	.5					
			.7				917	24	98	7	.2					
			1.4				1102	151		28.5	3.3					
		.018	1				938	47	184	34	1					1.42
			.5				104	82	221	91	.96					
			1				995	59	314	37	1					
		.007	.7		t		955	50	98	41	.5					1.25
			t				1051	26	103	29	.5					
			.5		t		512	148	246	158	1.4					
			1.5		1		941	149	270	29	1.5					
			.53	.878			1274	68	239	62	1.04					
0			1.2		12		970	34	230	15	.7	22	.27			.17
			1.2		t		998	43	77	14	.7					
		.015	1				1046	49	162	12	.7		.09			3.87
			1	.34			838	39	172	20	1	24	.32			1.8
			.054		.75		1	2	20	13	.13	3	*	*	.06	.02
0							t	9	30	14	.78	4				.11
0			.097		.86		t	7	48	30	.59	6	*	*		.08
0			.012		.28		t	1	3	5	.26	1	*	*		.02
0			.076				t	12	28	14	.34	5			.18	.12
0			.022				t	4	22	8	.28	5	*	*		.15
0					.34		3	11	28	35	.9	9	*	*		.14
0							t	3	28	8	.19	1				.05
0			.205		1.67		26	8	50	7	.37		4		.65	.07
0			.03		.65		1	1	11	28	.88	1	*	*	.5	.05
0			.031		1.7		5	2	23	14	.18	6	*	*		.02
0			.064		3.4		1	3	27	7	.25	4	*	*		
0			.038				1	7	23	13	.29	6	*	*		.08
0			.096		.16		4	10	38	20	1.39	8	*	*		.1
0			.069		.23		1	7	31	10	.59	5	.021			.08
0			.059				t	6	25	32	.34	5	*	*		.11
0			.029				2	5	32	18	.49	5	*	*		.03
0			.121				2	10	34	24	.37	8	*	*		.07
0		2.11	.061		.11		2	11	28	6	1.24	7				.09
0			.019				1	12	31	2	.08	2	*	*		.07
0			.093				1	3	24	2	.21	3	.01	*		.08
0			.023				1	2	8	4	.24	3	*	*		.04
0			.025		.31		t	2	9	12	.5	2	*	*		.02
0			.26				t	28	23	17	.33	10	*	*		.19
0			.029				t	5	8	4	.07	4	*	*	.4	.05
0			.014		.31		1	7	20	8	.05	3	*	*		.05
0			.093				t	3	25	24	.66	4	*	*		.07
0			.322		1.49		1	7	49	4	.5	4	*	*	.22	.08
0			.024		.37		1	1	11	4	.29	1	*	*		.01
0			.024				1	4	26	9	.61	4	.012	*	.02	.03
0			.157		1.38		1	5	36	3	.14	3	*	*		.05

Food Item	Measure	Weight g	Calories	Carbohydrate g	Protein g	Fiber g	Saturated fat g	Unsaturated fat g	Total fat g	Cholesterol mg	Vitamin A IU	Vitamin B1 mg	Vitamin B2 mg	Vitamin B6 mg
White	1 tsp	2.4	7	1.65	.25	.1			.05	0			.001	.003	
Poppy seed	1 tsp	2.8	15	.66	.5	.18	.14	1.04	1.25	0			.024	.005	.012
Poultry seasoning[36]	1 tsp	1.5	5	.98	.14	.17			.11	0	39	.004	.003	
Pumpkin pie spice[37]	1 tsp	1.7	6	1.17	.1	.25			.21	0	4	.002	.002	
Rosemary, dried	1 tsp	1.2	4	.77	.06	.21			.18	0	38	.006		
Saffron	1 tsp	.7	2	.46	.08	.03			.04	0				
Sage, grd	1 tsp	.7	2	.43	.07	.13	.05	.02	.09	0	41	.005	.002	
Salt	1 tsp	5.5	0	0	0				0	0	0	0	0	
Savory, grd	1 tsp	1.4	4	.96	.09	.21			.08	0	72		.005	
Tarragon, grd	1 tsp	1.6	5	.8	.36	.12			.12	0	67	.004	.021	
Thyme, grd	1 tsp	1.4	4	.89	.13	.26	.04	.03	.1	0	53	.007	.006	
Turmeric, grd	1 tsp	2.2	8	1.43	.17	.15			.22	0		.003	.005	

VEGETABLES, LEGUMES, SPROUTS, AND VEGETABLE JUICES[38]

Food Item	Measure	Weight g	Calories	Carbohydrate g	Protein g	Fiber g	Saturated fat g	Unsaturated fat g	Total fat g	Cholesterol mg	Vitamin A IU	Vitamin B1 mg	Vitamin B2 mg	Vitamin B6 mg
Alfalfa, sprouts, raw	1 cup	100	41		5.1	1.7			.6				.14	.21	
Artichoke, globe, boiled[39]	1 avg	100	44	9.9	2.8	2.4			.2		150	.07	.04	
Asparagus														
Cut pieces, raw	1 cup	135	35	6.8	3.4	.945			.3		1220	.24	.27	.2
Spears, ckd	4 lg	100	20	3.6	2.2	.7			.2		900	.16	.18	.1[40]
Spears, canned, drained	4 avg	80	17	2.7	1.9	.4			.3		640	.05	.08	.044
Bamboo shoots, raw	1 cup	125	36	6.9	3.47	.932			.4		26.7	.02	.093	
Beans														
Azuki, dry		100	326	58.4	21.5	4.3			1.6		6	.5	.1	
Black, dry	1 cup	200	678	122	44.6				3		60	1.1	.4	
Black-eye peas, ckd	1 cup	165	178	29.9	13.4				1.3		580	.5	.18	.18[40]
Canned w/pork	1 cup	250	304	47.6	15.2	3.6	2.3	3.3	6.4		324	.2	.08	
Canned w/o pork	1 cup	250	300	57.6	15.8	3.6			1.2		150	.18	.1	
Chickpeas (garbanzos), dry	1 cup	200	720	122	41	10	.9	8.3	9.6		100	.62	.3	
Green, snap, raw	1 cup	110	35	7.8	2.1	1.1			.2		660	.09	.12	.08
Green, snap, ckd	1 cup	125	31	6.8	2	1.2			.3		680	.09	.11	.087[40]
Green, snap, canned, drained	1 cup	135	32	7	1.9	1.2			.3		630	.04	.07	.054
Lentils, ckd	1 cup	200	212	38.6	15.6	2.4			t		40	.14	.12	
Lentil sprouts, raw	1 cup	100	104		8.4	1.1			.3			.21	.09	
Lima, ckd	1 cup	190	262	48.6	15.6	3			1.1			.25	.11	.3[40]
Lima, canned, drained	1 cup	170	163	31	9.2	3			.5		320	.05	.09	.15
Mung, sprouts, raw	1 cup	105	37	6.9	4	.7			.2		20	.14	.14	
Pinto, dry	1 cup	190	663	121	43.5	8			2.3			1.6	.4	1
Red kidney, ckd	1 cup	185	218	39.6	14.4	2.78			.9		10	.2	.11	
Red kidney, canned	1 cup	255	230	41.8	14.5	2.3			1		10	.13	.1	
Soybeans, ckd	1 cup	180	234	19.4	19.8	3			10.3		50	.38	.16	
Soybeans, canned, drained	1 cup	150	153	11.1	13.5	2.1			7.5		510	.09		
Soybean curd (tofu)	3.5 oz	100	72	2.4	7.8	.1			4.2		0	.06	.03	
Soybeans, fermented, miso		100	776	107	47.6				20.9		180	.29	.44	
Soybeans, fermented, natto		100	758	52.2	76.7				33.6		0	.32	2.27	
Soybean granules	1 cup	152	480	48	76				8		t	2.4	.68	
Soybean milk	1 cup	226	75	5	7.7				3.4		90	.18	.065	
Soybean sprouts, raw	1 cup	105	48	5.6	6.5	2.3			1.5		80	.24	.21	
Yellow wax, ckd	1 cup	125	28	5.8	1.8	1			.3		290	.09	.11	.098[40]
Yellow wax, canned, drained	1 cup	135	32	7	1.9	1			.4		140	.04	.07	.056
White, ckd	1 cup	190	224	40.3	14.8	3			1.1		0	.27	.13	

*Present, but approximate value in milligrams unavailable.

[36]Mixture of white pepper, sage, thyme, marjoram, savory, ginger, allspice, nutmeg.

[37]Mixture of cinnamon, ginger, nutmeg, allspice, cloves.

[38]Most of the vegetables are cooked, unsalted, in small amount of water for a short time.

[39]Base and soft ends of leaves.

[40]Based on frozen product.

Vitamin B12 mcg	Biotin mcg	Folic Acid mg	Niacin mg	Pantothenic Acid mg	Vitamin C mg	Vitamin E mg	Sodium mg	Phosphorus mg	Potassium mg	Calcium mg	Iron mg	Magnesium mg	Copper mg	Manganese mg	Selenium mg	Zinc mg
0		.005					t	4	2	6	.34	2	*	*		.03
0		.027					1	24	20	41	.26	9	*	*		.29
0		.045			.18		t	3	10	15	.53	3				.05
0		.038			.4		1	2	11	12	.34	2				.04
0		.012			.74		1	1	11	15	.35	3	*	*		.04
0							1	2	12	1	.08					
0		.04			.23		t	1	7	12	.2	3	*	*		.03
		0			0		2132		t	14	t		.022			.22
0		.057					t	2	15	30	.53	5	*	*		.06
0		.143					1	5	48	18	.52	6	*	*		.06
0		.069					1	3	11	26	1.73	3	*	*	.075	.09
0		.113			.57		1	6	56	4	.91	4	*	*		.1
			1.6		16					28	1.4					1
			.7		8		30	69	301	51	1.1		.2	.36		.35
0	.675	.086	2	.837	45	2.59	3	84	375	30	1.4	27	.148	.256		1.31
0			1.4	.4[40]	26		1	50	183	21	.6		.1			
0	1.6	.005	.6	.156	12		189	42	133	15	1.5		.12			
			.8		5.32			78.7	708	17.3	.667					
			2.5		0		7	350		75	4.8					
			4.4				50	840	2076	270	15.8					
0		.168	2.3	.66[40]	28		2	241	625	40	3.5	90.7				3
		.061	1.6	.23	4		1158	230	526	136	4.4	100	.55			
			1.6		4		844	302	670	170	5	146				
		.398	4		t		52	662	1594	300	13.8					5.4
0		.048	.6	.19	21	.1	8	48	267	62	.9	35	.26	.45	.66	.4
0		.05	.6	.168[40]	15		5	46	189	63	.8		.125			.4
0	1.35	.016	.4	.1	5		319	34	128	61	2	28	.054		1.2	.4
			1.2		0			238	498	50	4.2		.54			2
			1.1		24					12	3					1.5
0		.082	1.3	.48[40]			4	293	1163	55	5.9		.32			1.7
0		.022	.9	.22	10		401	119	377	48	4.1					
		.012	.8		20		5	67	234	20	1.4					.9
0		.41	4.2	1.23			19	868	1870	257	12.2					
		.068	1.3				6	259	629	70	4.4		.647			
			1.5				8	278	673	74	4.6					
			1.1		0		4	322	972	131	4.9					
					3		354	176		100	5.2					
			.1		0		7	126	42	128	1.9	111				
			1.3		0		13,381	1402	1515	308	7.7					
			5		0			826	1129	467	16.8					
			1.6		t		8			240	10.8					
			.5		0			109		47.5	1.8					
			.8		14			70		50	1.1					1.6
0		.042	.6	.172[40]	16		4	46	189	63	.8					
0			.4		7		319	34	128	61	2					
			1.3		0		13	281	790	95	5.1					1.8

Food Item	Measure	Weight g	Calories	Carbohydrate g	Protein g	Fiber g	Saturated fat g	Unsaturated fat g	Total fat g	Cholesterol mg	Vitamin A IU	Vitamin B₁ mg	Vitamin B₂ mg	Vitamin B₆ mg
Beets, diced														
Raw	1 cup	135	58	13.4	2.2	1.1			.1		30	.04	.07	.074
Cooked	1 cup	170	54	12.2	1.9	.94			.2		30	.05	.07	
Canned, drained	1 cup	170	63	15	1.7	.94			.2		30	.02	.05	.068
Beet greens														
Raw	3.5 oz	100	24	4.6	2.2	1.3			.3		6100	.1	.22	.05
Cooked	1 cup	145	26	4.8	2.5	1.4			.3		7400	.1	.22	
Broccoli														
Raw, 5½″ long	1 piece	100	32	5.9	3.6	1.5			.3		2500[41]	.1	.23	.195
Cooked	1 cup	155	40	7	4.8	2			.5		3800	.14	.31	
Brussels sprouts														
Raw	9 med	100	45	8.3	4.9	1.6			.4		550	.1	.16	.23
Cooked	1 cup	155	56	9.9	6.5	2.1			.6		810	.12	.22	.262[40]
Cabbage														
Common, sliced, raw	1 cup	70	17	3.8	.9	.8			.1		90	.04	.04	.112
Common, sliced, ckd	1 cup	145	29	6.2	1.6	1			.3		190	.06	.06	
Red, sliced, raw	1 cup	70	22	4.8	1.4	1			.1		30	.06	.04	.14
Savoy, sliced, raw	1 cup	70	17	3.2	1.7	.5			.1		140	.04	.06	.133
Chinese, raw	1 cup	75	11	2.3	.9	.6			.1		110	.04	.03	
Chinese, ckd	1 cup	160	16	2.6	2.4						80	.14	.14	
Carrots														
Raw	1 lg	100	42	9.7	1.1	1			.2		11,000	.06	.05	.15
Cooked	1 cup	155	48	11	1.4	1.5			.3		15,750	.08	.08	
Canned, drained	1 cup	155	47	10.4	1.2	1			.5		22,500	.03	.05	.045
Juice	1 cup	227	96	22.2	2.47						24,750	.13	.12	.5
Cauliflower, flower buds														
Raw	1 cup	100	27	5.2	2.7	1			.2		60	.11	.1	.21
Cooked	1 cup	125	28	5.1	2.9	1.25			.3		80	.11	.1	.22[40]
Celeriac root, raw	4 roots	100	40	8.5	1.8	1.3			.3			.05	.06	.165
Celery														
Raw	1 cup	120	20	4.7	1.1	.7			.1		320	.04	.04	.072
Cooked	1 cup	150	21	4.7	1.2	.9			.2		390	.03	.05	
Chard, Swiss														
Raw	3.5 oz	100	25	4.6	2.4	.8			.3		6500	.06	.17	
Cooked	1 cup	145	26	4.8	2.6	1			.3		7830	.06	.16	
Chives, chopped, raw	1 tbsp	10	3	.6	.2	.1			t		580	.008	.013	.018
Collards														
Raw	3 oz	100	40	7.2	3.6	.9			.7		6500	.2	.31	
Cooked	1 cup	145	42	7.1	3.9	1.15			.9		7830	.2	.29	
Corn														
Cooked	1 cup	165	137	31	5.3				1.7		660	.18	.17	.47[40]
Canned, drained	1 cup	165	139	32.7	4.3	1.1			1.3		580	.05	.08	.33
Cream-style canned	1 cup	256	210	51.2	5.4				1.5		840	.08	.13	.1
Cress, sprigs														
Raw	5–8	10	3	.6	.3	.1			.1		930	.008	.026	.025
Cooked	1 cup	135	31	5.1	2.6	1.2			.8		10,400	.08	.22	
Cucumber, sliced, un-pared, raw	1 cup	105	16	3.6	.9	.6			.1		260	.03	.04	.042
Dandelion greens														
Raw	3.5 oz	100	45	9.2	2.7	1.6			.7		14,000	.19	.26	
Cooked	1 cup	105	35	6.7	2.1	1.3			.6		12,290	.14	.17	
Dock (sorrel), raw	3.5 oz	100	28	5.6	2.1	.8			.3		12,900	.09	.22	
Eggplant														
Raw	1 cup	200	50	11.6	2.4	1.8			.4		20	.1	.1	.162
Cooked	1 cup	200	38	8.2	2	1.8			.4		20	.1	.08	
Endive, raw	1 cup	50	10	2.1	.9	.45			.1		1650	.04	.07	
Garlic, raw	1 clove	3	4	.9	.2				t		t	.01	t	
Ginger root, fresh	3.5 oz	100	49	9.5	1.4	1.1			1		10	.02	.04	

[41]Value for leaves is 16,000 IU/100 gr, flower clusters 3000 IU, stalks 400 IU.

Vitamin B$_{12}$ mcg	Biotin mcg	Folic Acid mg	Niacin mg	Pantothenic Acid mg	Vitamin C mg	Vitamin E mg	Sodium mg	Phosphorus mg	Potassium mg	Calcium mg	Iron mg	Magnesium mg	Copper mg	Manganese mg	Selenium mg	Zinc mg
0		.126	.5	.2	14		81	45	452	22	.9	31	.297	1.27		.068
		.133	.5		10		73	39	354	24	.9		.34			
0			.2	.17	5		401	31	284	32	1.2	25.5	.238			
0	3	.05	.4	.1	30		130	40	570	119	3.3	106	.09	1.3		
			.4		22		110	36	481	144	2.8					
0		.069	9	1.17	113		15	78	382	103	1.1	24	.03	.15		
		.073	1.2		140		16	96	414	136	1.2		.15			.23
0	.4	.078	.9	.723	102	1	14	80	390	36	1.5	29	.05	.27		.38
0		.056	1.2	.63[40]	135		16	112	423	50	1.7		.12			.54
0	.07	.046	.2	1.143	33	.2	14	20	163	34	.3	13	.091		1.54	.3
		.026	.4			.48		20	29	236	64	.4		.13			.6
0	1.4	.031	.3	.226	43	.14	18	25	188	29	.6	12.6	.042	.07		
0			.2		39		15	38	188	47	.6					
		.062	.5		19		17	30	190	32	.5	10.5				
			1.6		52			64		52	.4					
0	3	.032	.6	.28	8	.45	47	36	341	37	.7	23	.15	.1	2.2	.4
		.037	.8		9		51	48	344	51	.9		.12			.5
0	2	.002	.6	.195	3		366	34	186	47	1.1	7	.06		2.02	.5
.023	0		1.35		20		105	81	767	8.3	1.5	51				
0	1.5	.055	.7	1	78	.15	13	56	295	25	1.1	24	.13	.17	.7	.37
0		.042	.8	.64[40]	69		11	53	258	26	.9		.07			
0			.7		8		100	115	300	43	6					
0	.12	.014	.4	.514	11	.57	151	34	409	47	.4	26	17	.19		.16
			.5		9		132	33	359	47	.3		.18			
0		.03	.5	.172	32	1.5	147	39	550	88	3.2	65	.11	.3		
			.6		23		125	35	465	106	2.6					
0			.1		6		t	4	25	7	.2	3	.011			
		.102	1.7		92		43	63	401	203	1	57				
			1.7		67		36	57	339	220	.9					
0		.035	2.1	.725[40]	12		t	147	272	5	1					.7
0	1.95	.013	1.5	.363	7		389	81	160	8	.8	34			.495	.7
			2.6		13		604	143	248	8	1.5					1.06
0			1		7		1	8	61	8	.1					
			1.1		46		11	65	477	82	1.1					
0	1	.015	.2	.25	12	8.4	6	28	168	26	1.2	12	.09	.15		.22
					35		76	66	397	187	3.1	36	.15	.3		
					19		46	44	244	147	1.9					
			.5		119		5	41	338	66	1.6					
0		.062	1.2	.44	10		4	52	428	24	1.4	32	.2	.22		
		.032	1		6		2	42	300	22	1.2					
		.024	.3		5		7	27	147	41	.9	5	.045	.11		
			t		t		1	6	16	1	t	1.08	.008		.008	.038
			.7		4		6	36	264	23	2.1					

Food Item	Measure	Weight g	Calories	Carbohydrate g	Protein g	Fiber g	Saturated fat g	Unsaturated fat g	Total fat g	Cholesterol mg	Vitamin A IU	Vitamin B₁ mg	Vitamin B₂ mg	Vitamin B₆ mg
Jerusalem artichoke, raw	4 sm	100	42	16.7	2.3	.8			.1		20	.2	.06	.071
Kale														
Raw	3.5 oz	100	38	6	4.2	1.3			.8		8900	.16	.26	.3
Cooked	1 cup	110	43	6.7	5	1.4			.8		9130	.11	.2	.19⁴⁰
Kohlrabi, diced														
Raw	1 cup	150	43	9.9	3	1.5			.15		30	.09	.06	.22
Cooked	1 cup	165	40	8.7	2.8	1.5			.2		30	.1	.05	
Leeks, raw, 5″ long	3–4	100	52	11.2	2.2	1.3			.3		40	.11	.06	.2
Lettuce														
Boston or bib, raw	1 cup	55	8	1.4	.7	.25			.1		530	.03	.03	.028
Cos or romaine, raw	1 cup	55	10	1.9	.7	.35			.2					
Iceberg, raw	1 cup	75	10	2.2	.7	.35			.1		250	.05	.05	.028
Looseleaf, raw	1 cup	55	10	1.9	.7	.35			.2		1050	.03	.04	.028
Lotus root, 1 segment	⅔ avg	100	69	15.7	2.8				.1		0	.146	.011	
Mushrooms														
Raw	1 cup	70	20	3.1	1.9	.56			.2		t	.07	.32	.087
Canned, drained	1 cup	270	51	6.9	3.3				.6		0	.06	.66	.16
Sauteed	4 med	70	78	2.8	1.7	.7			7.4		173	.055	.275	
Mustard greens														
Raw	3.5 oz	100	31	5.6	3	1.1			.5		7000	.11	.22	
Cooked	1 cup	180	29	5	3.1	1.82			.4		14,760	.144	.25	.139⁴⁰
Okra														
Raw	1 cup	100	36	7.6	2.4	1			.3		520	.17	.21	.075
Cooked	1 cup	160	46	9.6	3.2	1.5			.5		780	.21	.29	.07⁴⁰
Onions														
Raw	1 cup	170	65	14.8	2.6	1			.2		70	.05	.07	.22
Cooked	1 cup	210	61	13.7	2.5	1.2			.2		80	.06	.06	
Dehydrated, flakes	3.5 oz	100	350	82	8.7	4.4			1.3		200	.25	.18	.5
Scallions, bulb and tops, raw	1 cup	100	36	8.2	1.5	1			.2		2000	.05	.05	
Parsley, chopped, raw	1 cup	60	26	5.1	2.2	.9			.4		5100	.07	.16	.098
Parsnips														
Raw	½ lg	100	76	17.5	1.7	2			.5		30	.08	.09	.09
Cooked	1 cup	155	102	23.1	2.3	3			.8		50	.11	.12	
Peas														
Raw	1 cup	145	122	20.9	9.1	2.9			.6		930	.51	.2	.23
Cooked	1 cup	160	114	19.4	8.6	3.2			.6		860	.45	.18	.24⁴⁰
Canned, drained	1 cup	170	150	28.6	8	3.9			.7		1170	.15	.1	.085
Split, ckd	1 cup	200	696	125	48.4	2.4			2		240	1.48	.58	
Peppers														
Green, sliced, raw	1 cup	80	18	3.8	1	1.12			.2		340	.06	.06	.208
Green, sliced, ckd	1 cup	135	24	5.1	1.4	1.89			.3		570	.08	.09	
Red, sliced, raw	1 cup	100	31	7.1	1.4				.3		4450	.08	.08	
Hot chili, green, canned	1 cup	245	49	12.3	1.7	3			.2		1490	.07	.07	
Hot chili, red, canned	1 cup	245	51	9.6	2.2				1.5		23,500	.02	.22	
Pickles														
Dill	1 lg	100	11	2.2	.7	.5			4		100	t	.02	.007
Sour	1 lg	105	10	2	.5	.5			.2		100	t	.02	
Sweet (gherkins)	1 lg	35	51	12.8	.2				.1		30	t	.01	
Pimientos, canned	3 med	100	27	5.8	.9	.6			.5		2300	.02	.06	
Potato														
Raw, diced	1 cup	150	114	25.7	3.2				.2		t	.15	.06	
Baked in skin	1 lg	202	145	32.8	4	1.2			.2		t	.15	.07	
Boiled in skin	1 med	100	76	17.1	2.1	.5			.1		t	.09	.04	
Dehydrated flakes, dry	1 cup	45	164	37.8	3.2	.5			.3		t	.1	.03	.216
Dehydrated flakes, prepared	1 cup	210	195	30.5	4				6.7		270	.08	.08	
French fries	10 pieces	50	137	18	2.1	.5	2	4	6.6		t	.06	.04	.09⁴⁰

⁴²Values range from 7/100 gm for freshly harvested to 75 after long storage.

Vitamin B₁₂ mcg	Biotin mcg	Folic Acid mg	Niacin mg	Pantothenic Acid mg	Vitamin C mg	Vitamin E mg	Sodium mg	Phosphorus mg	Potassium mg	Calcium mg	Iron mg	Magnesium mg	Copper mg	Manganese mg	Selenium mg	Zinc mg
0			1.3		4			78		14	3.4	11				
0	.5	.06	2.09	1	125	8	75	73	318	179	2.2	37	.09	.5		
0			1.8	.38⁴⁰	102		47	64	243	206	1.8	31				
0		.015	.45	.247	99		12	75	558	61	.53	55	.21		.16	
			.3		71		10	68	429	54	.5					
0	1.4		.5	.12	17	1	5	50	347	52	1.1	23	.09		.07	
0	.35	.02	.2	.1	4	.22	5	14	145	19	1.1	5	.08	.4		.3
0	.35	.02	.2	.1	5		7	17	131	15	.4	5	.035		.675	.3
0	.35	.02	.2	.1	10		5	14	145	37	.8		.035			.2
			.3		75			103		30	.6					
0	11.2	.016	2.9	1.54	2	.58	11	81	290	4	.6	7.7	1.08	.056	8.54	.91
0			5.4	2.7				243		21	2.1	21	.7		29.4	
			2.9		t			81		8	.7		.545			
0			.8	.21	97		32	50	377	183	3	27				
0			1.1	.295⁴⁰	117		32	32	396	284	1.4					
0		.024	1	.26	31		3	51	249	92	.6	41	.11			
0			1.4	.34⁴⁰	32		3	66	278	147	.8					
0	1.53	.042	.3	.22	17	.442	17	61	267	46	.9	20.4	.255	.61	2.55	.6
			.4		15		15	61	231	50	.8		.14			
			1.4	1.2	35		88	273	1383	166	2.9	106				
0		.036	.4	.144	32		5	39	231	51	1					.3
0	.24	.07	.7	.18	103		27	38	436	122	3.7	24.5	.293	.563		
0	.1	.067	.2	.6	16		12	77	541	50	.7	32	.1	.2		
			.2		16		12	96	587	70	.9					
0		.029	4.2	1.1	39	3.1	3	168	458	38	2.8	50.7	.33			1.2
0			3.7	.5⁴⁰	32		2	158	314	37	2.9		.24			1.2
0	3.4	.034	1.4	.255	14	.034	401	129	163	44	3.2	34	.289			1.3
			6				80	536	1790	66	10.2		.5			
0		.015	.4	.184	102		10	18	170	7	.6	14.4	.128		.48	.048
			.6		130		12	22	201	12	.7					
0			.5	.271	204			30		13	.6					
0			1.7	1.68	167		10.4	34	462	12	1	28	.26	.31		
0		.15	1.5	2.65	74			39		22	1.2	418				
0			t		6		1428	21	200	26	l	12				.27
			t		7		1353	15		17	3.2					
			t		2			6		4	.4		.35			.052
0			.4	.166	95			17		7	1.5		.6			
	2.3				30		5	80	611	11	.9					
			2.7		31		6	101	782	14	1.1		.26			
			1.5		16		3	53	407	7	.6		.1			.3
0			2.4	.065	14		40	78	720	16	.8	45	.08			
			1.9		11		485	99	601	65	.6					.76
0		.011	1.6	.27⁴⁰	10		3	56	427	8	.6					.14
			4.8		32		379	172	1318	26	1.9		.459			

Food Item	Measure	Weight g	Calories	Carbohydrate g	Protein g	Fiber g	Saturated fat g	Unsaturated fat g	Total fat g	Cholesterol mg	Vitamin A IU	Vitamin B₁ mg	Vitamin B₂ mg	Vitamin B₆ mg
Fried from raw	1 cup	170	456	55.4	6.8	1.6			24.1		t	.2	.12	
Hash browns	1 cup	155	355	45.1	4.8	1.2			18.1		t	.12	.08	
Mashed w/milk[43]	1 cup	210	137	27.3	4.4	.8			1.5		40	.17	.11	.13[40]
Scalloped and au gratin w/o cheese	1 cup	245	255	36	7.4				9.6	14	390	.15	.22	.18[40]
Scalloped and au gratin w/ cheese	1 cup	245	355	33.3	13				19.4	36	780	.15	.29	
Potato chips	10 chips	20	113	10	1.1	.3	2	6	8		t	.04	.014	
Pumpkin, canned	1 cup	245	81	19.4	2.5	3			.7		15,860	.07	.12	.139
Radish														
Red, raw	10 med	50	8	1.6	.5	.35			t		t	.01	.01	.037
Oriental, raw	3.5 oz	100	19	4.2	.9	.7			.1		10	.03	.02	
Rutabaga														
Raw	1 cup	140	64	15.4	1.5	1.4			.1		810	.1	.1	.14
Cooked	1 cup	170	60	13.9	1.5	2			.2		940	.1	.1	
Sauerkraut														
Canned	1 cup	235	42	9.4	2.4	1.6			.5		120	.07	.09	.31
Juice	1 cup	242	24	5.6	1.7				t			.07	.1	.605
Shallots, chopped, raw	1 tbsp	10	7	1.7	.3	1			t		t	.01	t	
Spinach														
Raw	1 cup	55	14	2.4	1.8	.3			.2		4460	.06	.11	.14
Cooked	1 cup	180	41	6.5	5.4	1			.5		14,580	.13	.25	.34[40]
Canned, drained	1 cup	205	49	7.4	5.5	1.6			1.2		16,400	.04	.25	.14
New Zealand, raw	3.5 oz	100	19	3.1	2.2	.7			.3		4300	.04	.17	
New Zealand, cooked	1 cup	180	23	3.8	3.1	1.1			.4		6480	.05	.18	
Squash														
Summer, raw	1 cup	130	25	5.5	1.4	.75			.1		530	.07	.12	.186
Summer, ckd	1 cup	180	25	5.6	1.6	.8			.2		700	.09	.14	.113[40]
Winter, baked	1 cup	205	129	31.6	3.7	2.6			.8		8610	.1	.27	.18[40]
Sweet potato														
Baked	1 avg	146	161	37	2.4	1.8			.6		9230[45]	.1	.08	
Candied, 2″ × 4″	2 halves	100	168	34.2	1.3	.6			3.3		6300[45]	06	.04	
Canned	1 cup	200	216	49.8	4	2			.4		15,600[45]	.1	.08	.132
Tomato														
Raw	1 med	150	33	7	1.6	.8			.3		1350	.09	.06	.15
Canned	1 cup	241	51	10.4	2.4	.8			.5		2170	.12	.07	.126
Juice	1 cup	243	46	10.4	2.2	.4			.2		1940	.12	.07	.366
Paste, canned	1 cup	262	215	48.7	8.9	2			1		8650	.52	.31	
Puree, canned	1 cup	249	97	22.2	4.2	1			.5		4000	.22	.12	.45
Turnips														
Raw	1 cup	130	39	8.6	1.3	1.15			.3		t	.05	.09	.117
Cooked	1 cup	155	36	7.6	1.2	1.35			.3		t	.06	.08	
Turnip greens														
Raw	3.5 oz	100	28	5	3	.8			.3		7600	.21	.39	.263
Cooked	1 cup	145	29	5.2	3.2	1			.3		9140	.22	.35	.14[40]
Vegetable juice cocktail	1 cup	242	41	8.7	2.2	.8			.2		1690	.12	.07	
Water chestnuts	4 avg	25	20	4.8	.4	.2			.1		0	.04	.05	
Watercress, raw	1 cup	35	7	1.1	.8	.35			.1		1720	.03	.06	.045
Yams, ckd in skin	1 cup	200	210	48.2	4.8	1.8			.4		t	.18	.8	
Yeast														
Bakers', dry (active)	1 oz	28	80	11	10.5	.1			.5		t	.66	1.53	.56
Bakers', compressed	1 oz	28	24	3.1	3.4				.1		t	.2	.47	.168
Brewer's, debittered	1 tbsp	8	23	3.1	3.1	.14			.1		t	1.25	.34	.2
Torula	1 oz	28	79	10.5	10.9	.92			.3		t	3.97	1.43	.84

[43] Made with 6 tbsp milk and ½ tsp salt added to four med. potatoes.

[44] Amounts may vary significantly between brands.

[45] Varies with color of flesh; deep orange varieties average 10,000 IU/100 gm; lt yellow about 600 IU.

Vitamin B₁₂ mcg	Biotin mcg	Folic Acid mg	Niacin mg	Pantothenic Acid mg	Vitamin C mg	Vitamin E mg	Sodium mg	Phosphorus mg	Potassium mg	Calcium mg	Iron mg	Magnesium mg	Copper mg	Manganese mg	Selenium mg	Zinc mg
0		.026	3.3	.47[40]	14		446	122	736	19	1.4					
0		.021	2.1	.48[40]	21		632	103	548	50	.8		.2			
			2.5		27		870	181	801	132	1					
			2.2		25		1095	299	750	311	1.2					
			1		3			28	226	8	.4	9.6	.06			.162
0		.047	1.5	1	12		5	64	588	61	1		.33			
0		.012	.1	.092	12		8	14	145	14	.5	7	.08	.025	2.1	.13
			.4		32			26	180	35	.6					
0		.038	1.5	.22	60		7	55	335	92	.6	20	.11	.056		
		.036	1.4		44		7	53	284	100	.5					
0			.5	.22	33		1755[44]	42	329	85	1.2		.235			1.88
0			.5	.29	44		1905[44]	34		90	2.7					
			t		t		1	6	33	4	.1					
0	3.5	.106	.3	.15	28	1.25	39	28	259	51	1.7	44	.32	.42		.5
0		.164	.9	.23[40]	50		90	68	583	167	4		.252			1.3
0	4	.1	.6	.13	29		484	53	513	242	5.3	112				1.6
0			.6	.312	30		159	46	795	58	2.6	40				
			.9		25		166	50	833	86	2.7					
0		.04	1.3	.468	29		1	38	263	36	.5	21	.22	.182		
0			1.4	.3[40]	18		2	45	254	45	.7					.324
0			1.4	.56[40]	27		2	98	945	57	1.6					.28
		.026	.8		25		14	66	342	46	1		.22			
			.4		10		42	43	190	37	.9					
0			1.2	.86	28		96	82	400	50	1.6		.12			
0	2	.012	1	.48	34	.54	4	40	366	20	.8	21	.24	.27	.75	.2
0	4.32	.007	1.7	.55	41		3.3	46	523	14	1.2	24	.5	.1	2.41	.5
0		.017	1.9	.607	39		486	44	552	17	2.2	20				.1
			8.1		128		100	183	2237	71	9.2	50				
0			3.2		82		1000	85	1060	32	4.2	50				
0	.13	.026	.8	.26	47	.026	64	39	348	51	.7	25	.09	.052	.78	
			.5		34		53	37	291	54	.6		.06			
0		.095	.8	.38	139	2.3	10	58	440	246	1.8	58	.09	1.4		
0			.9	.2[40]	100			54		267	1.6					
			1.9		22		484	53	535	29	1.2					
			.2		1		5	16	125	1	.2	2.4				
0	.14	.017	.3	.108	28		18	19	99	53	.6	6.5	.032	.189		
			1.2		18			100		8	1.2		.44			
		1.15	10.4	3.08	t		15	366	566	12	4.6		1.96			
	112	.14	3.2	.98	t		5	112	173	4	1.4	16.5				
	64	.192	3	1	t		10	140	152	17	1.4	18.5	.266	.042		
	28	.84	12.6	3.08	t		4	486	580	120	5.5	46				

REFERENCES

Composition of Foods, Agric. Handbook no. 8, Dept. of Agric.
Nutritive Value of American Foods, Agric. Handbook no. 456, Dept. of Agric.
Food Values, Bowes and Church, J.B. Lippincott, New York.
Scientific Tables, 6th ed., Geigy Pharmaceuticals, Ardsley, New York.
The Composition of Foods, McCance and Widdowson, Medical Research Council Special Report Series no. 297, Her Majesty's Stationery Office, London, England.
Selected articles from *The Journal of the American Dietetic Association*, *Cereal Chemistry*, *British Journal of Nutrition*, and the *Journal of Nutrition*.

WEIGHTS AND MEASURES

Weights

1 microgram	=	1/1,000,000 gram
1,000 micrograms	=	1 milligram
1 milligram	=	1/1,000 gram
1,000 milligrams	=	1 gram
1.00 ounce	=	28.35 grams
3.57 ounces	=	100.00 grams
0.25 pound	=	113.00 grams
0.50 pound	=	227.00 grams
1.00 pound	=	16.00 ounces
1.00 pound	=	453.00 grams

Capacity Measurements

1 quart	=	4 cups
1 pint	=	2 cups
1 cup	=	½ pint
1 cup	=	8 fluid ounces
1 cup	=	16 tablespoons
2 tablespoons	=	1 fluid ounce
1 tablespoon	=	½ fluid ounce
1 tablespoon	–	3 teaspoons

Approximate Equivalents

1 average serving	=	about 4 ounces
1 ounce fluid	=	about 28 grams
1 cup fluid		
Cooking oil	=	200 grams
Water	=	220 grams
Milk, soups	=	240 grams
Syrup, honey	=	325 grams

1 cup dry		
Cereal flakes	=	50 grams
Flours	=	100 grams
Sugars	=	200 grams
1 tablespoon fluid		
Cooking oil	=	14 grams
Milk, water	=	15 grams
Syrup, honey	=	20 grams
1 tablespoon dry	=	1/6 ounce
Flours	=	8 grams
Sugars	=	12 grams
1 pat butter	=	½ tablespoon
1 teaspoon fluid	=	about 5 grams
1 teaspoon dry	=	about 4 grams
1 grain	=	about 65 milligrams
1 minim	=	about 1 drop water

Abbreviations and Symbols Used in the Tables

avg	average		reg	regular
cal	calorie		sm	small
diam	diameter		svg	serving
enr	enriched		t	trace
g	gram		tbsp	tablespoon
IU	International Unit		tsp	teaspoon
lb	pound		w	with
lg	large		—	reliable data lacking
mcg	microgram		/	of; with
mg	milligram		"	inches
oz	ounce			

Essential Amino Acid Contents of Some Foods

One of the most important aspects of obtaining a good diet is the balancing of amino acids. There are approximately 22 amino acids that are the primary components of protein (see "Protein," p. 9). Eight of these amino acids, tryptophan, leucine, lysine, methionine, phenylalanine, isoleucine, valine, and threonine, are known to be "essential" because they cannot be manufactured by the body itself and must be supplied by foods in the diet.[1]

The amino acid content of every food differs. The amino acids in foods must be consumed in amounts and proportions that closely approximate the pattern required by the body. If *one* essential amino acid (EAA) is missing or present in a low amount, protein synthesis in the body will fall to a very low level or stop altogether. In most foods containing protein, all the EAAs are present, but in some foods one or more of the EAAs may be present in a substantially lower amount than the others, placing it out of proportion and deviating from the EAA pattern required by the body. The EAA that is absent or provides the lowest percentage of the daily Estimated Amino Acid Requirement (EAAR) (as established by the National Academy of Sciences) is known as the limiting amino acid (LAA) and is the factor

determining the amount and quality of protein utilized by the body. For example, a food containing 100 percent of a person's lysine requirement but only 20 percent of his methionine requirement results in only 20 percent of the protein in that food being used as protein by the body. The rest is used as fuel rather than for replenishing or building of tissue.

Foods such as meat, fish, poultry, and dairy products are high in protein content and have a good proportion of EAAs. Many vegetables and fruits are low in or missing some amino acids, thus rendering the amino acids present relatively useless. Foods low in or missing a particular amino acid (the LAA) will have increased protein quality when combined in a meal with foods high in this same LAA. Macaroni and cheese, vegetable stew, and chicken chow mein are examples of how foods high in certain amino acids can be balanced with foods low or missing one or more EAA. Supplements may be used to increase the protein quality of foods.

The following chart lists the EAA content of some foods. To date, available information is incomplete on the EAA content of many foods. However, foods listed here occur in the same order as those in the "Table of Food Composition," pp. 199–234, thus providing easy reference to other nutrients contained in these foods.

The amino acid content for each food is given in

[1]Histidine and arginine are necessary for growth in children, but it is debatable whether or not they perform this function in adults.

milligrams. The LAA supplied is given as percentage of daily EAAR for men and women of average weights.[2] For example, a breakfast of two poached eggs (supply 54 percent of the LAA), two pieces of dry whole wheat toast (supply 10 percent of the LAA), and a glass of orange juice (supplies 0.0 percent of the LAA) eaten together provides 64 percent of the total protein needs for that particular day for a 160-pound man. This leaves only 36 percent of his daily amino acid requirements to be fulfilled.

The body's protein requirements can be easily met if the foods eaten are properly combined in order to provide *usable* protein. This means that smaller quantities of food can be consumed and the body's nutritional needs will still be taken care of. *The importance of balancing the amino acids to obtain the best possible protein from foods cannot be overstressed.*

The calories shown in the following chart are given in relation to the weight of the food in grams. They are shown mainly for reference and have little effect on the

LAA percentage. To determine individual caloric needs, refer to the chart on page 245. It should be remembered that although some foods, such as fruits and vegetables, are low in EAA content, they may contain other nutrients such as vitamins and minerals, essential for good health.

The abbreviations and symbols that appear in the following chart have the same meaning as those that appear in the "Table of Food Composition" (see p. 234).

The percentages listed in the "amino acid" chart are based on the following conversion table, prepared by the Food and Nutrition Board of the National Academy of Sciences. To find exact individual amino acid requirements, simply divide body weight by 2.2 to find weight in kilograms. Then multiply this figure times the requirement for each amino acid listed under "infant," "child," or "adult." The results will appear as total milligrams of each amino acid required to carry on the daily body-building functions of protein.

REQUIREMENT (per kg of body wt), mg/day

Amino Acid	Infant (3–6 mo)	Child (10–12 yr)	Adult	Amino Acid Pattern for High Quality Proteins, mg/g of protein
Histidine	33	?	?	17
Isoleucine	80	28	12	42
Leucine	128	42	16	70
Lysine	97	44	12	51
Total S-containing amino acids (includes methionine)	45	22	10	26
Total aromatic amino acids (includes phenylalanine)	132	22	16	73
Threonine	63	28	8	35
Tryptophan	19	4	3	11
Valine	89	25	14	48

Source: National Academy of Sciences, *Recommended Dietary Allowances*, 1974, p. 44.

[2] For complete information, see National Academy of Sciences, *Recommended Dietary Allowances*, 1974, p. 44.

BREADS, CEREALS, GRAINS, AND GRAIN PRODUCTS

Food Item	Measure	Weight g	Calories	Protein g	Essential Amino Acids, mg								% of Limiting Amino Acid Supplied†	
					TRP	LEU	LYS	MET	PHA	ISL	VAL	THR	Men (160 lb)	Women (124 lb)
Bread														
Cracked wheat	1 slice	23	61	2	24	134	54	30*	98	86	92	58	4	5
Cracked wheat, toasted	1 slice	19	60	2	24	134	54	30*	98	86	92	58	4	5
French, enr flour	1 slice	20	58	1.8	22	139	41	23*	99	83	77	52	4	5
Italian, enr flour	1 slice	20	58	1.8	22	139	41	23*	99	83	77	52	3	4
Pumpernickel	1 slice	32	79	2.9	32	194	119	46*	136	125	151	107	6	8
Raisin	1 slice	23	60	1.5	18	100	40	22*	74	64	69	30	3	4
Raisin, toasted	1 slice	19	60	1.5	18	100	40	22*	74	64	69	30	3	4
Rye	1 slice	23	56	2.1	23	141	67	32*	101	90	109	67	4	6
Rye, toasted	1 slice	20	56	2.1	23	141	67	32*	101	90	109	67	4	6
White, enr	1 slice	23	62	2.0	24	159	60	29*	108	96	92	62	4	6
White, toasted	1 slice	23	62	2.0	24	159	60	29*	108	96	92	62	4	5
Whole wheat	1 slice	23	55	2.1	29	166	71	37*	117	106	113	72	5	7
Whole wheat, toasted	1 slice	19	55	2.4	29	166	71	37*	117	104	113	72	5	7
Bread stuffing, uncooked	1 cup	190	704	24	292	1,916	646	330*	1,330	1,146	1,086	732	46	58
Bread crumbs, dry	1 cup	88	345	11.0	133	871	294	150*	605	522	494	333	21	27
Buns, soft, enr flour (hamburger, hotdog)	1 avg	30	89	2.5	31	200	82	38*	134	124	121	82	5	7
Cornflakes	1 cup	25	93	1.98	14	272	40	35*	92	80	100	72	5	6
Corn grits, cooked	1 cup	242	123	2.9	17	377	84	55*	131	134	147	116	8	10
Cornmeal, cooked	1 cup	240	115	2.64	14	313	71	46*	108	111	122	96	6	8
Cracker														
Graham	1 med	7	28	0.56	10	54	22	12*	39	35	37	23	2	2
Standard, round, snack	1 med	3	17	0.24	3	22	7	4*	16	13	12	8	1	1
Soda	1 square	6	26	0.55	6	44	14	8*	32	26	22	16	1	1
Danish pastry	1 sm	35	148	2.6	33	205	77	42*	144	128	125	84	6	8
Farina, instant cooked	1 cup	38	131	4.1	—*	262	76	46	198	186	167	106	—	—
Flour														
Buckwheat, light	1 cup	110	382	7.0	119	437	416	134*	296	267	394	282	19	24
Potato	1 cup	110	386	8.8	97	442	468	115*	389	389	468	345	16	20
Rye, medium	1 cup	110	385	13.0	138	840	514	200*	197	1,201	652	464	28	36
Soy, full fat	1 cup	110	418	45.0	605	3,428	2,784	605*	2,179	2,380	2,339	1,734	84	108
Wheat, enr, all-purpose	1 cup	110	394	12.0	139	893	267	151*	638	534	499	336	21	27
Whole wheat	1 cup	120	410	15.0	192	1,072	432	240*	784	688	739	464	33	43
Macaroni, enr, salt-cooked	1 cup	140	155	5.3	58	317	154	72*	250	240	274	187	10	13
Muffin														
Plain, enr flour	1 med	48	139	3.7	49	312	157	68*	202	199	202	136	9	12
Blueberry	1 med	40	112	2.9	38	243	122	53*	157	155	157	106	7	9
Noodles, enr, salt-cooked	1 cup	160	200	6.6	73	436	218	112*	317	323	389	277	16	20
Oatmeal or rolled oats, cooked	1 cup	236	130	4.7	76	501	221	86*	275	275	319	205	12	15

*Limiting amino acid.

†Percentages are based on Recommended Dietary Allowances for limiting amino acid of each particular food.

Food Item	Measure	Weight g	Calories	Protein g	Essential Amino Acids, mg								% of Limiting Amino Acid Supplied[†]	
					TRP	LEU	LYS	MET	PHA	ISL	VAL	THR	Men (160 lb)	Women (124 lb)
Pancake, buckwheat	1 med	45	90	3.1	46	258	189	68*	153	168	192	131	9	12
Rice														
Brown, cooked	1 cup	150	178	3.8	41	327	148	68*	190	179	266	148	9	12
Brown, raw	1 cup	190	744	14.3	159	1,233	558	260*	717	675	1,004	558	36	47
Instant	1 cup	148	161	3.3	36	284	129	59*	165	155	231	129	8	11
Parboiled, cooked, long gr.	1 cup	150	155	3.2	35	275	125	58*	160	150	224	125	8	10
White, cooked	1 cup	150	158	3	33	258	117	54*	150	141	210	117	8	10
White, raw	1 cup	191	675	13	140	1,107	503	230*	643	604	900	503	32	41
Rice flakes	1 cup	30	111	1.77	15	—*	19	—*	96	—*	—*	—*	—	—
Roll														
Sweet	1 avg.	50	158	4.25	54	349	155	71*	232	218	215	145	10	13
Dinner, enr flour	1 med	38	113	3.12	38	249	102	47*	166	153	149	102	7	8
Popcorn, with oil and salt	1 cup	14	66	1.4	9	182	40	26*	63	65	72	56	4	5
Tortilla, yellow corn	6" diam cake	30	63	1.5	8	242	38	28*	64	88	78	60	4	5
Waffle	1 avg	75	206	6.98	94	598	331	144*	379	391	404	272	20	26
Wheat														
Bran	1 oz	29	62	4.6	74	273	190	56*	167	185	213	130	8	10
Flakes	1 cup	36	125	4.4	49	363	147	52*	195	202	233	145	7	9
Germ	1 tbsp	6	24	1.8	16	110	99	26*	58	76	88	86	4	5
DAIRY PRODUCTS														
Cheese														
Brick	1 svg	28	103	6.2	87	608	453	161*	335	415	446	229	22	29
Camembert, domestic	1 svg	28	84	4.9	69	475	358	127*	265	328	353	181	18	23
Cheddar, American	1 piece	17	68	4.3	60	417	310	111*	230	285	306	157	15	20
Cheddar, American, grated	1 tbsp	7	28	1.75	25	176	131	47*	97	121	129	67	7	8
Cottage, creamed	1 cup	225	235	31.0	336	3,294	2,562	854*	1,647	1,769	1,769	1,434	119	153
Cottage, uncreamed	1 cup	260	223	44.2	469	4,608	3,584	1,195*	2,304	2,475	2,475	2,005	166	209
Edam	1 oz	28	87	7.7	108	755	562	200*	416	516	555	285	28	36
Gruyere	1 oz	28	115	8.1	105	778	591	211*	429	543	575	300	29	38
Limberger	1 oz	28	69	5.9	83	578	431	153*	319	395	425	218	21	27
Parmesan	1 oz	28	110	10.0	140	980	730	260*	540	670	720	370	36	47
Pasteurized, processed, American	1 oz	28	103	6.5	91	631	475	169*	351	436	468	240	23	30
Pasteurized, processed, pimento (American)														
Roquefort	1 oz	28	103	6	81	601	453	161*	329	415	441	227	22	29
Swiss, domestic	1 oz	28	99	7.8	123	884	665	235*	485	609	650	336	33	42
Cream														
Half and half	1 tbsp	15	20	0.48	7	50	39	12*	24	32	35	23	2	2
Half and half	1 cup	240	322	7.68	106	752	592	182*	364	486	524	350	25	33
Heavy or whipping	1 cup	238	861	5.24	71	512	401	123*	246	329	357	238	17	22

* Limiting amino acid.

†Percentages are based on Recommended Dietary Allowances for limiting amino acid of each particular food.

Food Item	Measure	Weight g	Calories	Protein g	Essential Amino Acids, mg								% of Limiting Amino Acid Supplied[†]	
					TRP	LEU	LYS	MET	PHA	ISL	VAL	THR	Men (160 lb)	Women (124 lb)
Cream (Cont.)														
Sour	1 oz	30	57	0.8	12	83	65	20*	40	53	58	39	3	4
Egg														
Boiled, poached, or raw	1 med	50	79	6.5	102	559	406	197*	369	420	470	318	27	35
Fried	1 med	50	108	6.2	99	546	397	192*	360	409	459	310	27	34
Scrambled or omelet	1 med	64	116	7.6	112	644	476	215*	407	472	527	355	30	39
White	1 med	31	16	3.4	51	296	204	133*	214	218	262	150	18	24
Yolk	1 med	17	58	2.72	39	235	185	70*	123	171	190	140	10	13
Milk, cow's														
Buttermilk	1 cup	246	90	8.9	90	809	678	188*	433	514	613	384	26	34
Skim, dry, instant	1 cup	64	228	23	320	2,260	1,780	570*	1,095	1,461	1,575	1,073	79	102
Skim, fortified	1 cup	246	89	8.9	137	970	764	235*	470	627	676	451	33	42
Whole, fortified	1 cup	244	159	8.54	118	832	655	202*	403	538	580	386	28	36
Milk, goat, fresh	1 cup	244	163	7.7	94	663	741	156*	289	203	328	515	22	28
Milk, human, fresh	1 oz	30	23	0.3	5	27	19	6*	13	16	18	13	t	t
Yogurt, part skim	1 cup	250	125	4.3	93	842	706	196*	450	536	638	400	27	35
DESSERTS AND SWEETS														
Banana bread	1 slice	49	134	2.4	33	178	92	45*	123	117	119	81	6	8
Doughnut														
Cake	1 avg	33	129	1.52	20	126	55	27*	85	79	78	53	4	5
Raised or yeast	1 avg	33	136	2.1	26	169	74	35*	114	107	106	72	5	6
Raised, jelly-filled	1 avg	65	226	3.4	44	276	120	58*	186	174	172	116	8	10
FISH AND SEAFOODS														
Anchovy														
Canned	3 fillet	12	21	2.3	23	175	202	67*	85	117	122	99	9	12
Paste	1 tsp	7	14	1.4	14	106	123	41*	52	71	74	60	6	7
Bass, fried	1 lb	453	756	96	857	6,513	7,542	2,485*	3,171	4,371	4,542	3,685	345	445
Cod, canned	1 lb	453	385	87	870	6,609	7,655	2,523*	3,216	4,435	4,611	3,742	345	450
Flounder, baked	1 lb	453	915	135	1,359	10,125	11,880	3,915*	4,995	6,885	7,155	5,805	536	699
Haddock, fried	1 lb	453	742	88	888	6,709	7,762	2,556*	3,262	4,530	4,675	3,793	350	456
Herring, pickled	1 lb	453	1,003	91	924	6,930	8,040	2,681*	3,420	4,711	4,896	3,973	367	478
Mackerel, canned	1 lb	453	789	87	957	7,178	8,326	2,775*	3,541	4,785	5,072	4,115	385	497
Perch, yellow, raw	1 lb	453	412	87	883	6,459	7,773	2,563*	3,266	4,502	4,684	3,796	351	457
Pike														
Blue and northern, flesh only	1 lb	453	403	82	830	6,225	7,304	2,407*	3,071	4,233	4,399	3,569	334	431
Walleye, flesh only	1 lb	453	392	86	875	6,562	7,700	2,538*	3,238	4,462	4,638	3,762	353	455
Salmon, pink, canned	1 lb	453	639	93	929	6,967	8,081	2,695*	3,433	4,643	4,919	3,995	374	481
Shrimp														
Canned	1 lb	453	525	110	1,098	8,345	9,662	3,184*	4,063	5,600	5,819	4,721	442	571
Cooked	1 lb	453	989	92	821	6,240	7,225	2,381*	3,038	4,187	4,351	3,530	331	427

*Limiting amino acid.
†Percentages are based on Recommended Dietary Allowances for limiting amino acid of each particular food.

Food Item	Measure	Weight g	Calories	Protein g	Essential Amino Acids, mg								% of Limiting Amino Acid Supplied[†]	
					TRP	LEU	LYS	MET	PHA	ISL	VAL	THR	Men (160 lb)	Women (124 lb)
Smelt, raw	4-5 med	100	98	18.6	186	1,395	1,637	539*	688	949	986	800	75	97
Swordfish, broiled	1 lb	453	764	129	1,268	9,513	11,161	3,678*	4,693	6,469	6,722	5,454	504	657
Trout, rainbow, raw	1 lb	453	883	97	974	7,302	8,571	2,827*	3,606	6,654	5,164	4,186	387	505
Tuna, canned in oil, drained	1 lb	453	892	130	1,307	9,804	11,504	3,791*	4,837	6,667	6,930	5,621	527	679
FOOD SUBSTITUTES														
Cream substitute, liquid	1 tbsp	14	24	0.12	1	11	9	3*	6	8	8	5	†	†
FRUITS														
Apple, raw, whole	1 med	130	76	0.26	-*	17	14	5	12	19	12	10	-	-
Apricot, raw	1 med	38	19	0.38	-*	68	68	13	38	41	56	48	-	-
Avocado	1 lg	216	361	4.54	46	-*	240	38	-*	-*	-*	-*	-	-
Banana, raw	1 med	150	128	1.65	28	-*	82	16	-*	-*	-*	-*	-	-
Cantaloupe, raw	1/4	100	30	0.7	1	-*	18	2	-*	-*	-*	-*	-	-
Dates														
Dried	1 med	10	27	0.22	6	8	7	3*	6	7	9	6	†	†
Dried and pitted	1 cup	178	488	3.92	109	136	117	47*	113	133	168	109	7	8
Fig, raw	1 med	38	30	0.46	20	103	95	20*	57	72	91	76	3	4
Grapefruit:														
Canned	1 cup	250	175	1.5	1	-*	9	-*	-*	-*	-*	-*	-	-
Red flesh	1 med	260	180	1.3	1	-*	9	-*	-*	-*	-*	-*	-	-
Orange, fresh	1 med	180	88	1.8	5	-*	48	5	-*	-*	-*	-*	-	-
Papaya, raw	1 lg	400	156	2.4	16	-*	51	3	-*	-*	-*	-*	-	-
Peach, fresh	1 med	100	38	0.68	4*	29	30	31	18	13	40	27	1	2
Pear, Japanese	1 med	182	111	1.27	7	36	25	9*	21	25	36	23	1	1
Persimmon, raw	1 med	100	96	0.88	14	52	42	8*	38	36	38	49	1	1
Pineapple, canned in heavy syrup	1 slice	122	90	0.37	5	-*	9	1	-*	-*	-*	-*	-	-
Strawberries, raw	1 cup	149	55	1.04	13	63	48	1.5*	34	27	34	37	†	†
MEATS, POULTRY, AND GAME														
Beef														
Chuck roast	1 lb	453	1481	108	1,154	7,888	8,369	2,405*	3,944	5,002	5,291	4,233	334	431
Corned beef	1 lb	453	1685	72	836	5,864	6,254	1,775*	2,944	3,746	3,976	3,160	247	318
Dried beef, uncooked	3 oz	85	173	29.1	341	2,388	2,547	723*	1,199	1,526	1,618	1,288	100	130
Heart, lean	1 lb	453	490	78	1,009	6,906	6,363	1,862*	3,492	3,880	4,423	3,570	259	334
Liver, fried	1 lb	453	635	120	1,354	8,398	6,772	2,167*	4,515	3,786	5,689	4,334	301	388
Rump roast	1 lb	453	1571	107	1,176	8,036	8,526	1,752*	4,018	5,096	5,390	3,084	243	314
Round steak	1 lb	453	856	141	1,062	7,257	7,700	2,212*	3,628	4,602	4,868	3,894	307	395
Short ribs	1 lb	453	1092	128	1,148	7,847	8,326	2,392*	3,924	4,976	4,264	4,211	332	429
Sirloin steak, broiled	1 lb	453	1848	101	1,187	8,110	8,604	2,472*	4,055	5,143	5,440	4,352	343	443
Beef and vegetable stew	1 lb	453	403	29	305	1,936	2,083	573*	1,069	1,281	1,398	1,096	80	103
Brains, cooked, all kinds	1 lb	453	566	47	625	3,828	3,443	997*	2,292	2,283	2,428	2,238	138	179
Calf														
Liver, fried	1 lb	453	1182	134	1,306	8,100	6,532	2,090*	4,355	4,529	5,487	4,181	290	315

*Limiting amino acid.
†Percentages are based on Recommended Dietary Allowances for limiting amino acid of each particular food.

Food Item	Measure	Weight g	Calories	Protein g	Essential Amino Acids, mg								% of Limiting Amino Acid Supplied[†]	
					TRP	LEU	LYS	MET	PHA	ISL	VAL	THR	Men (160 lb)	Women (124 lb)
Sweetbread (pancreas), braised	1 lb	453	760	87	1,132	6,794	6,445	1,568*	3,658	4,442	4,703	4,007	218	281
Lamb														
Leg, roast	1 lb	453	1264	80	1,525	9,075	9,543	2,824*	4,832	6,131	5,768	5,421	392	506
Shoulder	1 lb	453	1531	98	902	5,413	5,621	1,666*	2,845	3,609	3,401	3,192	231	299
Pork														
Bacon, broiled, drained	1 lb	453	2767	137	381	3,048	2,476	610*	1,829	1,676	1,829	1,295	85	109
Canadian bacon, cooked, drained	1 lb	453	1255	125	907	7,256	5,896	1,451*	4,354	3,991	4,354	3,084	202	260
Ham, cured, roasted	1 lb	453	1309	95	1,238	7,037	7,807	2,386*	3,715	4,847	4,953	4,379	331	428
Liver, fried	1 lb	453	594	93	1,410	8,686	7,005	2,242*	4,670	4,950	5,884	4,484	311	402
Spareribs, cooked	1 lb	453	1993	94	509	2,901	3,214	980*	1,529	1,999	2,030	1,803	136	176
Veal, rump roast	1 lb	453	1064	126	1,150	6,460	7,346	2,036*	3,540	4,690	4,514	2,806	283	365
Chicken														
Fryers, ready to cook	1 lb	308	382	57.4	689	4,190	5,109	1,492	2,296	3,042	2,813	2,468	199	256
Breasts	1 lb	358	394	74.5	894	5,438	6,630	1,937	2,980	3,948	3,800	3,204	259	332
Drumsticks	1 lb	272	313	51.22	614	3,738	4,457	1,331	2,048	2,714	2,509	2,202	178	228
Thighs	1 lb	340	435	61.6	739	4,497	5,482	1,602	2,464	3,265	3,018	2,649	213	275
Liver	1 lb	453	585	89.4	1,252	8,225	6,705	2,056	4,470	4,649	5,632	4,202	285	365
Turkey														
Raw, ready to cook	1 lb	330	722	66.6	-	5,128	6,061	1,865	2,664	3530	3330	2,864	-	-
Duck														
Domestic, ready to cook	1 lb	371	1213	59.5	-	4,641	5,176	1,488	2,320	3,094	2,856	2,618	-	-
NUTS AND SEEDS														
Almonds, dried	1 cup	133	760	25	234	1,934	774	344*	1,524	1,161	1,495	811	47	61
Brazil nuts, unsalted	1 cup	167	1,079	23	312	1,885	740	1,571	1,030	990	1,374	705	85	110
Cashews, unsalted	1 cup	100	569	15	430	1,410	740	327*	877	1,135	1,479	688	45	59
Coconut														
Fresh	1 cup	100	346	3.5	33	269	151	71*	174	180	212	129	10	13
Shredded	1 cup	62	344	2.2	21	175	98	46*	113	117	138	84	6	8
Hazelnuts	11 avg	15	97	1.6	27	118	53	18*	68	107	118	52	3	3
Peanuts														
Roasted with skin	1 cup	240	1397	60	800	4,432	2,592	640*	3,680	2,992	3,616	1,952	89	115
Salted, roasted	1 cup	240	1418	62	800	4,800	2,816	704*	4,000	3,248	3,936	2,128	98	126
Pecans, raw halves	1 cup	104	715	10	144	804	452	159*	587	575	546	405	22	28
Pistachios	1 cup	100	594	19	-*	1,523	1,080	367	1,088	881	1,344	613	-	-
Pumpkin and squash kernels	1 cup	230	1271	67	1,201	5,269	3,068	1,267*	3,735	3,735	3,602	2,001	176	227
Sesame seeds	1 cup	230	1339	42	711	3,641	1,256	1,382*	3,181	2,052	1,925	1,548	192	248
Sunflower seeds, dry	1 cup	100	560	24	85	401	225	119*	278	267	317	230	17	21
Walnuts, English	1 cup	100	651	15	175	1,228	441	306*	767	767	974	589	43	55
SAUSAGE, COLD CUTS, AND LUNCHEON MEATS														
Braunschweiger	1 lb	453	1447	67.1	738	5,636	5,234	1,409*	3,020	3,288	4,160	2,885	196	253

*Limiting amino acid.
†Percentages are based on Recommended Dietary Allowances for limiting amino acid of each particular food.

Food Item	Measure	Weight g	Calories	Protein g	Essential Amino Acids, mg								% of Limiting Amino Acid Supplied[†]	
					TRP	LEU	LYS	MET	PHA	ISL	VAL	THR	Men (160 lb)	Women (124 lb)
Frankfurters, cooked	1 lb	453	1377	56	454	4,026	4,536	1,191*	2,041	2,722	2,835	2,325	165	213
Headcheese	1 lb	453	1216	70.3	351	4,429	4,288	1,195*	2,671	2,390	2,882	1,968	166	214
Liverwurst	1 lb	453	1393	73.5	808	6,174	5,733	1,544*	3,381	3,602	4,557	3,160	214	277
Salami	1 lb	453	1411	79.4	972	7,776	8,748	2,268*	3,996	5,292	5,400	4,428	315	406
Sausage, bologna	1 lb	453	1379	54.9	439	3,953	4,447	1,153*	1,976	2,690	2,745	2,251	160	207
Vienna sausage, canned	1 lb	453	1089	63.5	572	4,572	5,144	1,334*	2,286	3,048	3,175	2,604	185	239
VEGETABLES														
Asparagus, raw	1 spear	16	44	2.9	5	18	20	6*	13	15	20	13	1	1
Beans														
Green, cooked	1 cup	125	31	2	28	116	104	30*	48	90	96	76	4	5
Lima, raw	1 cup	100	346	20	202	1,628	1,488	250	1,212	992	1,030	836	34	44
Yellow or wax, cooked	1 cup	100	22	1.4	20	81	73	21*	34	63	67	57	3	4
Bean sprouts (mung beans)	1 cup	100	28	3.2	22	291	218	35*	154	179	189	99	5	6
Broccoli	1 cup	150	39	4.65	45	202	181	61*	149	157	210	153	8	11
Cabbage														
Red, raw	1 cup	100	31	2.0	16	80	94	18*	42	78	60	56	3	3
Shredded	1 cup	105	25	1.4	11	55	64	13*	28	54	41	38	2	2
Carrots														
Diced, cooked	1 cup	150	47	1.35	11	77	62	11*	50	54	66	51	2	2
Raw	1 lg	100	42	1.1	9	59	48	9*	38	42	51	40	1	2
Cauliflower, raw	1 cup	100	27	2.7	35	181	151	54*	84	116	162	113	8	10
Celery, raw	1 lg stalk	50	8	0.45	4	—*	6	5	—*	—*	—*	—*	—	—
Chick-peas (garbanzos), dry, raw	1/2 cup	100	360	20.5	164	1,517	1,415	266*	1,004	1,189	1,004	738	37	48
Collards, leaves, steamed	1 cup	200	66	7.2	76	302	280	64*	172	168	270	156	9	11
Sweet corn														
Cream style	1 cup	200	164	4.2	32	572	192	98*	292	192	328	214	14	18
Whole kernel	1 cup	200	132	3.8	22	418	140	72*	212	140	240	156	10	13
Cucumber, raw	1/2 med	50	8	0.5	4	23	22	5*	12	16	17	14	1	1
Eggplant, cooked	1 cup	180	34	1.8	16	112	49	9*	79	92	106	63	1	2
Kale, raw w/stems	1 cup	125	47	5.25	57.5	341	162.5	47.5*	215	179	246	189	6.25	8.75
Lentils, dry, whole	1 cup	200	680	49.4	444	3,508	3,014	346*	2,272	2,618	2,668	1,728	48	60
cooked	1 cup	200	212	15.6	140	954	898	100*	654	540	626	496	13	17
Lettuce														
Iceberg	3 1/2 oz	100	13	0.9	12	—*	70	4	—*	—*	—*	—*	—	—
Leaf	3 1/2 oz	100	18	0.3	13	—*	75	4	—*	—*	—*	—*	—	—
Romaine	3 1/2 oz	100	18	0.3	13	—*	75	4	—*	—*	—*	—*	—	—
Mushrooms, canned	1 cup	200	34	3.8	12	444	—*	266	—*	840	596	—*	—	—
Onions														

*Limiting amino acid.
†Percentages are based on Recommended Dietary Allowances for limiting amino acid of each particular food.

Food Item	Measure	Weight g	Calories	Protein g	TRP	LEU	LYS	MET	PHA	ISL	VAL	THR	Men (160 lb)	Women (124 lb)
													% of Limiting Amino Acid Supplied[†]	
						Essential Amino Acids, mg								
Cooked, mature	1 cup	210	61	2.5	33	65	116	23*	71	38	55	40	3	4
Dry, mature	1 med	100	38	1.5	22	39	69	14*	42	22	23	24	2	3
Flakes	1 oz	29	100	2.5	33	65	117	23*	71	38	55	40	3	4
Peas, green, cooked	1 cup	133	94	7.2	53	452	338	51*	281	330	294	114	6.65	7.98
Pepper, green, raw	1 lg	100	22	1.2	3	46	50	16*	55	46	32	50	2	3
Potato														
Baked with skin	1 med	100	93	2.6	26	130	138	31*	114	114	138	107	4	6
Mashed with butter and milk	1 cup	200	188	4.2	42	210	222	50*	184	184	222	172	7	9
Pan fried	1 cup	133	356	5.32	53	266	282	64*	235	235	282	217	8	11
Pumpkin, canned	2/5 cup	100	33	1.0	13	79	46	19*	56	56	54	30	3	3
Radish, red, raw	1 sm	10	1.7	0.1	0.04	—*	0.28	0.02	—*	—*	0.25	0.49	—	—
Soybeans														
Immature, raw	1 cup	200	268	21.8	320	1,944	1,596	316	1,236	1,136	1,200	964	44	56
Mature, cooked	1 cup	200	260	22	330	1,870	1,518	330*	1,188	1,298	1,276	846	46	59
Spinach, steamed	1 cup	180	42	6	86	416	334	92*	232	254	296	238	12	16
Squash														
Summer, cooked	1 cup	200	28	1.8	14	82	68	24*	48	58	66	42	3	4
Summer, raw	1 cup	200	38	2.2	18	100	84	28*	60	70	82	50	4	5
Winter, cooked	1 cup	200	76	2.2	22	126	106	36*	76	90	104	64	5	6
Sweet potato, baked	1 sm	100	141	2.1	36	120	99	38*	116	101	157	99	5	7
Tomato														
Canned, whole	1 cup	240	50	2.4	22	98	101	17*	67	70	67	79	2	3
Cooked, boiled	1 cup	200	52	2.6	24	106	110	18*	72	76	72	86	2	2
Juice, canned	1 cup	200	38	1.8	16	74	76	12	50	52	50	60	2	2
Puree, canned	1 cup	249	97	4.2	38	172	176	29	118	122	118	139	4	5
Raw	1 med	150	33	1.65	15	68	69	12	46	48	46	54	2	2
Turnip														
Greens, steamed	1 cup	133	26.6	2.93	46.5	207	132	53*	146	108	149	126	6.65	9.3
Sliced, steamed	1 cup	133	31	1.06	—*	—*	56	12	19	19	—*	—*	—	—
Watercress, raw	1 cup	50	10	1.1	17	84	58	7*	40	50	54	54	1	1

* Limiting amino acid.

† Percentages are based on Recommended Dietary Allowances for limiting amino acid of each particular food.

References:

Amino Acid Content of Foods (Rome, Italy: Food and Agriculture Organization of the United Nations, 1972.)

Church, Charles F. and N. Helen: Food Values of Portions Commonly Used, 11th ed. (Philadelphia: J.B. Lippincott Co., 1970.)

Heinz Nutritional Data, 6th ed. (Pittsburgh: Heinz International Research Center, 1972.)

Krause, Marie V. and Martha A. Hunscher: Food, Nutrition and Diet Therapy, 5th ed. (Philadelphia: W.B. Saunders Co., 1972.)

SECTION IX

Nutrient Allowance Chart

The following chart is designed to give you a better understanding of the calories and nutrients your body requires daily. The figures are based on the Recommended Dietary Allowances (RDA) of the National Research Council.[1] RDA should not be confused with United States Recommended Daily Allowances (USRDA), a set of values derived from RDA by the Food and Drug Administration as standards for nutritional labeling.

The chart is divided into three categories: children, girls and women, and boys and men. The sections are further divided into different ages and weights.

Level of Activity

Resting Metabolic Rate. Represents the minimum energy needs for day and night with no exercise or exposure to cold.

Sedentary. Includes occupations that involve sitting most of the day, such as secretarial work and studying.

Light. Includes activities that involve standing most of the day, such as teaching or laboratory work.

Moderate. May include walking, gardening, and housework.

[1] National Academy of Sciences, *Recommended Dietary Allowances*, 1974.

Active. May include dancing, skating, and manual labor such as farm or construction work.

The Nutrient Allowance Chart includes the requirements for resting metabolic rate and for light activity. The chart below is included to allow calculation of calories for requirements for sedentary, moderate, and active levels. Although calorie requirements vary with the level of activity, nutrient requirements, as stated under an individual's desirable weight in the Nutrient Allowance Chart remain the same.

DAILY CALORIE REQUIREMENTS FOR LEVELS OF ACTIVITY

Metabolic Rate	Men	Women
Resting	See "Nutrient Allowance Chart"	See "Nutrient Allowance Chart"
Sedentary	16 cal/lb body weight	14 cal/lb body weight
Light	See "Nutrient Allowance Chart"	See "Nutrient Allowance Chart"
Moderate	21 cal/lb body weight	18 cal/lb body weight
Active	26 cal/lb body weight	22 cal/lb body weight

It can be seen from the above chart that a moderately active man of 180 pounds requires approximately 3780 calories per day. This figure is obtained by multiplying 180 pounds by 21 calories. These estimates do not take into account body build and height, which also affect calorie requirements.

The "Desirable Height and Weight Chart" is included so that dieters may estimate their ideal weight, based on sex, height, and body frame. This information should be used in connection with the "Nutrient Allowance Chart" so that one may determine what nutrients and calories are required and cut calories accordingly. If a popular fad diet is used, there is greater risk of illness occurring, due to any one of the nutrient deficiencies. For further information about dieting, see "Overweight and Obesity," page 155.

The carbohydrate, fat, and protein allowances given in the "Nutrient Allowance Chart" apply to only those persons with light activity patterns. The amount of protein should not fall below the figure given, since this is considered the amount needed by the average healthy person in order to repair and build the body. However, the utilization of nutrients varies among individuals; these amounts are not required by everyone.

DESIRABLE HEIGHT AND WEIGHT CHART

DESIRABLE WEIGHTS FOR MEN AGED 25 AND OVER*

Height with Shoes (1-in. heels)		Small Frame	Medium Frame	Large Frame
Ft	In.			
5	2	112-120	118-129	126-141
5	3	115-123	121-133	129-144
5	4	118-126	124-136	132-148
5	5	121-129	127-139	135-152
5	6	124-133	130-143	138-156
5	7	128-137	134-147	142-161
5	8	132-141	138-152	147-166
5	9	136-145	142-156	151-170
5	10	140-150	146-160	155-174
5	11	144-154	150-165	159-179
6	0	148-158	154-170	164-184
6	1	152-162	158-175	168-189
6	2	156-167	162-180	173-194
6	3	160-171	167-185	178-199
6	4	164-175	172-190	182-204

*Weight in pounds according to frame (in indoor clothing). For nude weight, deduct 5 to 7 lb. This chart prepared by Metropolitan Life Insurance Company.

DESIRABLE WEIGHTS FOR WOMEN AGED 25 AND OVER*

Height with Shoes (2-in. heels)		Small Frame	Medium Frame	Large Frame
Ft	In.			
4	10	92-98	96-107	104-119
4	11	94-101	98-110	106-122
5	0	96-104	101-113	109-125
5	1	99-107	104-116	112-128
5	2	102-110	107-119	115-131
5	3	105-113	110-122	118-134
5	4	108-116	113-126	121-138
5	5	111-119	116-130	125-142
5	6	114-123	120-135	129-146
5	7	118-127	124-139	133-150
5	8	122-131	128-143	137-154
5	9	126-135	132-147	141-158
5	10	130-140	136-151	145-163
5	11	134-144	140-155	149-168
6	0	138-148	144-159	153-173

*Weight in pounds according to frame (in indoor clothing). For nude weight, deduct 2 to 4 lb. This chart prepared by Metropolitan Life Insurance Company.

If there is a need to reduce the intake of calories, it is more desirable to reduce the intake of carbohydrates and fats rather than that of protein. In the case of the heavily active person, an increase in the amount of carbohydrates, fats, and possibly protein will help to meet the higher caloric need. For the sedentary person, the carbohydrate and fat intake may be decreased to meet the lower caloric need.

Nutrient	Approximate Calorie Yield
1 g protein	4
1 g carbohydrate	4
1 g fat	9

When adjustments are made in calorie intake, it should be kept in mind that the total number of calories consumed as fats should not exceed one-third of the daily calorie allowance. An easy way to check is to multiply nine times the number of grams of fat consumed, as this will give the total calories consumed as fat. The result should not exceed one-third of the daily calorie allowance. For further discussion of calories, see "Calories," page 7.

The age categories used in the "Nutrient Allowance Chart" are the same as those used in RDA. Requirements or adequate intakes are not listed by the RDA for potassium, sodium, biotin, choline, folic acid, inositol, PABA, pantothenic acid, and vitamin K; these figures were obtained from other sources.

NUTRIENT ALLOWANCE CHART

	Children (Boys and Girls)				Girls			Women
Age	0-6 mo	1-3 yr	4-6 yr	7-10 yr	11-14 yr	15-18 yr	19-22 yr	23-50 yr
Weight, lb	14	28	44	66	97	119	128	128
Weight, kg	6	13	20	30	44	54	58	58
Calories required for								
Resting metabolic rate								1620
Light activity	770	1100	1600	2200	2300	2300	2000	2000
Carbohydrates, g	115	165	240	330	345	345	346	300
Fats, g	28	38	58	80	80	78	79	66
Protein, g	14	23	30	36	44	48	46	46
MINERALS								
Calcium, mg	360	800	800	800	1,200	1,200	800	800
Iodine, mcg*	35	60	80	110	115	115	100	100
Iron, mg*	10	15	10	10	18	18	18	18
Magnesium, mg	60	150	200	250	300	300	300	300
Phosphorus, mg	240	800	800	800	1,200	1,200	800	800
Potassium, mg	Average daily intake 1,950-5,850 mg							
Sodium, mg	Average daily intake 2,300-6,900 mg							
VITAMINS								
Vitamin A, IU	1,400	2,000	2,500	3,300	4,000	4,000	4,000	4,000
Vitamin B complex								
Thiamine (B_1), mg	0.3	0.7	0.9	1.2	1.2	1.1	1.1	1.0
Riboflavin (B_2), mg	0.4	0.8	1.1	1.2	1.3	1.4	1.4	1.2
Pyridoxine (B_6), mg	0.3	0.6	0.9	1.2	1.6	2.0	2.0	2.0
Cyanocobalamin (B_{12}), mcg*	0.3	1.0	1.5	2.0	3.0	3.0	3.0	3.0
Biotin, mcg	Adequate daily intake 150-300 mcg				Adequate daily intake 150-300 mg			
Choline, mg*	Average daily intake 500-900 mg				Average daily intake 500-900 mg			
Folic acid, mg	0.5	0.1	0.2	0.3	0.4	0.4	0.4	0.4
Inositol, mg*					Average daily intake 1,000 mg			
Niacin, mg	5.0	9.0	12	16	16	14	14	13
Para-aminobenzoic acid (PABA), mg	No Recommended Dietary Allowance				No RDA			
Pantothenic acid, mg	No Recommended Dietary Allowance				Adequate daily intake 5-10 mg			
Vitamin C (ascorbic acid), mg	35	40	40	40	45	45	55	45
Vitamin D, IU	400	400	400	400	Adequate daily intake 400 IU			
Vitamin E, IU	4.0	7.0	9.0	10	12	12	12	12
Vitamin K, mcg†					Adequate daily intake 300-500 mcg			

*Robert S. Goodhart and Maurice E. Shils, *Modern Nutrition in Health and Disease*, 5th ed. (Philadelphia: Lea and Febiger, 1973), p. 263.
†Goodhart and Shils, *Modern Nutrition in Health and Disease*, 5th ed., p. 172.

	Women			Boys			Men	
Age	Pregnant	Lactating	51 and over	11-14 yr	15-18 yr	19-22 yr	23-50 yr	51 and over
Weight, lb			128	97	134	147	154	154
Weight, kg			58	44	61	67	70	70
Calories required for								
Resting metabolic rate								
Light activity	+300	+500	1850	2800	3000	3000	2600	2600
Carbohydrates, g			277	–	–	–	390	390
Fats, g			59				87	87
Protein, g	+30 g	+20 g	46	44	54	54	56	56
MINERALS								
Calcium, mg	1,200	1,200	800	1,200	1,200	800	800	800
Iodine, mcg*	125	150	80	130	150	140	110	110
Iron, mg*	18+	18	10	18	18	10	10	10
Magnesium, mg	450	450	300	350	400	350	350	350
Phosphorus, mg	1,200	1,200	800	1,200	1,200	800	800	800
Potassium, mg	Average daily intake 1,950-5,850 mg			Average daily intake 1,950-5,850 mg				
Sodium, mg	Average daily intake 2,300-6,900 mg			Average daily intake 2,300-6,900 mg				
VITAMINS								
Vitamin A, IU	5,000	6,000	4,000	5,000	5,000	5,000	5,000	5,000
Vitamin B complex								
Thiamine (B_1), mg	+.3	0.3	1.0	1.4	1.5	1.5	1.2	1.2
Riboflavin (B_2), mg	+.3	0.5	1.1	1.5	1.8	1.8	1.5	1.5
Pyridoxine (B_6), mg		2.5	2.0	1.6	2.0	2.0	2.0	2.0
Cyanocobalamin (B_{12}), mcg*	4.0	4.0	3.0	3.0	3.0	3.0	3.0	3.0
Biotin, mcg	Adequate daily intake 150-300 mcg			Adequate daily intake 150-300 mg				
Choline, mg*	Average daily intake 500-900 mg			Average daily intake 500-900 mg				
Folic acid, mg	0.8	0.5	0.4	0.4	0.4	0.4	0.4	0.4
Inositol, mg*	Average daily intake 1,000 mg			Average daily intake 1,000 mg				
Niacin, mg	+2	+4	12	18	20	18	16	16
Para-aminobenzoic acid (PABA), mg	No RDA			No RDA				
Pantothenic acid, mg	Adequate daily intake 5-10 mg			Adequate daily intake 5-10 mg				
Vitamin C (ascorbic acid), mg	60	80	45	45	45	45	45	45
Vitamin D, IU	Adequate daily intake 400 IU			Adequate daily intake 400 IU				
Vitamin E, IU	15	15	12	12	15	15	15	15
Vitamin K, mcg†	Adequate daily intake 300-500 mcg			Adequate daily intake 300-500 mcg				

*Goodhart and Shils, *Modern Nutrition in Health and Disease,* 5th ed., p 263.
†Goodhart and Shils, *Modern Nutrition in Health and Disease,* 5th ed., p. 172.

SECTION X

Diet Analysis

By now you probably have many questions about your own diet and its effect on your health.

* How many calories do I consume each day?
* How many nutrients does my body need?
* Which nutrients are present in my normal diet?
* Do I receive adequate amounts of these nutrients?
* Which nutrients are lacking in my normal diet?
* Should I supplement my diet?
* Can I improve my health by improving my diet?

Learning the answers to these questions through individual effort can result in mental as well as physical enlightenment. To help the individual answer these questions we have developed a "Diet Analysis" program that will enable anyone to evaluate and balance a diet.

Analyzing a diet is the most reliable, educational and effective way to become aware of one's own eating habits. Using the "Table of Food Composition" (pages 199–234) to help keep a written record of all foods/nutrients consumed and comparing actual daily nutrient intake with the minimum amounts established by the National Research Council's Recommended Dietary Allowances (RDA) allows one to accurately determine what nutrients are deficient, in excess, or absent from the diet altogether.

Diet analysis allows the individual to examine nutrient intake for one meal, one day or one week. Information provided by such analysis can be most valuable in helping prepare nutritionally balanced meals in the future; in fact, learning to balance meals should eventually become second nature to the individual. Diet analysis can be an important first step in gaining knowledge of the individual diet.

diet analysis

Food Item	Measure	Weight g	Calories	Protein g	Fats g	Carbohy-drates g	Water g	Calcium mg	Iodine mg	Iron mg	Magne-sium mg	Phos-phorus mg	Potas-sium mg
Breakfast													
egg, fried.	1 med.	50	108	6.2	8.6	0.4	34.0	30.0	—	1.20	5.0	111.0	70
whole wheat toast	1 slice	19	55	2.4	0.6	11.0	5.6	22.0	—	0.50	18.0	52.0	62
honey	1 tbsp.	21	64	0.1	—	16.0	3.6	1.0	—	0.11	0.6	1.3	11
skim milk	1 cup	246	89	8.9	0.2	13.0	223.0	298.0	—	—	35.0	234.0	357
orange juice	1 med.	180	88	1.8	0.4	20.0	154.0	74.0	—	0.72	19.8	36.0	360
Sub total		516	404	19.4	9.8	60.4	420.2	425.0	—	2.53	78.4	434.3	860.0
Lunch													
Sub total													
Dinner													
Sub total													
Snacks													
Sub total													
Total													
RDA													
+ or −													

Sample

Sodium mg	Copper mg	Vitamin A IU	(Thia-mine) B₁ mg	(Ribo-flavin) B₂ mg	Vitamin B₆ mg	Vitamin B₁₂ mcg	Biotin mcg	Choline mg	Folic Acid mg	Inositol g	Niacin mg	Panto-thenic Acid mg	Vitamin C mg	Vitamin D IU	Vitamin E mg	Vitamin K mg
169.0	0.03	71.0	0.05	0.15	—	—	—	—	—		0.10	—	0	27.0	—	—
119.0	—	—	0.04	0.02	—	—	—	—	0.010	0.01	0.60	—	—	—	—	—
1.1	0.04	0	—	0.01	0.004	0	—	—	0.001	—	0.06	0.04	0.21	—	—	—
118.0	0.01	998	0.10	0.44	0.100	1	—	—	—	—	.25	0.90	2.50	100.0	—	—
1.8	0.14	360	0.18	0.05	0.108	0	—	—	0.010	0.38	0.72	0.45	90.0	—	0.43	0.002
408.9	0.22	2,068	0.37	0.67	0.212	1	—	—	0.021	0.39	1.73	1.39	92.71	127.0	0.43	0.002

Sample

amino acids-protein

Food Item	Measure	Weight g	Calories	Protein g	Essential Amino Acids, mg								% of Limiting Amino Acid Supplied†	
					TRP	LEU	LYS	MET	PHA	ISL	VAL	THR	Men (160 lb)	Women (124 lb)
Breakfast														
egg, fried	1 med.	50	108	6.2	99	546	397	192	360	409	459	310	27	34
whole wheat toast	1 slice	19	55	2.4	29	166	71	37	117	104	113	72	5	7
honey	1 tbsp.	21	64	0.1	—	—	—							
skim milk	1 cup	246	89	8.9	137	970	764	235	470	627	676	451	33	42
orange juice	1 med.	180	88	1.8	—	—	—	—	—	—	—	—	—	—
Sub total		516	404	19.4	265	1682	1232	464	947	1140	1248	833	65	83
Lunch														
Sub total														
Dinner														
Sub total														
Snacks														
Sub total														
Total														
RDA														
+ or −														

sample

†Percentages are based on Recommended Dietary Allowances for limiting amino acid of each particular food.

Bibliography

Adams, Ruth and Frank Murray: *Body, Mind, and the B Vitamins.* (New York: Larchmont Books, 1972.)

_____ and _____ : *Vitamin E, Wonder Worker of the 70's.* (New York: Larchmont Books, 1972.)

Airola, Paavo: *Cancer Causes, Prevention, and Treatment.* (Phoenix, Ariz.: Health Plus, 1972.)

_____ : *Are You Confused?* (Phoenix, Ariz.: Health Plus, 1974.)

_____ : *How to Get Well.* (Phoenix, Ariz.: Health Plus, 1974.)

Altschul, A.M.: *Proteins, Their Chemistry and Politics.* (New York: Basic Books, 1965.)

American Journal of Obstetrics and Gynecology, Vol. 61, June 1951.

Anderson, Linnea, Marjorie Dibble, Helen S. Mitchell, and Hendrika Rynbergen: *Nutrition in Nursing.* (Philadelphia: J. B. Lippincott Co., 1972.)

Art of Nutritious Cooking, The. (Bismarck, N.Dak.: Nutrition Search, 1974.)

Bailey, Herbert: *Vitamin E: Your Key to a Healthy Heart.* (New York: Arc Books, 1970.)

Basu, T.K.: *About Mothers, Children and Their Nutrition.* (London: Thorsons Publ., 1971.)

Bender, A.E.: *Dietetic Foods.* (New York: Chemical Publ. Co., 1967.)

Benjamin, Harry: *Your Diet in Health and Disease.* (Croyden, Great Britain: Health for All Publ. Co., 1931.)

Bieler, Henry G.: *Food Is Your Best Medicine.* (New York: Random House, 1965.)

Bogert, L.J., George M. Briggs, and Doris H. Calloway: *Nutrition and Physical Fitness*, 9th ed. (Philadelphia: W.B. Saunders Co., 1973.)

Borsaak, Henry: *Vitamins.* (New York: Pyramid Books, 1940.)

Bowerman, William J. and W.E. Harris: *Jogging.* (New York: Grosset & Dunlap, 1967.)

Brunner, L.W., C.P. Emerson, Jr., L.K. Ferguson, and D.S. Suddarth: *Textbook of Medical-Surgical Nursing*, 2d ed. (Philadelphia: J.B. Lippincott Co., 1970.)

"Cancer News Journal." *Prevention*, December 1971.

Carey, Ruth L., Irma B. Vyhmeister, and Jennie S. Hudson: *Commonsense Nutrition.* (Omaha: Pacific Press, 1971.)

Carroll-Clark, E.H.: *How to Save Your Teeth.* (London: Thorsons Publ., 1968.)

Chaney, Margaret S. and Margaret L. Ross: *Nutrition*, 8th ed. (Boston: Houghton Mifflin Co., 1971.)

Cheraskin, E., W.M. Ringsdorf, and J.W. Clark: *Diet and Disease.* (Emmaus, Pa.: Rodale Books, 1968.)

Clark, Linda: *Get Well Naturally.* (New York: Devin-Adair Co., 1965.)

_____ : *Know Your Nutrition.* (New Canaan, Conn.: Keats Publ. Co., 1973.)

Clark, Michael: "Vitamin E—The Better Treatment for Angina." *Prevention.* December 1972.

Clarke, J.H.: *The Prescriber*, 8th ed. (Rustington, England: Health Science Press, 1968.)

Clymer, R. Swinburne: *Nature's Healing Agents*. (Philadelphia: Dorrance Co., 1963.)

Collins, Daniel A.: *Your Teeth, a Handbook of Dental Care for the Whole Family*. (Garden City, N.Y.: Doubleday & Co., 1967.)

Corrigan, A.B.: *Living with Arthritis*. (New York: Grosset & Dunlap, 1971.)

Crain, Lloyd: *Magic Vitamins and Organic Foods*. (Los Angeles: Crandrich Studios, 1971.)

Darling, Mary: *Natural, Organic, and Health Foods*. USDA Extention Folder No. 280. (St. Paul: University of Minnesota, 1973.)

Davidson, Stanley, R. Passmore, and J.F. Brack: *Human Nutrition and Dietetics*, 5th ed. (Baltimore: Williams and Wilkins Co., 1972.)

Davis, Adelle: *Let's Eat Right to Keep Fit*. (New York: Harcourt, Brace & World, 1954.)

_____: *Let's Have Healthy Children*, 2d ed. (New York: Harcourt, Brace & World, 1959.)

_____: *Let's Get Well*. (New York: Harcourt, Brace & World, 1965.)

Deutsch, Ronald M.: *The Family Guide to Better Food and Better Health*. (Des Moines, Iowa.: Meredith Corp., 1971.)

Dubos, Rene and Maya Pines: *Health and Disease*. (New York: Time-Life Books, 1965.)

Ebon, Martin: *The Truth about Vitamin E*. (New York: Bantam Books, 1972.)

Ellis, John M. and James Presley: *Vitamin B_6: The Doctor's Report*. (New York: Harper & Row, 1973.)

Fleck, Henrietta: *Introduction to Nutrition*, 2d ed. (New York: Macmillan Co., 1971.)

Fredericks, Carlton: *Nutrition–Your Key to Good Health*. (North Hollywood, Calif.: London Press, 1964.)

_____: *Eating Right for You*. (New York: Grosset & Dunlap, 1972.)

_____ and Herbert Bailey: *Food Facts and Fallacies*. (New York: Arco Publ. Co., 1965.)

Garrison, Omar V.: *The Dictocrats' Attack on Health Foods and Vitamins*. (New York: Arc Books, 1971.)

Gomez, Joan: *A Dictionary of Symptoms*. (New York: Bantam Books, 1967.)

Goodhart, Robert S. and Maurice E. Shils: *Modern Nutrition in Health and Disease*, 5th ed. (Philadelphia: Lea & Febiger, 1973.)

_____ and Michael G. Wohl: *Manual of Clinical Nutrition*. (Philadelphia: Lea & Febiger, 1964.)

Guthrie, Helen A.: *Introductory Nutrition*, 2d ed. (St. Louis: C.V. Mosby Co., 1971.)

Heinz Nutritional Data, 6th ed. (Pittsburgh: Heinz International Research Center, 1972.)

Heritage, Ford: *Composition and Facts about Food*. (Mokelumne Hill, Calif.: Health Research Center, 1968.)

Herting, David C: "Perspective on Vitamin E." *American Journal of Clinical Nutrition*, Vol. 19, pp. 210-216, September 1966.

Hill, Howard E.: *Introduction to Lecithin*. (Los Angeles: Nash Publ., 1972.)

Holvey, David (ed.): *The Merck Manual*, 12th ed. (Rahway, N.J.: Merck & Co., 1972.)

Hoover, John E. (ed.): *Remington's Pharmaceutical Sciences*, 14th ed. (Easton, Pa.: Mack Publ. Co., 1970.)

Howe, Phyllis S.: *Basic Nutrition in Health and Disease*, 5th ed. (Philadelphia: W.B. Saunders Co., 1971.)

Hunter, Beatrice T.: *The Natural Foods Primer*. (New York: Simon and Schuster, 1972).

Illustrated Medical and Health Encyclopedia. (New York: H.S. Stuttman Co., 1959.)

Industrial Medicine and Surgery, Vol. 21, June 1952.

Jensen, Bernard: *Seeds and Sprouts for Life*. (Escondido, Calif.: Jensen's Nutrition & Health Products, undated.)

Johnson, Harry J.: *Creative Walking for Physical Fitness*. (New York: Grosset & Dunlap, 1970.)

Jolliffe, Norman (ed.): *Clinical Nutrition*, 2d ed. (New York: Harper & Brothers, 1962.)

Journal of the American Dental Association, August 1955.

Kloss, Jethro: *Back to Eden*. (New York: Beneficial Books, 1972.)

Kotschevar, Lendal H. and Margaret McWilliams: *Understanding Food*. (New York: John Wiley and Sons, 1969.)

Krause, Marie V. and Martha A. Hunscher: *Food, Nutrition and Diet Therapy*, 5th ed. (Philadelphia: W.B. Saunders Co., 1972.)

Kuhne, Paul: *Home Medical Encyclopedia*. (Greenwich, Conn.: Fawcett, 1960.)

Kuntzleman, Charles T. (ed.): *The Physical Fitness*

Encyclopedia. (Emmaus Pa.: Rodale Books, 1970.)

Lappé, Francis L.: *Diet for a Small Planet.* (New York: Ballantine Books, 1971.)

Locke, David M.: *Enzymes–The Agents of Life.* (New York: Crown Press, 1971.)

Macia, Rafael: *The Natural Foods and Nutrition Handbook.* (New York: Harper & Row, 1972.)

Marsh, Dorothy B. (ed.): *The Good Housekeeping Cookbook.* (New York: Good Housekeeping Book Division, 1963.)

Martin, Ethel A.: *Nutrition in Action*, 2d ed. (New York: Holt, Rinehart, & Winston, 1967.)

McDermott, Irene E., Mabel B. Trilling, and Florence W. Nicolas: *Food for Better Living*, 3d ed. (Chicago: J.B. Lippincott Co., 1960.)

Mitchell, Helen S., Hendrika J. Rynbergen, Linnea Anderson, and Marjorie V. Dibble: *Cooper's Nutrition in Health and Disease.* (Philadelphia: J.B. Lippincott Co., 1972.)

Morales, Betty Lee: *Cancer Control Journal*, March 1973.

Moyer, William C.: *Buying Guide for Fresh Fruits, Vegetables and Nuts*, 4th ed. (Fullerton, Calif.: Blue Goose, 1971.)

Moyle, Alan: *Nature Cure for Asthma and Hay Fever.* (Croyden, Great Britain: Health for All Publ. Co., 1951.)

"New in Print/Sound/Film," *Journal of the American Dietetic Association*, September 1972, p. 340.

Norris, P.E.: *About Vitamins.* (London: Thorson's Publ., 1967.)

Null, Gary and Steve Null: *The Complete Handbook of Nutrition.* (New York: Robert Speller & Sons, 1972.)

Nutrition Almanac, 2d ed. (Minneapolis, Minn.: Nutrition Search, 1973.)

"Nutritive Value of Foods," *USDA Home and Garden Bull.* 72, 1971.

O'Brien, Edward J.: *Cigarettes: Slow Suicide!* (New York: Exposition Press, 1968.)

Page, M.E. and H.L. Abrams: *Your Body Is Your Best Doctor.* (New Canaan, Conn.: Keats Publ. Co., 1972.)

Pauling, Linus: *Vitamin C and the Common Cold.* (New York: Bantam Books, 1971.)

Pfeiffer, Carl C., Ph.D., M.D.: *Mental and Elemental Nutrients.* (New Canaan, Connecticut: Keats

Publishing, 1975.)

Pike, Ruth L. and Myrtle L. Brown: *Nutrition: An Integrated Approach.* (New York: John Wiley & Sons, 1967.)

"Potassium: The Neglected Mineral," *Let's Live*, October 1973.

Price, Joseph M.: *Coronaries Cholesterol Chlorine.* (New York: Pyramid Books, 1969.)

"Problem: Lead and What To Do About It," *Prevention*, October 1973.

Rainey, Jean: *How to Shop for Food.* (New York: Barnes & Noble, 1972.)

Recommended Dietary Allowances, 7th ed. (Washington, D.C.: National Academy of Sciences, 1974.)

Reuben, David, M.D.: *The Save Your Life Diet.* (New York: Ballantine, 1975.)

Robinson, Corinne H.: *Basic Nutrition and Diet Therapy*, 2d ed. (New York: Macmillan Co., 1970.)

_____ : *Normal and Therapeutic Nutrition*, 14th ed. (New York: Macmillan Co., 1972.)

Robley, Spencer H.: *Emphysema and Common Sense.* (West Nyack, N.Y.: Parker Publ. Co., 1968.)

Rodale, J.I.: *The Health Builder.* (Emmaus, Pa.: Rodale Books, 1957).

_____ : *The Complete Book of Food and Nutrition.* (Emmaus, Pa.: Rodale Books, 1961.)

_____ : *The Health Seeker.* (Emmaus, Pa.: Rodale Books, 1962.)

_____ : *Best Articles from* Prevention. (Emmaus, Pa.: Rodale Books, 1967.)

_____ : *The Complete Book of Vitamins.* (Emmaus, Pa.: Rodale Books, 1968.)

_____ : *The* Prevention *Method for Better Health.* (Emmaus, Pa.: Rodale Books, 1968.)

_____ : *Cancer Facts and Fallacies.* (Emmaus, Pa.: Rodale Books, 1969.)

_____ : *The Encyclopedia of Common Diseases.* (Emmaus, Pa.: Rodale Books, 1969.)

_____ : *My Own Technique of Eating for Health.* (Emmaus, Pa.: Rodale Press, 1969.)

_____ : *The Encyclopedia for Healthful Living.* (Emmaus, Pa.: Rodale Books, 1970.)

_____ : *Magnesium: That Nutrient that Could Change Your Life.* (New York: Pyramid Books, 1971.)

_____ : *Complete Book of Minerals for Health.* (Emmaus, Pa.: Rodale Books, 1972.)

_____ : *Vitamin A: Everyone's Basic Bodyguard.* (Emmaus, Pa.: Rodale Press, 1972.)

_____: *Be a Healthy Mother, Have a Healthy Baby.* (Emmaus, Pa.: Rodale Press, 1973.)

Rosenberg, Harold and A.N. Feldzamen: *The Doctor's Book of Vitamin Therapy: Megavitamins for Health.* (New York: G.P. Putnam's Sons, 1974.)

Rothenberg, Robert E.: *The New American Medical Dictionary and Health Manual.* (New York: New American Library, 1968.)

_____: *Health in the Later Years*, rev. (New York: Signet Books, 1972.)

Samuels, Mike and Hal Bennett: *The Well Body Book.* (New York: Random House, 1973.)

Shackelton, Alberta D.: *Practical Nurse Nutrition Education*, 3d ed. (Philadelphia: W. B. Saunders Co., 1972.)

Shute, Evan: *The Heart and Vitamin E.* (London, Canada: Evan Shute Foundation, 1963.)

Shute, Wilfrid E. and Harold J. Taub: *Vitamin E for Ailing and Healthy Hearts.* (New York: Pyramid House, 1969.)

Sidhwa, Kekir: *Fit for Anything.* (Lewes, Sussex, England: Health for All Publ. Co., 1964.)

Smith, Dorothy W., Carol P. Hanley Germain, and Claudia D. Gips: *Care of the Adult Patient.* (Philadelphia: J.B. Lippincott Co., 1971.)

"Smoking Depletes Vitamin C," *Prevention*, February 1971.

Sokoloff, Boris: *Cancer: New Approaches, New Hope.* (New York: Devin-Adair)

Stein, Mendel: *Vitamins.* (Edinburgh: Churchill, Livingstone, 1971.)

Stone, Irwin: *The Healing Factor: "Vitamin C" Against Disease.* (New York: Grosset & Dunlap, 1970.)

"Summer Cold; Vitamin C . . . ," *Prevention*, July 1970.

Swan, Dr. Roy: *The Multiple Sclerosis Diet Book.* (New York: Doubleday, 1977.)

Synder, Arthur W.: *Vitamins and Minerals.* (Los Angeles: Hansens, 1969.)

Thomas, Clayton L. (ed.): *Taber's Cyclopedia Medical Dictionary*, 12th ed. (Philadelphia: F.A. Davis Co., 1973.)

Toxicants Occurring Naturally in Foods. (Washington, D.C.: National Academy of Sciences, 1973.)

Vitamins Explained Simply, The, 5th ed. (Melbourne: Science of Life Books, 1972.)

Wade, Carlson: *Magic Minerals.* (West Nyack, N.Y.: Parker Publ. Co., 1967.)

_____: *Health Food Recipes for Gourmet Cooking.* (New York: Arco Publ. Co., 1969.)

_____: *Helping Your Health with Enzymes.* (New York: Universal—Award House, 1971.)

Watt, B.K. and A.L. Merill: "Composition of Foods—Raw, Processed, Prepared," *USDA Handbook* 8, 1963.

Wayler, Thelma J. and Rose S. Klein: *Applied Nutrition.* (New York: Macmillan Co., 1965.)

Webster, James: *Vitamin C, The Protective Vitamin.* (New York: Universal-Award House, 1971.)

Wheatley, Michael: *About Nutrition.* (London: Thorsons, 1971.)

White, Philip (ed.): *Let's Talk about Food*, 2d ed. (Chicago: American Medical Association, 1970.)

Williams, Roger J.: *Nutrition against Disease.* (New York: Pitman Publ., 1971.)

Williams, Sue R.: *Review of Nutrition and Diet Therapy.* (St. Louis: C.V. Mosby Co., 1973.)

Wilson, Eva D., Katherine H. Fischer, and Mary E. Fugue: *Principles of Nutrition*, 2d ed. (New York: John Wiley & Sons, 1965.)

Winter, Ruth: *Beware of the Food You Eat*, rev. ed. (New York: Signet Books, 1971.)

_____: *Vitamin E: the Miracle Worker.* (New York: Arco Publ. Co., 1972.)

Wintrobe, M.M. et al.: *Harrison's Principles of Internal Medicine*, 6th ed. (New York: McGraw-Hill Book Co., 1970.)

Yudkin, John: *Sweet and Dangerous.* (New York: Peter H. Wyden, 1972.)

Glossary

ABSORPTION The process by which nutrients are taken up by the intestines and are passed into the bloodstream.

ACID A water-soluble, sour substance (e.g., vinegar).

ACUTE Having a sudden onset, sharp rise, and short course.

ADRENAL GLAND A triangular-shaped organ located on the top of each kidney, which produces the hormone adrenalin.

ALKALI A substance that will neutralize an acid to form a salt; a base.

ALLERGY A reaction of body tissues to a specific substance.

AMINO ACIDS A class of organic compounds known as the "building blocks of the protein molecule."

ANTIBODY A substance produced in the body which reacts against bacteria, disease, or other foreign material in the bloodstream.

ANTICOAGULANT An agent that prevents or delays blood clotting.

ANTIOXIDANT A substance capable of protecting other substances from oxidation.

ANTITOXIN An antibody formed in the body which neutralizes a specific poison.

ASSIMILATE Absorb into the system; transform food into living tissues.

ATROPHY A wasting away of a cell, tissue, organ, or part.

AVIDIN A proteinlike substance isolated from egg white; an antagonist of biotin.

AVITAMINOSIS A condition due to the lack or the deficiency of a vitamin in the diet or to the lack of absorption or utilization of it.

BACTERIA One-celled organisms that may be either harmless, beneficial, or harmful to the body.

BILE A substance produced by the liver which aids in the digestion of fats by breaking them up in the intestine.

CAFFEINE A stimulant found in coffee, tea, and carbonated beverages.

CALCIFICATION Process by which organic tissue becomes hardened by a deposit of calcium salts.

CALORIE A measure of a unit of heat or energy.

CAPILLARY A minute, thin-walled blood vessel.

CARCINOGENIC Cancer-producing.

CAROTENE A yellow pigment that exists in several forms; alpha, beta, and gamma carotene are provitamins that may be converted into vitamin A in the body.

CATABOLISM That aspect of metabolism which converts nutrients or complex substances in living cells into simpler compounds, with the release of energy.

CELL The smallest structural unit of living material.

CELLULOSE A nondigestible carbohydrate found in the skins of fruits and vegetables.

CENTRAL NERVOUS SYSTEM The brain and spinal cord.

CHOLESTEROL A fatlike substance found in all animal fats, bile, skin, blood, and brain tissue.

CHRONIC   Long and drawn-out in reference to disease.

CHYME   The thick, grayish, semiliquid mass into which food is converted by gastric digestion. In this form it passes into the small intestine.

CIRCULATORY SYSTEM   The means of transportation of fluids within the body (e.g., blood is transported by the veins, arteries, and heart).

COAGULATION   The process of clotting in the blood.

COENZYME   As assistant, or helper, usually a vitamin or mineral, which is necessary for the enzyme to do its work.

COLD-PRESS   To use pressure without heat; a method used to extract certain oils from foods, helps preserve nutrient content.

COLLAGEN   The main organic constituent of connective tissue and of the organic substance of bones; changed into gelatin by boiling.

COLON   The large intestine.

COMPOUND   Made up of two or more parts.

CONGENITAL   Existing at or before birth.

CYANOSIS   Slightly blue or dark-purple discoloration of the skin due to abnormal amounts of reduced hemoglobin in the blood.

CYTOPLASM   The protoplasm of a cell outside the nucleus.

DEFICIENCY   The lack of a specific nutrient or nutrients.

DEGENERATION   Passage from a higher to a lower condition; decay.

DEHYDRATION   The abnormal depletion of body fluids from food or tissue; or the condition that results from undue loss of water.

DENTAL CARIES   Decay of the teeth.

DESICCATED LIVER   The dried liver of cattle used as a dietary supplement.

DETOXIFICATION   Reduction of the toxic or poisonous properties of a substance.

DISORDER   A disturbance of regular or normal functions.

DNA   Abbreviation for "deoxyribonucleic acid"; nucleic acid present in chromosomes in nuclei of cells; chemical basis of heredity and carrier of genetic information.

DYSTROPHY   Progressive weakening of a muscle.

ECLAMPSIA   A severe manifestation of toxemia of pregnancy, accompanied by convulsions.

EDEMA   Retention of fluids within the body, causing swelling.

EMULSION   A finely divided mixture or suspension of two liquids not mutually soluble.

ENZYME   A substance, usually protein in nature and formed in living cells, which brings about chemical changes.

EPITHELIAL TISSUE   Membrane that lines body canals, passages, and cavities.

ESTERS   Compounds formed by the combination of an organic acid with an alcohol.

EXCRETION   The process of eliminating waste products from the body.

FAO   Food and Agriculture Organization of the United Nations, headquarters in Rome, Italy.

FAT-SOLUBLE VITAMIN   Vitamin able to dissolve in fats or oils.

FATTY ACIDS   Substances that give fats their different flavors, textures, and melting points.

FIBRIN   Protein formed by action of thrombin and fibrogen; basis for blood clotting.

FLUORIDATION   The addition of fluoride to a water supply as part of a public health program to reduce the incidence of dental caries.

FODDER   Coarse feed for livestock.

GASTROINTESTINAL   Pertaining to the stomach and intestine.

GESTATION   Period of fetal development; pregnancy.

GINGIVITIS   Inflammation of the gums.

GLUCOSE   The simplest form of sugar in which a carbohydrate is assimilated in the body; blood sugar.

GLYCOGEN   Form in which carbohydrates are stored in the body.

GOITROGEN   A substance that increases susceptibility to goiter.

GRAM   A measurement of weight equal to about 1/28 ounce.

HEINZ BODIES   Granules in red blood cells due to damage of hemoglobin molecules.

HEME   The colored, insoluble component of hemoglobin, containing iron.

HEMICELLULOSE   A complex carbohydrate similar to cellulose found in the cell walls of plants; indigestible but absorbs water, thereby stimulating laxation.

HEMOGLOBIN   The iron-containing pigment of red blood cells.

HEMOLYSIS   Destruction of red blood cells.

HEMORRHAGE Abnormal internal or external discharge of blood.

HOMOGENIZED Made homogeneous. Usually applied to dispersing milk fat in such fine globules that cream will not rise to the top.

HORMONE A chemical substance that is secreted into body fluids and transported to another organ, where it produces a specific effect on metabolism.

HYDROCHLORIC ACID An acid that is a normal part of gastric juice.

HYDROGENATION The process of introducing hydrogen into a compound, as when oils are hydrogenated to produce solid fats.

HYPERVITAMINOSIS A condition due to an excess of one of more vitamins in the diet.

HYPOVITAMINOSIS A condition caused by lack of vitamins in the diet.

INFECTION A condition resulting from the invasion of tissue by harmful bacteria.

INFLAMMATION The reaction of tissue to any type of injury.

INORGANIC Occurring independently of living things.

INSULIN A hormone produced by the pancreas which is essential in regulating the metabolism of sugar.

INTESTINAL FLORA Bacteria present in the intestines, necessary for digestion and metabolism of certain nutrients.

KILOGRAM A measurement of weight equal to about 2.2 pounds.

LACTATION Production of milk in a mammal.

LACTOBACILLUS ACIDOPHILUS The bacteria found in yogurt.

LEGUMES Plants having seed-containing pods that are used as food.

LEINER'S DISEASE A widespread form of seborrheic dermatitis in infants.

LIPID A fat or fatlike substance.

LYMPH A clear, alkaline body fluid found in the lymph vessels and tissue spaces.

MALNUTRITION The condition of a person who does not receive a proper proportion of all essential nutrients.

MEGAVITAMIN Term used to describe massive quantities of a specific nutrient when given for therapeutic purposes.

METABOLISM The chemical changes in living cells by which energy is produced and new material is assimilated for the repair and replacement of tissues.

MICROGRAM A measure of weight; 1/1000 of a milligram.

MILLIGRAM A measure of weight; 1/1000 of a gram.

MINERAL An inorganic substance.

NERVOUS SYSTEM A network of nerve cells, brain, and spinal cord which regulates and coordinates body activities.

NUCLEOPROTEIN The main constituent of hereditary material.

NUTRIENT A substance needed by a living thing to maintain life, health, and reproduction.

ORGANIC Being composed of, or containing, matter of plant or animal origin.

ORGAN MEATS Those parts of an animal such as the liver, kidneys, sweetbreads, and brains.

OXALIC ACID A toxic acid that occurs in various plants and is found in chocolate.

OXIDATION The chemical process by which a substance combines with oxygen, resulting in a change to another form.

PARASITE An organism living off another organism.

PERIDENTITIS Inflammation of tissues surrounding a tooth.

PERISTALSIS The wavelike movement by which the alimentary tract propels its contents.

PERNICIOUS Tending to be serious or fatal.

PHOSPHOLIPID A fat in which one fatty acid is replaced by phosphorus and a nitrogenous compound.

PHOSPHORYLATION Enzymatic conversion of carbohydrates into phosphoric esters in metabolic processes.

PIGMENT A substance that gives color to other substances; e.g., to the eyes and skin.

PITUITARY GLAND Small gland in the brain which secretes substances necessary for basic life processes, such as growth.

PLACEBO An inactive substance used in place of the active substance; often used as a control in experiments.

PLATELET A small, round disk that plays an important role in blood coagulation.

POLYUNSATURATED Being in an organic compound such as a fatty acid in which there is more than one double bond.

PRESERVATIVES Substances added to medicines or foods to prevent spoilage.

PROTEIN A nutrient that is necessary for the building and repair of body tissues.

PROTOPLASM A thick, mucuslike substance that constitutes the physical basis of all living activities.

RECOMMENDED DIETARY ALLOWANCE The amount of nutrients suggested by the National Research Council as being necessary to maintain life processes in most healthy persons.

REMISSION The period of abatement of symptoms or the lessening of their severity.

RESPIRATORY SYSTEM The system of breathing apparatus including the nose, pharynx, larynx, tonsils, bronchi, and lungs.

RNA The abbreviation for "ribonucleic acid," which carries information from the nucleus to cytoplasmic sites.

ROSE HIPS The fruit of the rose, which consists of a fleshy bulblike receptacle located at the base of the rose.

ROUGHAGE A coarse, bulky food, high in fiber, which is nondigestible and stimulates bowel movement; e.g., cellulose.

SACCHARINE An intensely sweet, white, crystalline compound used as a substitute for ordinary sugar. It has no food or energy value.

SATURATED FATTY ACID Those fats that are solid at room temperature, with the exception of coconut oil.

STOMATITIS Inflammation of the mouth.

STRESS Anything that places undue strain upon the nervous and glandular systems of the body. Stress may be internal (from disease of malnutrition) or external (from environmental factors).

STRONTIUM 90 A radioactive isotope that emits beta rays; it is a radiation hazard.

SULFA DRUG A synthetic drug that inhibits or prevents the production of intestinal bacteria.

SUPPLEMENT Nutrient taken in addition to regular food in one of many forms, such as pills, powder, or liquid.

SYMPTOM Something that indicates the presence of a body disorder.

SYNERGIST A remedy that stimulates the action of another.

SYNTHESIS Process of building up, producing.

SYNTHETIC Artificially produced.

TETANY A condition, often due to body calcium imbalances or a vitamin D deficiency, which is marked by muscular spasms and tingling sensations.

THYROID GLAND Gland located at the base of the neck which produces hormones.

TISSUE A group of cells of a particular kind which form part of the structural material of an organism.

TISSUE RESPIRATION The process of using oxygen and other substances to build cells and release energy.

TOCOPHEROL Vitamin E, in forms such as alpha, beta, gamma, and delta.

TOXICITY Poisonous effect produced when a person ingests an amount of a substance that is above his or her level of tolerance.

TRACE MINERAL An element present in minute quantities which is essential to the life of an organism.

ULTRAVIOLET LIGHT Light that has rays of shorter wavelength than visible light.

UNSATURATED FATTY ACIDS Those fats that are liquid at room temperature.

URINARY TRACT Organs and ducts that secrete and eliminate urine; the kidneys, ureters, urinary bladder, and urethra.

VIRAL Caused by a virus.

VIRUS An infective agent capable of growth and reproduction only in living cells.

VITAMIN An organic substance found in foods which performs specific and vital functions in the cells and tissues of the body.

WATER BALANCE The ratio between the water absorbed by the body and that which is excreted.

WATER-SOLUBLE VITAMINS Vitamins able to dissolve in water.

WHITE BLOOD CELL Cell that does not contain hemoglobin and which helps defend the body against disease.

Index

An asterisk (*) following an entry refers to the "Table of Food Composition."

Abalone, 210*
Abdomen:
  anemia, 110
  congestive heart failure, 126
  constipation, 126
  diarrhea, 130
  diverticulitis, 131
  dyspepsia, 145
  gallstones, 136–137
  gastritis, 137
  gastroenteritis, 138
  hemorrhoids, 142
  leukemia, 148
  phlebitis, 157
Abscess, 108
Absorption, 2
  aging, 172
  anemia, 110
  calcium, 63
  celiac disease, 121
  cirrhosis of the liver, 124
  copper, 67
  cystic fibrosis, 127
  fats, 8
  gallstones, 136
  pernicious anemia, 157
  vitamin B₁₂, 27
  zinc, 83
Acerola cherries, 186, 212*
  food supplement, 195
  vitamin C, 43
Acne, 108
  vitamin A, 15–16
Adolescence, 171
  acne, 108
  anemia, 110
  milk, 190–191
  nutrient allowance:
    girls, 247
    boys, 248
Agar-agar, 210*
  diverticulitis, 131
Aging, 172–173
  arteriosclerosis, 111
  arthritis, 112
  cataracts, 121
  cerebrovascular accident, 122
  diverticulitis, 131
  gallstones, 136–137
  gout, 138
  influenza, 145
  leg cramp, 147
  osteoporosis, 155
  senility, 162
  vitamin B complex, 19
  vitamin B₁, 22
  vitamin B₆, 25
  vitamin E, 52–53
Air pollution:
  asthma, 114
  bronchitis, 117
  headache, 140

Ak-mak crackers, 200*
Alcohol, 200*
  alcoholism, 109
  beverages, 193
  drug abuse, 132
  dyspepsia, 145
  epilepsy, 134
  gastritis, 137
  gastroenteritis, 138
  gout, 138
  headache, 140
  hyperthyroidism, 143
  neuritis, 154
  peptic ulcer, 163
  pneumonia, 158
  prostatitis, 159
Alcoholism, 109
  magnesium, 73–75
  vitamin B complex, 18–19
Aldosterone:
  sodium, 81
Alfalfa, 176, 194, 226*
Allergies, 110
  common cold, 125–126
  conjunctivitis, 126
  dermatitis, 128–129
  edema, 133
  gastroenteritis, 138
  glaucoma, 138
  hay fever, 140
  "masked food," 150
  mental illness, 150
  pneumonia, 158
  rhinitis, 140
  vitamin C, 43
Allspice, 224*
Almonds, 220*
  meal, 220*
Aluminum, 61–62
Amblyopia, 110
American cheese, 204*
Amino acid:
  content of foods, 235–243
  eggs, 186
  essential, 9, 235–243
  niacin, 36
  protein, 9–10
Anchovy, 210*
Anemia, 110
  aging, 173
  alcoholism, 109
  arthritis, 112–113
  bruising, 118
  cancer, 119–120
  carbohydrates, 8
  celiac disease, 122
  colitis, 125
  copper, 68–69
  drug abuse, 132
  fatigue, 135
  folic acid, 32
  hemorrhagic, 72

  hypocromic, 71
  iron, 71–72
  leukemia, 148
  meats, 189
  nephritis, 154
  pernicious, 157
    cobalt, 67
    gastritis, 137
    vitamin B₁₂, 28
  pregnancy, 170
  scurvy, 161
  stomach ulcer, 163
  vitamin B₆, 26
Angel food cake, 206*
Angelica, 176–177
Angina pectoris, 111, 141
Anise seed, 224*
Antibiotics:
  abscess, 108
  venereal disease, 168
  vitamin C, 43
Antibodies:
  fever, 135
  mononucleosis, 151
  protein, 9
Anxiety:
  colitis, 124
  constipation, 126
  diarrhea, 130
  dyspepsia, 145
  glaucoma, 138
  insomnia, 145–146
  pellagra, 157
  stress, 163
Apple, 212*
  brown betty, 206*
  butter, 206*
  dried, 212*
  fruits, 186–187
  juice, 212*
  pie, 208*
"Approximate Nutrient Composition of the Body," 106
Apricot, 212*
  nectar, 212*
Arachidonic acid fats, 8
Arteries:
  arteriosclerosis and atherosclerosis, 111–112
  myocardial infarction, 152
Arteriosclerosis and atherosclerosis, 111–112
  aging, 173
  cerebrovascular accident, 122
  congestive heart failure, 126
  hypertension, 141
  leg cramp, 147
  stomach ulcer, 163
  vitamin E, 52
Arthritis, 112–114
  aging, 173
  backache, 115
  osteoarthritis, 112
  rheumatoid, 112–113

Artichoke, 226*
  Jerusalem, 230*
Ascorbic acid (*see* Vitamin C)
Asparagus, 226*
  soup, 222*
Aspirin:
  drug abuse, 132
  gastritis, 137
  vitamin C, 43
Asthma, 114
  bronchitis, 117–118
  emphysema, 133–134
Athlete's foot, 114–115
Autism, 115
  pangamic acid, 115
"Available Forms of Nutrient Supplements,"
    100–105
Avocado, 212*
Azuki beans, 226*

Backache, 115–116
  cystitis, 128
  fatigue, 135
  lumbago, 115
  menopause, 172
Bacon, 218*
  Canadian, 218*
  fat, 222*
Bacteria:
  abscess, 108
  burns, 119
  carbuncle, 121
  conjunctivitis, 126
  cystic fibrosis, 127
  cystitis, 128
  diarrhea, 130
  diverticulitis, 131
  ear infection, 132
  eggs, 186
  gastritis, 137
  halitosis, 139
  impetigo, 144
  meats, 190
  milk, 190
  mononucleosis, 151
  nephritis, 154
  pneumonia, 158
  prostatitis, 159
  swollen glands, 164
  tuberculosis, 166
  vaginitis, 167
Baldness, 116
  hair problems, 139
Bamboo shoots, 226*
Banana, 212*
  baking (plantain), 216*
  fruits, 186–187
Barbeque sauce, 222*
Barbados cherries, 212*
Barley, 200*
  celiac disease, 121–122
  coffee substitutes, 194
  grains, 187–188
  pearled, 200*
  Scotch, 200*

Basil, 224*
Bass, 210*
Bay leaf, 224*
Beans, 226*
  bean and pork soup, 222*
  chili, 218*
  legumes, 188–189
  sprouts, 226*
Bedsores, 116
Beef, 216–220*
  corned, 216*
  dried, chipped, 216*
  ground, 216*
  heart, 216*
  kidney, 216*
  liver, 216*
  meats, 189
  roast, 218*
  soup, 222*
  steak, 216–218*
  tongue, 200*
  worms, 169
Beer, 200*
Beets, 228*
  greens, 228*
  sugar, 192, 208*
Bell's palsy, 116–117
Beriberi, 117
  congestive heart failure, 125
  vitamin B_1, 22
Berries, 212–216* (*see also* Fruits)
Beryllium, 62
Beverages, 185, 194–195, 200*
Bibb lettuce, 230*
Bile:
  digestion, 2
  gallstones, 136–137
  vitamin D, 48
Bioflavonoids, 59–61
  labyrinthitis, 61
  rheumatoid arthritis, 60
  rose hips, 195
  ulcers, 60–61
Biotin, 30
  "Available Forms of Nutrient
    Supplements," 102
  eggs, 186
  leg cramp, 147
  mononucleosis, 151
  "Nutrients That Function Together," 95
  sulfur, 82
  "Summary Chart of Nutrients," 87
  vitamin B complex, 18–21
Biscuit, 200*
Bitot's spots, 117
Black beans, 226*
Blackberries, 212*
  juice, 212*
Black-eye peas, 226*
Blackheads (*see* Acne)
Blackstrap molasses, 208*
Black walnuts, 220*
Bladder:
  cystitis, 128
  multiple sclerosis, 151
  nephritis, 154

Blindness:
  cataracts, 121
  glaucoma, 138
  vitamin A, 15
Blood:
  absorption, 2–3
  anemia, 110–111
  arteriosclerosis and atherosclerosis,
    111–112
  bedsores, 116
  calcium, 63–65
  cataracts, 121
  cerebrovascular accident, 122–123
  childhood, 171
  chlorine, 65
  congestive heart failure, 126
  copper, 67
  cystitis, 128
  diabetes, 129
  fats, 8
  folic acid, 32–33
  gastritis, 137
  hypoglycemia, 144
  iron, 71–72
  leukemia, 146
  magnesium, 73–75
  manganese, 75–76
  menstruation, 171
  nephritis, 154
  para-aminobenzoic acid, 37–38
  peptic ulcer, 163
  potassium, 78–80
  pregnancy, 169–170
  pressure:
    carbohydrates, 8
    cerebrovascular accident, 122–123
    dizziness, 131
    hypertension, 143
    overweight and obesity, 155–156
    sodium, 81–82
  protein, 9
  renal calculi, 146
  sausage, 218*
  sodium, 81–82
  tuberculosis, 166
  varicose veins, 167–168
  vitamin B_6, 25–26
  vitamin B_{12}, 27–29
  vitamin C, 43–44, 46
  zinc, 83–84
Blueberries, 212*
Blue cheese, 204*
  salad dressing, 222*
Bluefish, 210*
Boil, 117
  carbuncle, 121
  impetigo, 144
Bologna, 218*
Bone:
  arthritis, 112–114
  backache, 115–116
  bedsores, 116
  bursitis, 119
  calcium, 63–65

childhood, 171
ear infection, 132
fats, 8
fluorine, 68–69
fracture, 136
iron, 71–72
magnesium, 73–75
osteoporosis, 155
phosphorus, 77–78
pregnancy, 170
rickets and osteomalacia, 160–161
scurvy, 161
sinusitis, 162
sodium, 81–82
vitamin B₁₂, 27
vitamin D, 47–49
Bone meal:
  calcium, 63–64
  supplementary foods, 194
Boron, 85
Boston cream pie, 206*
Boston lettuce, 230*
Bouillon, 222*
  chicken, 224*
Bowel:
  constipation, 126–127
  diverticulitis, 131
  multiple sclerosis, 151
Boysenberries, 212*
Brain, 218*
  alcoholism, 109
  anemia, 110
  arteriosclerosis and atherosclerosis,
    111 112
  cerebrovascular accident, 122–123
  cholesterol, 8
  copper, 68
  dizziness, 131
  drug abuse, 132
  ear infection, 132
  epilepsy, 134
  headache, 140
  meats, 189
  multiple sclerosis, 151–152
  protein, 9
  vitamin B₁, 21
Bran:
  flakes, 200*
  grains, 187–188
  muffins, 202*
  raw wheat, 200*
Braunschweiger, 218*
Brazil nuts, 220*
Breads, 200–204*
  crumbs, 200*
  grains, 187
  pudding w/raisins, 208*
  rolls, 202*
  tooth and gum disorders, 165
Brewer's yeast, 232*
  supplementary foods, 195
  vitamin B complex, 18
Brick cheese, 204*
Brie cheese, 204*
Broccoli, 228*

Brown sugar, 208*
Brownie, 206*
Bronchitis, 117–118
  emphysema, 133–134
Bruises, 118
Brussels sprouts, 228*
Bruxism, 118
Buckwheat flour, 202*
  pancakes, 202*
Bulgur, 200*
Buns, 200*
Burns, 118–119
  vitamin C, 43
  vitamin E, 51, 53
Bursitis, 119
Butter, 222*
  apple, 206*
  oils, 191
  vitamin A, 13
Buttermilk, 206*
  milk, 190

Cabbage, 228*
  iodine, 70
Cadmium, 62–63
  zinc, 84
Caesar salad dressing, 222*
Caffeine:
  beverages, 193–194
  hyperthyroidism, 143
  insomnia, 145
Cake, 206–208*
  icings, 208*
Calcium, 63–65
  adolescence, 171
  aging, 173
  anemia, 110
  arteriosclerosis and atherosclerosis,
    111–112
  "Available Forms of Nutrient
    Supplements," 104
  bone meal, 194
  bruxism, 118
  bursitis, 119
  cataracts, 121
  celiac disease, 121–122
  colitis, 124
  diabetes, 130
  fats, 8
  fever, 135
  fluorine, 68–69
  fracture, 136
  gallstones, 136
  insomnia, 146
  lactation, 171
  leg cramp, 147–148
  magnesium, 73–75
  menopause, 172
  mental illness, 149–151
  milk, 190–191
  nails, 153
  nuts, 191
  "Nutrients That Function Together," 94,
    96–99
  osteomalacia, 160

osteoporosis, 155
phosphorous, 77–78
polio, 158
pregnancy, 170
renal calculi, 146–147
"Rich Sources of Nutrients," 196
rickets, 160–161
scurvy, 161
seaweed, 195
seeds, 192
"Summary Chart of Nutrients," 90
sweeteners, 192
tooth and gum disorders, 165
tuberculosis, 166
vegetables, 193
vitamin D, 47–50
worms, 169
zinc, 83
Calcium orotate (vitamin B₁₃), 29
Calf (see Veal)
Calories, 7
  abscess, 108
  adolescence, 171
  alcoholism, 109
  bedsores, 116
  burns, 119
  cancer, 120
  carbohydrates, 7–8
  celiac disease, 122
  cerebrovascular accident, 123
  childhood, 171
  congestive heart failure, 126
  cystic fibrosis, 127
  diabetes, 129
  fats, 8–9
  fever, 135
  influenza, 145
  kwashiorkor, 147
  myocardial infarction, 153
  neuritis, 154
  overweight and obesity, 155–
    156
  Parkinson's disease, 156
  polio, 158
  prostatitis, 159
  protein, 9
  sweeteners, 192
  swollen glands, 164
  underweight, 167
Calisthenics, 4
Camembert cheese, 204*
Cancer, 119–120
  carbohydrates, 8
  laetrile, 35–36
  pangamic acid, 39–41
  swollen glands, 164
Candy, 208*
  acne, 108
  candied citron, 208*
  cane sugar, 208*
  diabetes, 128
Canker sores, 120–121
Cantaloupe, 212*
Caramel, 208*
Caraway seed, 224*

Carbohydrates, 7–8
  arteriosclerosis and atherosclerosis, 112
  biotin, 30
  diabetes, 129
  diarrhea, 130
  dyspepsia, 145
  fruits, 186
  gallstones, 137
  grains, 187
  halitosis, 140
  hypoglycemia, 144
  kwashiorkor, 147
  magnesium, 73–74
  manganese, 75
  mental illness, 150
  myocardial infarction, 153
  neuritis, 154
  niacin, 36
  overweight and obesity, 155–156
  phosphorous, 77
  protein, 9–10
  "Rich Sources of Nutrients," 196
  stress, 163
  sweeteners, 192
  tonsilitis, 165
  tooth and gum disorders, 165
  tuberculosis, 166
  vegetables, 193
  vitamin B complex, 18
  vitamin B_1, 21
  vitamin B_2, 23
  vitamin B_6, 25
  vitamin B_{12}, 27
Carbonated beverages, 193, 200*
Carbuncle, 121
Cardamom, 224*
Carob: flour, 202*
  sweeteners, 192
Carotene:
  diabetes, 129
  fats, 8
  fruits, 186
  tuberculosis, 166
  vitamin A, 13–15
Carp, 210*
Carrots, 228*
Casaba melon, 212*
Cashews, 220*
Cataracts, 120
  vitamin B_2, 24
Catfish, 210*
Catsup, 222*
Cauliflower, 228*
Caviar, 210*
Celeriac root, 228*
Celery, 228*
  seed, 224*
  soup, 224*
Celiac disease, 121–122
  vitamin K, 59
Cellulose:
  bran, 188
  carbohydrates, 7
  fruits, 186
  grains, 187–188

legumes, 188–189
  vegetables, 193
Cereals, 200–204*
Cerebrovascular accident, 122–123
  arteriosclerosis and atherosclerosis,
    111–112
Cervelat, 218*
Chamomile, 177
Chard, Swiss, 228*
Charley horse, 147–148
Cheddar cheese, 204*
Cheese, 204*
  milk, 190
  souffle, 204*
  spread, 204*
Cherries, 212*
  syrup, 212*
Chestnuts, 220*
  water chestnuts, 232*
Chickpeas, 226*
Chicken, 218*
  fat, 222*
  gizzard, 218*
  heart, 218*
  poultry, 189–190
  soups, 224*
Chicken pox, 123
Chicory, 194
Children:
  calcium, 63–65
  croup, 127
  impetigo, 144
  infancy and childhood, 171
  kwashiorkor, 147
  leukemia, 148
  nephritis, 154
  "Nutrient Allowance Chart," 247–248
  rickets, 48, 160–161
  tooth and gum disorders, 165–166
  vitamin D, 48
  worms, 169
Chili:
  beef soup, 224*
  con carne w/beans, 218*
  powder, 224*
  sauce, 222*
Chills:
  abscess, 108
  carbuncle, 121
  gastroenteritis, 138
  influenza, 145
  pneumonia, 158
  renal calculi, 144
  tonsilitis, 165
Chipped beef, 216*
Chives, 228*
Chloride (see Chlorine)
Chlorine, 65–66
  "Nutrients That Function Together," 97
  "Rich Sources of Nutrients," 197
  sodium, 81
  "Summary Chart of Nutrients," 90
  vitamin E, 51
Chocolate:
  acne, 108

baking, 208*
  bittersweet, 208*
  cake, 206*
  calcium, 64
  candy, 208*
  cookies, 208*
  fudge, 208*
  milk, 208*
  mint patty, 208*
  pudding, 208*
  semisweet, 208*
  sweeteners, 192
  syrup, 208*
Cholesterol, 8–9
  arteriosclerosis and atherosclerosis,
    111–112
  cerebrovascular accident, 122
  eggs, 186
  fish, 186
  gallstones, 136
  inositol, 34
  lecithin, 195
  level, high, 123–124
  vitamin B_6, 25–26
  vitamin D, 47–49
Choline, 30–32
  alcoholism, 109
  "Available Forms of Nutrient
    Supplements," 102
  inositol, 33–34
  lecithin, 195
  "Nutrients That Function Together," 93–96
  "Rich Sources of Nutrients," 196
  "Summary Chart of Nutrients," 88
  vitamin B complex, 18–21
Chromium, 66–67
  "Available Forms of Nutrient
    Supplements," 104
  diabetes, 129–130
  "Nutrients That Function Together," 97
  "Rich Sources of Nutrients," 197
  "Summary Chart of Nutrients," 90
Chuck roast, 216*
Chyme, 2
Cinnamon, 224*
Cirrhosis of the liver, 124
  alcoholism, 109
  cancer, 120
  gastritis, 137
  iron, 71
Citron, candied, 208*
Clams, 210*
  chowder, 224*
Cloves, 224*
Club soda, 200*
Club steak, 216*
Cobalamin (see vitamin B_{12})
Cobalt, 67
  "Available Forms of Nutrient
    Supplements," 104
  fish, 186
  "Rich Sources of Nutrients," 197
  "Summary Chart of Nutrients," 90
Cocktail: alcoholic, 200*
  fruit, 214*

Cocoa, 192
Coconut, 220*
  milk, 220*
Cod, 210*
  cod-liver oil, 222*
    vitamin A, 13–14
    vitamin D, 47–48
Coenzymes:
  folic acid, 32
  metabolism, 3
  niacin, 36
  pantothenic acid, 41
  para-aminobenzoic acid,
    37–38
  potassium, 78
  vitamin B$_1$, 21
Coffee, 200*
  beverages, 194
  dyspepsia, 145
  gastritis, 137
  hypertension, 143
  hyperthyroidism, 143
  hypoglycemia, 144
  peptic ulcer, 163
  substitutes, 194
Colby cheese, 204*
Cold (see Common cold)
Cola, 200*
  beverages, 193
  insomnia, 145
Colitis, 124–125
Collagen and vitamin C, 43
Collards, 228*
Colon:
  colitis, 124
  constipation, 126
  diarrhea, 130
  diverticulitis, 131
Coma:
  diabetes, 129
  meningitis, 149
Comfrey, 177–178
Common cold, 125–126
  pneumonia, 158
  sinusitis, 162
  vitamin C, 43
Condensed milk, 206*
Congestive heart failure, 126
  edema, 133
Conjunctivitis, 126
Consomme, 222–224*
Constipation, 126–127
  beriberi, 117
  carbohydrates, 7
  diverticulitis, 131
  hemorrhoids, 142
  Parkinson's disease, 156
Convulsions:
  beriberi, 117
  epilepsy, 134
  fever, 135
  vitamin B$_6$, 26
Cookies, 208*
Copper, 67–68
  anemia, 110–111

eggs, 186
fish, 186
meats, 189
nuts, 191
"Rich Sources of Nutrients," 197
vitamin C, 44
zinc, 84
Coriander:
  leaf, 224*
  seed, 224*
Corn, 228*
  bread, 200*
  flakes, 200*
  flour, 202*
  grits, 200*
  meal, 200*
  muffins, 202*
  oil, 222*
  popcorn, 202*
  starch, 200*
  syrup, 208*
  tortilla, 202*
Corned beef, 216*
  hash w/potato, 218*
Coronary occlusion, 141
Coronary sclerosis, 141
Coronary thrombosis, 141
Cos lettuce, 230*
Cottage cheese, 204*
Cottonseed oil, 222*
Crab, 210*
Crabapple, 212*
Cracked wheat bread, 200*
Crackers, 200*
Cramp:
  calcium, 64
  gastroenteritis, 138
  leg cramp, 147–148
  menstruation, 171
Cranberry, 212*
  sauce, 212*
Cream, 204*
  cheese, 204*
  of wheat, 202*
  soups, 222–224*
  sour, 204*
  whipping, 204*
Cress, 228*
Cretinism and iodine, 70
Croup, 127
Cucumber, 228*
Cumin seed, 224*
Currants, 212*
Curry powder, 224*
Custard, 208*
Cystic fibrosis, 127–128
Cystitis, 128
  prostatitis, 159

Daiquiri, 200*
Dairy products, 204–206*
Damson plums, 216*
Dancing, 4
Dandelion, 178
  greens, 228*

Dandruff, 128
Danish pastry, 202*
Dates, 212*
Deer (venison), 220*
Delirium in alcoholism, 109
Dermatitis, 128–129
  biotin, 30
  niacin, 36–37
  pellagra, 157
  vitamin A, 15
  vitamin B$_6$, 25–27
Desserts and sweets, 206*
Diabetes, 129–130
  carbohydrates, 8
  cataracts, 121
  cerebrovascular accident, 122
  gallstones, 136–137
  magnesium, 74–75
  neuritis, 154
  vitamin E, 53
Diarrhea, 130–131
  anemia, pernicious, 157
  beriberi, 117
  celiac disease, 122
  colitis, 124–125
  fever, 135
  gastritis, 137
  gastroenteritis, 138
  kwashiorkor, 147
  leg cramp, 147
  magnesium, 74–75
  niacin, 36–37
  pellagra, 157
  polio, 158
  potassium, 79–80
Diet Analysis, 249–252
Diet drinks, 200*
Digestion, 2
  carbohydrates, 7
  digestive juice:
    cystic fibrosis, 127
    gastritis, 137
    nuts, 191
    seasoning, 191
  digestive system:
    colitis, 124–125
    headache, 140
    niacin, 36–37
  fats, 9
  peptic ulcer, 163
Dill:
  seed, 224*
  weed, 224*
Diphtheria and croup, 127
Diverticulitis, 131
Dizziness, 131
  anemia, 110
  carbohydrates, 8
  drug abuse, 132
  ear infection, 132
Dock, 228*
Doughnuts, 208*
Dressings:
  salad, 222*
Dried beef, 216*

Dried milk, 206*
Drug addiction and vitamin C, 44
Drugs:
  abuse, 132
  cancer, 120
  epilepsy, 134
  gastroenteritis, 138
  gout, 139
  headache, 140
  hypertension, 143
  hypoglycemia, 144
  insomnia, 146
  Parkinson's disease, 156
Duck, 218*
Dulse, 195–196, 210*
Dyspepsia, 145
  cancer, 120
  fatigue, 135
  gastritis, 137

Ear:
  dizziness, 131
  gout, 139
  infection, 132
  influenza, 145
  tonsilitis, 165
Eclair, 208*
Eczema, 132–133
  dermatitis, 128
  fats, 9
Edam cheese, 204*
Edema, 133
  beriberi, 117
  hypertension, 143
  kwashiorkor, 147
  menstruation, 171
  nephritis, 154
  sodium, 81
  vitamin E, 52
Eel, 210*
Eggs, 186, 204–206*
  amino acid chart, 239
  fats, 8
  protein, 236, 239
Eggnog, 206*
Eggplant, 228*
Elderberries, 212*
Emphysema, 133–134
  vitamin E, 55
Endive, 228*
English muffin, 200*
English walnuts, 220*
Enzymes, 2
  calcium, 63
  copper, 68
  digestion, 2
  manganese, 75
  protein, 9
  vitamin B$_2$, 23
  vitamins, 11
Epilepsy, 134
"Essential Amino Acid Contents of Some
  Foods," 235–243
Estrogen and vitamin E, 51, 53
Eucalyptus, 178

Evaporated milk, 206*
Exercise, 4–5
  acne, 108
  arthritis, 113
  atherosclerosis, 112
  backache, 115
  congestive heart failure, 126
  constipation, 126
  diabetes, 129
  edema, 133
  epilepsy, 134
  fatigue, 135
  gout, 139
  hemorrhoids, 142
  hypertension, 142
  mononucleosis, 151
  multiple sclerosis, 151
  myocardial infarction, 153
  nutrition and health, 1
  osteoporosis, 155
  overweight and obesity, 155
  phlebitis, 158
  underweight, 167
  varicose veins, 167
"Expenditure of Caloric Energy Per Hour," 4
Extracts, 191–192
Eyes:
  cataracts, 121
  common cold, 125
  conjunctivitis, 126
  edema, 133
  eyestrain, 134–135
  gallstones, 137
  glaucoma, 138
  headache, 140
  shingles, 162
  sinusitis, 162
  vision and focus disorders, 168–169
  vitamin A, 14–15
  vitamin B complex, 18–20
  vitamin B$_2$, 23–24
  vitamin E, 50, 55

Farina, 202*
Fasting, 1
Fatigue, 135
  aging, 173
  anemia, 110
  arthritis, 113
  beriberi, 117
  bronchitis, 117
  carbuncle, 121
  congestive heart failure, 126
  constipation, 126
  dermatitis, 128
  epilepsy, 134
  hypoglycemia, 144
  iron, 71
  menopause, 172
  mental illness, 149
  mononucleosis, 151
  nephritis, 154
  night blindness, 155
  para-aminobenzoic acid, 38
  pneumonia, 158

  pregnancy, 170
  sinusitis, 162
  stress, 163
  tuberculosis, 166
  underweight, 167
  vitamin B$_1$, 22
  vitamin B complex, 19–21
Fats, 7, 8–9, 222*
  acne, 108
  alcoholism, 109
  angina pectoris, 111
  arteriosclerosis and atherosclerosis,
    111–112
  beverages, 193
  calcium, 64
  carbohydrates, 7–8
  celiac disease, 122
  chocolate, 192
  choline, 31
  cocoa, 192
  congestive heart failure, 126
  constipation, 126
  cystic fibrosis, 127
  dermatitis, 128
  diabetes, 129
  digestion, 2
  dyspepsia, 145
  eggs, 186
  epilepsy, 134
  fish, 186
  gallstones, 136–137
  gout, 139
  hypoglycemia, 144
  inositol, 33–34
  kwashiorkor, 147
  lecithin, 195
  manganese, 75
  margarine, 191
  meats, 189
  milk, 190
  myocardial infarction, 152–153
  niacin, 36
  nutrition and health, 1
  nuts, 191
  oils, 191
  overweight and obesity, 155–156
  pantothenic acid, 41
  phosphorus, 77
  poultry, 189
  psoriasis, 159
  seeds, 192
  source of calories, 7
  stress, 163
  underweight, 167
  vitamin A, 14
  vitamin B$_2$, 23
  vitamin D, 47
  vitamin E, 50–53
  vitamin K, 58–59
  vitamins, 12
Fatty acids, 8, 55–58
  absorption, 2
  fats, 8–9
  fish, 186
  margarine, 191

metabolism, 3
oils, 191
phosphorus, 77
sunflower seeds, 192
vitamin E, 50–51
wheat germ, 196
Fennel seed, 224*
Fenugreek seed, 224*
Fever, 135
abscess, 108
arthritis, 113
backache, 115
bronchitis, 117
carbuncle, 121
cirrhosis of the liver, 124
common cold, 125
croup, 127
cystitis, 128
diverticulitis, 131
ear infection, 132
epilepsy, 134
gastroenteritis, 138
headache, 140
influenza, 145
leukemia, 148
meningitis, 149
mononucleosis, 151
myocardial infarction, 152
nephritis, 154
phlebitis, 157
pneumonia, 158
polio, 158
prostatitis, 159
renal calculi, 147
sinusitis, 162
swollen glands, 165
tonsilitis, 165
tuberculosis, 166
venereal disease, 168
Fiber, 186–187
Fig, 212–214*
bar, 208*
Filberts, 220*
nuts, 191
Fish, 210–212*
foods, 186
phosphorus, 77
sulfur, 82
vitamin A, 13
vitamin B12, 27
vitamin D, 47
worms, 169
Flank steak, 216*
Flavonals, 59
Flavons:
"Available Forms of Nutrient Supplements," 104
bioflavonoids, 59
Flounder, 210*
Flour, 202*
grains, 187–188
Flu:
gastroenteritis, 138
influenza, 145

Fluorides:
fluorine, 68–69
osteoporosis, 155
"Rich Sources of Nutrients," 197
Fluorine, 68–69
"Available Forms of Nutrient Supplements," 104
fish, 186
"Nutrients That Function Together," 97
"Summary Chart of Nutrients," 91
water, 85
Folic acid, 32–33
alcoholism, 109
anemia, 110
pernicious, 157
arthritis, 113–114
"Available Forms of Nutrient Supplements," 102
celiac disease, 122
"Nutrients That Function Together, 94–97
para-aminobenzoic acid, 37
pellagra, 151
"Rich Sources of Nutrients," 196
"Summary Chart of Nutrients," 88
vitamin B complex, 18–21
vitamin C, 43
Food poisoning:
diarrhea, 130
foods, beverages, and supplementary foods, 185
gastroenteritis, 138
zinc, 83–84
Food preparation:
foods, beverages, and supplementary foods, 185
meats, 189–190
oils, 191
vegetables, 193
worms, 169
Food storage:
eggs, 186
fish, 186
foods, beverages, and supplementary foods, 185
fruits, 187
grains, 188
legumes, 188–189
meats, 189–190
milk, 190–191
nuts, 191
oils, 191
seasonings, herbs, spices, and extracts, 191–192
seeds, 192
sweeteners, 192
vegetables, 193
Fracture, 136
neuritis, 154
osteoporosis, 155
vitamin C, 44, 46
Frankfurter, 218*
French bread, 200*
French fries, 230*
French salad dressing, 222*
Frog's legs, 210*

Fruits, 212–216*
acerola cherries, 195
bioflavonoids, 59
carbohydrates, 7
cocktail, 214*
colitis, 125
constipation, 126
diabetes, 129
drinks, 200*
foods, beverages, supplementary foods, 185
hypoglycemia, 144
jams, 208*
jellies, 208*
juices, 212–216*
diverticulitis, 131
foods, 187
peptic ulcer, 163
pie, 208*
potassium, 79
preserves, 208*
"Rich Sources of Nutrients," 196–198
seasonings, herbs, spices, and extracts, 191
sherbet, 206*
tooth and gum disorders, 165
vitamin C, 43
Fudge, 208*
Furuncle (see Boil)

Gallbladder:
calcium, 63
choline, 31
cystic fibrosis, 127
digestion, 2
gallstones, 136–137
Gallstones, 136–137
polio, 158
Garbanzos, 226*
Garlic, 228*
powder, 224*
Gastritis, 137
Gastroenteritis, 138
Gastrointestinal tract:
beriberi, 117
carbohydrates, 7
pellagra, 156–157
vitamin A, 14, 16
vitamin B complex, 18
vitamin B12, 27
vitamin E, 50
Gherkins, 230*
Gin, 200*
Ginger, 224*
ale, 200*
root, 228*
Gingerbread, 208*
Gingersnap, 208*
Gingivitis, 160, 165
Ginseng, 178–179
Gjetost cheese, 204*
Gland:
cystic fibrosis, 127
goiter, 138
hyperthyroidism, 143
hypothyroidism, 144
iodine, 69–70

mononucleosis, 151
swollen glands, 164–165
Glaucoma, 138
Glomerulonephritis, 154
Glucose, 7
absorption, 2
carbohydrates, 7
diabetes, 128
hypoglycemia, 144
potassium, 78
vitamin B₁, 21
Gluten:
celiac disease, 120
wheat flour, 202*
Glycerol absorption, 2
Glycogen:
carbohydrates, 7
potassium, 78
Goat milk, 206*
Goiter, 138
hyperthyroidism, 143
iodine, 69–70
Golden seal, 179
Gonorrhea, 168
Goose, 218*
Gooseberries, 214*
Gout, 138–139
neuritis, 155
Graham crackers, 200*
Grains, 200–204*
amino acid chart, 237–243
calcium, 64
carbohydrates, 7
celiac disease, 121–122
foods, 187–188
magnesium, 73
manganese, 75
phosphorus, 77
potassium, 79
vitamin B complex, 18
Granadilla, 214*
Granola, 202*
Grapefruit, 214*
juice, 214*
Grapes, 214*
Green beans, 226*
Green goddess salad dressing, 222*
Gruyere cheese, 204*
Guava, 214*
Gums:
halitosis, 139–140
leukemia, 148
scurvy, 161–162
tooth and gum disorders, 165–166

Haddock, 210*
Hair problems, 139
copper, 68
kwashiorkor, 147
para-aminobenzoic acid, 38
protein, 10
sulfur, 81–82
venereal disease, 168
vitamin A, 15, 17
vitamin B complex, 18–20

Half and half cream, 204*
Halibut, 210*
Halitosis, 139–140
Ham, 218*
Hash: corned beef, 218*
Hawthorn, 179–180
Hay fever, 140
(see also Allergies)
Hazelnuts, 220*
Headache, 140
backache, 115
carbohydrates, 8
common cold, 125
dizziness, 131
drug abuse, 132
fatigue, 135
fever, 135
gastritis, 137
hypertension, 143
influenza, 145
insomnia, 145
menopause, 172
meningitis, 149
menstruation, 171
mononucleosis, 151
para-aminobenzoic acid, 38
polio, 158
sinusitis, 162
tonsilitis, 165
venereal disease, 168
Head cheese, 218*
Hearing and ear infection, 132
Heart disease, 141–143
aging, 173
angina pectoris, 111, 141
attack (see Myocardial infarction)
beriberi, 117
calcium, 63–64
carbohydrates, 8
cerebrovascular accident, 122
congestive heart failure, 126
edema, 133
fats, 8
hypertension, 143
influenza, 145
magnesium, 73–74
overweight and obesity, 155
phosphorus, 77
potassium, 78
protein, 9
thiamine, 21–23
vitamin E, 50–55
Hemoglobin:
anemia, 110
copper, 67
folic acid, 32
iron, 70
Hemophilia, 142
Hemorrhage:
arteriosclerosis and atheriosclerosis, 112
cerebrovascular accident, 122
iron, 71
protein, 10
vitamin C, 43
vitamin K, 58–59

Hemorrhoids, 140–141
Hepatitis, 141
choline, 31
cirrhosis of the liver, 124
Herb glossary, 182
Herbal preparations, 182
Herbs, 175–183
as seasonings, 191, 224–226*
Herpes zoster, 162
vitamin B₁, 22–23
Hesperidan (see Bioflavonoids)
Hickory nuts, 220*
Hijiki, 210*
Hollandaise sauce, 222*
Honey, 208*
sweeteners, 192–193
Honeydew melon, 214*
Hormones:
adrenal, 163
hyperthyroidism, 143
hypoglycemia, 144
iodine, 69–70
phosphorus, 77
vitamin D, 48
Horseradish, 222*
Hot dog, 218*
meats, 189
How vitamins and minerals are explained in
this book, 12–13
Human milk, 206*
Hydrogenated fats, 8
Hypercalcemia and vitamin D, 48
Hypertension, 143
arteriosclerosis and arterio-
sclerosis, 112
overweight and obesity, 155
Hyperthyroidism, 143
Hypoglycemia, 144
epilepsy, 134
Hypothyroidism, 144
congestive heart failure, 125
iodine, 69

Iceberg lettuce, 230*
Ice cream, 206*
sherbet, 206*
Ice milk, 206*
Icing, cake, 208*
Impetigo, 144
Indigestion, 145
vitamin B₁, 22
Infancy, 171
Infants:
anemia, 110
croup, 127
cystic fibrosis, 127–128
dermatitis, 128
normal life cycle, 171
nutrient allowances, 247
scurvy, 161
vitamin A, 14
vitamin B₁₂, 27
vitamin E, 51–52

Infection:
    abscess, 108
    aging, 173
    backache, 115
    beriberi, 117
    boil, 117
    bronchitis, 117
    burns, 119
    bursitis, 119
    carbuncle, 121
    common cold, 125–126
    diverticulitis, 131
    dizziness, 131
    ear infection, 132
    gallstones, 137
    glaucoma, 138
    goiter, 139
    halitosis, 139
    headache, 140
    herpes zoster, 162
    impetigo, 144
    kwashiorkor, 147
    meningitis, 149
    mononucleosis, 151
    multiple sclerosis, 151
    neuritis, 154
    phlebitis, 157–158
    polio, 158
    prostatitis, 159
    renal calculi, 146
    scurvy, 161
    sinusitis, 162
    swollen glands, 164
    tonsilitis, 165
    tuberculosis, 166
    vaginitis, 167
    venereal disease, 168
    vitamin A, 14–15
    vitamin C, 43–44
Influenza, 145
Inositol, 33–35
    "Available Forms of Nutrient
        Supplements," 102
    "Nutrients That Function Together," 95
    "Rich Sources of Nutrients," 196
    "Summary Chart of Nutrients," 88
    vitamin B complex, 18–21
Insomnia, 145–146
    drug abuse, 132
    hypertension, 143
Insulin:
    diabetes, 129
    zinc, 83
Intestines:
    carbohydrates, 7
    celiac disease, 121–122
    colitis, 124–125
    constipation, 126–127
    diarrhea, 130
    digestion, 2
    diverticulitis, 131
    drug abuse, 132
    dyspepsia, 145
    gallstones, 136
    magnesium, 73–74
    manganese, 75

osteoporosis, 155
    vitamin B_{12}, 27, 29
    worms, 169
Intrinsic factor:
    anemia, pernicious, 157
    gastritis, 137
    vitamin B_{12}, 27
Iodide (see Iodine)
Iodine, 69–70
    "Available Forms of Nutrient
        Supplements," 104
    fish, 186
    goiter, 138
    hypothyroidism, 144
    salt, 226*
    seasonings, 191
    seaweed, 195
    sex, 172
    "Summary Chart of Nutrients," 97
Irish moss, 195–196
Iron, 71–72
    adolescence, 171
    alcoholism, 109
    anemia, 110–111
    "Available Forms of Nutrient
        Supplements," 105
    calcium, 63
    cancer, 120
    celiac disease, 122
    colitis, 125
    copper, 67
    eggs, 186
    fatigue, 135
    fish, 186
    folic acid, 32
    gastritis, 137
    grains, 187
    headache, 140
    legumes, 188
    leukemia, 148
    meats, 189
    menstruation, 171
    milk, 190
    "Nutrients That Function Together,"
        97–98
    nuts, 191
    peptic ulcer, 163
    pregnancy, 170
    "Rich Sources of Nutrients," 197
    "Summary Chart of Nutrients," 91
    tooth and gum disorders, 165
    tuberculosis, 166
    vegetables, 193
    vitamin C, 45
    vitamin E, 51
    wheat germ, 196
    worms, 169
    zinc, 84
Isometrics, 4
Italian:
    bread, 200*
    salad dressing, 222*

Jam, 208*
Jaundice, 146
    cirrhosis of the liver, 124

Jelly, 208*
Joints:
    aging, 173
    arthritis, 112–114
    gout, 138–139
    leg cramp, 147
Jogging, 4
Juices (see Fruits, Vegetables)

Kale, 230*
Kelp, 195–196, 210*
Kernicterus and vitamin K, 59
Kidney, 216*
    beans, 226*
    copper, 68
    cystitis, 128
    edema, 133
    fats, 8
    hypertension, 143
    influenza, 145
    magnesium, 73–75
    meats, 189
    nephritis, 154
    overweight and obesity, 155
    potassium, 78
    prostatitis, 159
    rickets, 161
    sodium, 81
    stones, 146–147
    thiamine, 21
Kidney stones (renal calculi), 146–147
    fracture, 136
    polio, 158
Knockwurst, 218*
Kohlrabi, 230*
Kombu, 210*
Kumquat, 214*
Kwashiorkor, 147
    magnesium, 74
    protein, 10

Lactation, 170–171
Laetrile, 35–36
Lamb, 218*
Lard, 222*
Lead, 72–73
Lecithin:
    choline, 30
    eggs, 186
    inositol, 33–34
    phosphorus, 77
    supplementary foods, 195
Leeks, 228*
Leg cramp, 147–148
    calcium, 64
Legumes, 188–189
    copper, 68
    "Rich Sources of Nutrients,"
        196–197
    sulfur, 82
Lemon, 214*
    juice, 214*
    meringue pie, 208*
Lemonade, 214*
Lemon grass (see "Available Forms of
    Nutrient Supplements")

Lentils, 226*
  legumes, 188–189
  sprouts, 226*
Lettuce, 228*
Leukemia, 148
  bruises, 118
  neuritis, 154
  swollen glands, 164
  zinc, 84
Licorice, 180
Life cycle, 169–173
Lima beans, 226*
Limberger cheese, 204*
Lime, 214*
  juice, 214*
Limiting amino acid, 235–236
Linoleic acid: dermatitis, 128
  fats, 8–9
  oils, 191
  vitamin F, 55
Lipids, 8–9
Lithium, 84
Liver:
  alcoholism, 109
  beef, 216*
  calf, 220*
  cancer, 120
  carbohydrates, 7
  chicken, 216*
  choline, 31–32
  cirrhosis of the liver, 124
  copper, 68
  dessicated, 195
  fats, 8
  gallstones, 136
  gastritis, 137
  iron, 71
  lamb, 218*
  liverwurst, 218*
  manganese, 75
  pate, 218*
  protein, 9
  vitamin A, 13–18
  vitamin B complex, 18–19, 21
  vitamin B₁₂, 27, 29
  vitamin D, 47–48, 50
  vitamin E, 51
Lobster, 210*
Loganberries, 214*
Looseleaf lettuce, 230*
Loquats, 214*
Lotus root, 230*
Low-fat milk, 206*
Lumbago (see Backache)
Lungs:
  asthma, 114
  bronchitis, 117–118
  cystic fibrosis, 127–128
  emphysema, 133–134
  influenza, 145
  iron, 71–72
  pneumonia, 158
  tuberculosis, 166
  vitamin A, 14, 17
  vitamin D, 48, 50

Lychees, 214*
  nuts, 220*
Lymph glands:
  mononucleosis, 151
  swollen glands, 164–165
  tonsilitis, 165

Macadamia nuts, 220*
Macaroni, 202*
Macaroons, 208*
Mace, 224*
Mackerel, 210*
Magnesium, 73–75
  alcoholism, 109
  "Available Forms of Nutrient
    Supplements," 105
  fish, 186
  leg cramp, 147
  "Nutrients That Function Together," 94,
    96–98
  nuts, 191
  renal calculi, 147
  "Rich Sources of Nutrients," 197
  "Summary Chart of Nutrients," 91
  tooth and gum disorders, 165–166
Malnutrition:
  bronchitis, 117
  celiac disease, 122
  cystic fibrosis, 127
  epilepsy, 134
  kwashiorkor, 147
  multiple sclerosis, 151
  Parkinson's disease, 156
  pneumonia, 158
  rickets, 160
  scurvy, 161
  tuberculosis, 166
Malt:
  dried, 212*
  milk, 206*
Manganese, 75–76
  "Available Forms of Nutrient
    Supplements," 105
  diabetes, 129–130
  "Nutrients That Function Together," 94,
    96–98
  "Rich Sources of Nutrients,"
    197
  "Summary Chart of Nutrients," 91
Mango, 214*
Maple syrup, 208*
Margarine, 222*
  fats, 8–9
  oils, 191
Marjoram, 224*
Martini, 200*
Mayonnaise, 222*
Measles, 148–149
  swollen glands, 164
Meat, 216–220*
  amino acid chart, 240–241
  beef, 216–218*
  calf, 220*
  foods, 189–190
  frankfurter, 218*

  gout, 139
  iron, 70
  niacin, 36
  peptic ulcer, 163
  phosphorus, 77
  pork, 218*
  potted, 218*
  protein, 9
  rabbit, 218*
  sausage, 218–220*
  soups, 222–224*
  substitutes, 188
  sweetbreads, 220*
  tongue, 218*
  tooth and gum disorders, 165
  veal, 220*
  venison, 220*
  vitamin B₂, 23
  vitamin B₁₂, 27
  worms, 169
Ménièrè's syndrome, 149
Meningitis, 149
  epilepsy, 134
Menopause, 172
Menstruation, 171
Mental illness, 149–151
Mercury, 76
Meringue pie, 208*
Metabolism, 3
  arteriosclerosis and atherosclerosis,
    111–112
  calories, 7
  carbohydrates, 7
  copper, 68
  fats, 9
  fever, 135
  goiter, 138
  gout, 138–139
  hyperthyroidism, 143
  inositol, 34
  minerals, 12
  nutrient allowances, 245
  protein, 9
  vitamin B₁₂, 27
Migraine (see Headache)
Milk, 206*
  bone meal, 194
  calcium, 63
  colitis, 125
  fats, 8
  foods, 190–191
  insomnia, 146
  kwashiorkor, 147
  lactation, 170–171
  peptic ulcer, 163
  pregnancy, 170
  protein, 9–10
  vitamin K, 58
Millet, 202*
Minerals, 12
  alcoholism, 109
  carbohydrates, 8
  diabetes, 129
  diarrhea, 130
  diverticulitis, 131

foods, 185
fruits, 186
grains, 187
meats, 189
nutrients, 11
oil:
    constipation, 126
    vitamin K, 58
peptic ulcer, 163
renal calculi, 146
seeds, 192
supplementary foods, 194
sweeteners, 192
tooth and gum disorders, 165
tonsilitis, 165
vegetables, 193
Minestrone soup, 224*
Mint patty, 208*
Miso, 222,* 226*
Molasses, 208*
sweeteners, 193
Molybdenum, 76–77
    "Nutrients That Function Together," 98
    "Rich Sources of Nutrients," 197
    "Summary Chart of Nutrients," 91
Mononucleosis, 151
swollen glands, 164
Monterey cheese, 204*
Mouth:
    canker sores, 120–121
    digestion, 2
    tooth and gum disorders, 165
    vitamin A, 13–14, 18
    vitamin B complex, 18–19, 21
    vitamin B$_2$, 24
    vitamin B$_6$, 25, 27
Mozzarella cheese, 204*
Muenster cheese, 204*
Muffin, 202*
Multiple sclerosis, 151–152
Mung beans, 226*
Muscle:
    aging, 173
    alcoholism, 109
    backache, 115
    bronchitis, 117
    bursitis, 119
    calcium, 63, 65
    childhood, 171
    common cold, 125
    constipation, 126
    diabetes, 129
    exercise, 4–5
    iron, 70
    leg cramp, 147–148
    magnesium, 73–74
    muscular dystrophy, 152
    phosphorus, 77
    potassium, 78–79
    protein, 9
    scurvy, 161
    vitamin B$_1$, 21–22
    vitamin E, 50–51, 53–55
Mushrooms, 230*
soup, 224*

Mustard, 222*
greens, 230*
seed, 224*
Mutton (see Lamb)
Myocardial infarction, 152–153
Myoglobin, 70

Nail problems, 153
protein, 9
sulfur, 82
vitamin B$_2$, 23
Natto, 226*
Nausea:
    beriberi, 117
    congestive heart failure, 126
    dizziness, 131
    ear infection, 132
    fever, 135
    gallstones, 137
    headache, 140
    indigestion, 145
    meningitis, 149
    nephritis, 154
    pantothenic acid, 42–43
    polio, 158
    sodium, 81
    tonsilitis, 165
Nectarine, 214*
Nephritis, 154
vitamin E, 52
Nerves:
    backache, 115–116
    epilepsy, 134
    multiple sclerosis, 151–152
    neuritis, 154
    niacin, 36–37
    pangamic acid, 39, 41
    Parkinson's disease, 156
    polio, 158–159
    sciatica, 161
    shingles, 162
    vitamin B complex, 18–20
    vitamin B$_1$, 21–23
    vitamin B$_2$, 24
Neuritis, 154
alcoholism, 109
Niacin, 36–37
    alcoholism, 109
    "Available Forms of Nutrient
      Supplements," 103
    backache, 115–116
    cancer, 120
    dizziness, 131
    headache, 140
    indigestion, 145
    legumes, 199
    mental illness, 149–150
    night blindness, 155
    "Nutrients That Function Together," 94–95
    pellagra, 156–157
    phlebitis, 158
    poultry, 189
    "Summary Chart of Nutrients," 88
    vitamin B complex, 18–21
    vitamin B$_6$, 25

Niacinamide (see Niacin)
Nicotine:
    hyperthyroidism, 143
Nicotinamide (see Niacin)
Nicotinic acid (see Niacin)
Nickel, 77
Night blindness, 155
vitamin A, 14–15, 17
Nitrogen and burns, 117
Noodles, 202*
soups, 222–224*
Nori, 195–196, 210*
Nose:
    allergies, 110
    common cold, 125
    ear infection, 132
    halitosis, 139
    headache, 140
    leukemia, 148
    sinusitis, 162–163
Nucleic acid:
    DNA, 83
    folic acid, 32
    RNA, 14
    zinc, 83
Nutmeg, 224*
Nuts, 220*
    acne, 108
    fats, 8
    foods, 191
    sulfur, 82

Oats:
    flakes, 202*
    grains, 188
    oatmeal, 202*
    oatmeal cookies w/raisins, 208*
Obesity, 155–156
    arteriosclerosis and atherosclerosis, 112
    arthritis, 113
    bruising, 118
    carbohydrates, 8
    cerebrovascular accident, 122
    diabetes, 129
    fatigue, 135
    fats, 9
    gallstones, 136–137
    gout, 139
    hemorrhoids, 142
    hypertension, 143
    myocardial infarction, 153
    peptic ulcer, 163
    varicose veins, 167
Oils, 191, 222*
    cod-liver oil, 222*
    fats, 8–9
    soybeans, 189
    vitamin A, 13–14
    vitamin D, 47
    vitamin E, 50–51
    vitamin K, 58
    wheat germ, 196
Okra, 230*
Olives, 214*
oil, 222*

Omelet, 206*
Onions, 230*
    powder, 224*
    soup, 224*
Orange, 214*
    juice, 214*
Oregano, 224*
Organic supplements, 100
Orotic acid (see vitamin B₁₃)
Osteoarthritis (see Arthritis)
Osteomalacia, 160–161
    calcium, 64
    phosphorus, 77–78
    vitamin D, 48–49
Osteoporosis, 155
    backache, 115
    calcium, 64
    fluorine, 69
    fracture, 136
    phosphorus, 77–78
    vitamin D, 48
Overweight (see Obesity)
Oysters, 210*
    fish, 186
    stew, 224*
Oxalic acid:
    calcium, 64
    chocolate, 192
Oxygen:
    anemia, 110
    angina pectoris, 111
    cerebrovascular accident, 122
    emphysema, 133
    iron, 71
    metabolism, 3
    myocardial infarction, 153
    pangamic acid, 39–40
    sulfur, 82
    vitamin E, 50, 52
Oxidation:
    fats, 8–9
    nuts, 191
    soybeans, 189

Pancakes, 202*
Pancreas:
    alcoholism, 109
    cystic fibrosis, 127
    diabetes, 129
    digestion, 2
    hypoglycemia, 144
    iron, 71
    manganese, 75
    sweetbreads, 220*
    zinc, 83–84
Pangamic acid, 39–41
    autism, 115
    "Available Forms of Nutrient
        Supplements," 103
    "Nutrients That Function Together," 94–96
    "Rich Sources of Nutrients," 197
    "Summary Chart of Nutrients," 88
Pantothenic acid, 41–43
    "Available Forms of Nutrient
        Supplements," 103

bruxism, 118
cancer, 120
headache, 140
insomnia, 146
leg cramp, 147–148
mental illness, 149, 151
"Nutrients That Function Together," 95, 99
"Rich Sources of Nutrients," 197
stress, 164
"Summary Chart of Nutrients," 88
worms, 169
Papaya, 214*
    juice, 214*
Paprika, 224*
Para-aminobenzoic acid (PABA), 37–38
    "Available Forms of Nutrient
        Supplements," 103
    "Nutrients That Function Together," 96
    "Rich Sources of Nutrients," 197
    "Summary Chart of Nutrients," 88
Paralysis:
    arteriosclerosis and atherosclerosis, 112
    beriberi, 117
    cerebrovascular accident, 122
    multiple sclerosis, 151
    muscular dystrophy, 152
    pantothenic acid, 42
    polio, 158
    vitamin B₁₂, 28
Parathyroid:
    calcium, 64
    magnesium, 73
    renal calculi, 146
Parkinson's disease, 156
Parmesan cheese, 204*
Parsley, 224,* 230*
Parsnips, 230*
Passion fruit, 214*
Pasta, 202*
Pasteurization, 190
Peach, 214*
Peanuts, 202*
    brittle, 208*
    butter, 202*
    flour, 202*
    oil, 222*
Pear, 214*
Peas, 230*
    soup, 224*
Pecans, 220*
    pie, 208*
Pellagra, 156–157
    alcoholism, 109
    niacin, 36–37
Pepper, 224–225*
    seasonings, 191
Peppermint, 180
Peppers:
    green, 230*
    hot chili, 230*
    red, 230*
Peptic ulcer, 163–164
    anemia, 110
    backache, 115
    gastritis, 137

Perch, 210*
Periodontitis, 165
Pernicious anemia, 157
    vitamin B₁₂, 28
Persimmon, 216
Perspiration:
    cystic fibrosis, 127
    fever, 135
Pheasant, 218*
Phlebitis, 157–158
    edema, 133
Phosphorus, 77–78
    "Available Forms of Nutrient
        Supplements," 105
    calcium, 63–64
    eggs, 186
    fish, 186
    fracture, 136
    magnesium, 73–74
    meats, 189
    milk, 190
    nuts, 191
    "Nutrients That Function Together," 94,
        96–99
    osteoporosis, 155
    polio, 158
    pregnancy, 170
    "Rich Sources of Nutrients," 197
    rickets, 160–161
    scurvy, 161
    seeds, 192
    stress, 163–164
    "Summary Chart of Nutrients, 91–92
    tooth and gum disorders, 165–166
    zinc, 83
Phytic acid:
    calcium, 64
    zinc, 83
Pickles:
    dill, 230*
    sour, 230*
    sweet, 230*
Pie, 208*
    crust, 208*
    fruit, 208*
Pigs' feet, 218*
Pike, 210*
Piles (see Hemorrhoids)
Pimientos, 230*
Pimples (see Acne)
Pineapple, 216*
    juice, 216*
Pine nuts, 220*
Pinto beans, 226*
Pistachio nuts, 220*
Pita bread, 200*
Pizza, 202*
Plantain, 216*
Plums, 216*
Pneumonia, 158
    alcoholism, 109
    influenza, 145
    worms, 169
Polio, 158–159
Polish sausage, 220*

Pollack, 210*
Pollution, environmental:
    vitamin A, 13–14
    vitamin C, 44
Polyneuritis (see Neuritis)
Pomegranate, 216*
Popcorn, 202*
Poppy seed, 226*
Pork, 218*
    bacon, 218*
    bean and pork soup, 222*
    Boston butt, 218*
    chops, 218*
    feet, 218*
    ham, 218*
    lard, 222*
    picnic, 218*
    sausage, 218–220*
    spareribs, 218*
    worms, 169
Port du Salut cheese, 204*
Porterhouse steak, 218*
Potassium, 78–80
    alcoholism, 109
    "Available Forms of Nutrient
        Supplements," 105
    burns, 119
    cancer, 120
    chlorine, 65–66
    congestive heart failure, 126
    diarrhea, 130
    fever, 135
    fracture, 136
    gastroenteritis, 138
    hypertension, 143
    insomnia, 146
    magnesium, 73
    meats, 189
    nephritis, 154
    "Nutrients That Function Together,"
        94–95, 98
    nuts, 191
    polio, 158–159
    "Rich Sources of Nutrients," 197
    "Summary Chart of Nutrients," 92
    tooth and gum disorders, 165–166
Potato, 230–232*
    chips, 232*
    flour, 202*
    foods, 193
    soup, 224*
    sweet, 232*
Poultry, 218–220*
    niacin, 36
    meats, 189–190
    seasoning, 226*
Pound cake, 208*
Pregnancy, 169–170
    anemia, 110
    beriberi, 117
    biotin, 30
    diabetes, 129
    edema, 133
    folic acid, 32
    hemorrhoids, 142

iodine, 70
iron, 71–72
menstruation, 171
nephritis, 154
nutritional requirements, 248
overweight and obesity, 155
rickets, 161
stress, 163
vaginitis, 167
varicose veins, 167
vitamin A, 14, 18
vitamin B complex, 18, 21
vitamin B_2, 24
vitamin B_6, 25, 27
vitamin D, 48, 50
vitamin K, 58–59
Preserves, 208*
Pretzel, 202*
Pricklypear, 216*
Prostate, 159
Prostatitis, 159
Protein, 9–10
    absorption, 2
    alcoholism, 109
    amino acids, 235–236
    anemia, pernicious, 157
    angina pectoris, 111
    backache, 115–116
    bedsores, 116
    beverages, 193
    bronchitis, 117–118
    burns, 118–119
    bursitis, 119
    cancer, 120
    calories, 7
    carbohydrates, 7
    celiac disease, 122
    cirrhosis of the liver, 124
    croup, 127
    cystic fibrosis, 127–128
    dermatitis, 128–129
    diabetes, 129–130
    diarrhea, 130–131
    digestion, 2
    ear infection, 132
    edema, 133
    eggs, 186
    emphysema, 133–134
    epilepsy, 134
    fever, 135
    fish, 186
    fracture, 136
    folic acid, 32
    gallstones, 137
    grains, 187–188
    hair problems, 139
    hyperthyroidism, 143
    hypoglycemia, 144
    influenza, 145
    insomnia, 146
    kwashiorkor, 147
    legumes, 188–189
    magnesium, 73–74
    meats, 189
    milk, 190

mononucleosis, 151
muscular dystrophy, 152
myocardial infarction, 152–153
nail problems, 153
nephritis, 154
neuritis, 154
niacin, 36
nuts, 191
nutrient allowance, 245–248
nutrients, 11
osteoporosis, 155
overweight and obesity, 156
pellagra, 157
phosphorus, 77
pneumonia, 158
polio, 158–159
potassium, 78
pregnancy, 170
prostatitis, 159
psoriasis, 159–160
"Rich Sources of Nutrients," 196
scurvy, 161–162
seeds, 192
sinusitis, 162–163
stress, 163–164
supplementary foods, 194–196
sweeteners, 192
swollen glands, 164–165
tonsilitis, 165
tuberculosis, 166
vegetables, 193
venereal disease, 168
vitamin B_2, 23
vitamin B_6, 25
vitamin B_{12}, 27–28
vitamin C, 43
worms, 169
Provolone cheese, 204*
Prune, 216*
    juice, 216*
Psoriasis, 159–160
Ptyalin in digestion, 2
Puberty, 171
Pudding, 208*
Pumpernickel bread, 200*
Pumpkin:
    canned, 232*
    pie, 208*
        spice, 226*
    seeds, 220*
Pyelonephritis (see Nephritis)
Pyorrhea, 160
    tooth and gum disorders, 165–166
Pyridoxine (see Vitamin B_6)

Quince, 216*

Rabbit, 218*
Rabies and epilepsy, 134
Radiation and leukemia, 148
Radish:
    Oriental, 232*
    Red, 232*
Raised doughnut, 208*

Raisin, 216*
  bread, 200*
  cookie w/oatmeal, 208*
  pudding w/rice, 208*
Raspberries, 216*
  juice, 216*
Recommended Dietary Allowances:
  "Nutrient Allowance Chart," 245–248
Renal calculi (kidney stones), 146–147
Reproduction:
  childhood, 171
  female system:
    iron, 71–72
    menopause, 172
    menstruation, 171
    pregnancy, 169–170
    vaginitis, 167
  folic acid, 32
  male system:
    prostatitis, 159
    zinc, 83–84
  manganese, 75
  niacin, 36
  sex, 171–172
Respiratory system:
  alcoholism, 109
  asthma, 114
  beriberi, 117
  bronchitis, 117–118
  common cold, 125
  emphysema, 133–134
  influenza, 145
  pneumonia, 158
  potassium, 70–80
Rest:
  acne, 108
  angina pectoris, 111
  boil, 117
  bronchitis, 117
  bursitis, 119
  carbuncle, 121
  common cold, 125
  congestive heart failure, 126
  constipation, 126
  ear infection, 132
  epilepsy, 134
  fatigue, 135
  gastroenteritis, 138
  gout, 139
  mononucleosis, 151
  multiple sclerosis, 151
  myocardial infarction, 152–153
  nephritis, 154
  tuberculosis, 166
  vaginitis, 167
  varicose veins, 167–168
Rheumatic fever, 160
  congestive heart failure, 126
Rheumatoid arthritis, 112–113
Rheumatism, 160
  arthritis, 112–114
Rhinitis, 161
Rhubarb, 216*
Rib roast, 218*
Riboflavin (see Vitamin B₂)
Ribs, pork, 218*

Rice, 202*
  bran, 202*
  brown, 187, 202*
  flour, 202*
  grains, 187
  instant, 202*
  parboiled, 202*
  pudding, 208*
  puffed, 202*
  white, 187, 202*
  wild, 202*
Rickets, 160–161
  calcium, 64
  epilepsy, 134
  vitamin D, 48
Ricotta cheese, 204*
RNA and vitamin A, 14
Roast:
  beef chuck, 216*
  beef rump, 218*
  veal rib, 220*
  veal rump, 220*
Rolls, 202*
Romaine lettuce, 230*
Root beer, 200*
Roquefort cheese, 204*
  salad dressing, 222*
Rose hips, 180
  supplementary foods, 195
  vitamin C, 43
Rosemary, 226*
Round steak, 218*
Rum, 200*
Rump roast:
  beef, 218*
  veal, 220*
Russian salad dressing, 222*
Rutabaga, 232*
Rutin (see Bioflavonoids)
Rye:
  bread, 200*
  celiac disease, 121–122
  cracker, 200*
  flour, 202*
  grains, 187–188

Saccharine (sweeteners), 192
Safflower oil, 222*
Saffron, 226*
Sage, 226*
Salad dressings, 222*
Salami, 220*
Salmon, 210*
Salt, 226*
  arteriosclerosis and atherosclerosis, 112
  chlorine, 65–66
  cerebrovascular accident, 122–123
  cystic fibrosis, 127–128
  diarrhea, 130–131
  edema, 133
  fever, 135
  hypertension, 143
  iodine, 70
  leg cramp, 147–148
  nephritis, 154

  polio, 158–159
  seasoning, 191
  sodium, 81–82
Sandabs, 210*
Sardines, 210*
Sarsaparilla, 180–181
Sauces, 222*
Sauerkraut, 232*
Sausage, 218–220*
Savory, 226*
Scallops, 210*
Scurvy, 161–162
  alcoholism, 109
  halitosis, 140
  iron, 72
  vitamin C, 44, 47
Seafood, 210–212*
  copper, 68
  fish, 186
  fluorine, 69
  iodine, 70
  sodium, 81
Seaweed, 210–212*
  agar-agar, 210*
  diverticulitis, 131
  dulse, 210*
  hijiki, 210*
  kelp, 210*
  kombu, 210*
  supplementary foods,
    195–196
Seasonings, 224–226*
  dyspepsia, 145
  foods, 191–192
  gastritis, 137
  prostatitis, 159
  seeds, 192
  sinusitis, 162
Seeds, 220*
  fats, 8
  foods, 192
Selenium, 80–81
Senility, 162
Sesame:
  oil, 222*
  seeds, 220
    foods, 192
Sex, 171–172
Shad, 210*
Shallots, 232*
Shellfish (see Seafood)
Sherbet, 206*
Shingles, 162
Shock in burns, 119
Shortening, 222*
Shredded wheat, 202*
Shrimp, 210*
Silicon, 85
Sinuses and influenza, 145
Sinusitis, 162–163
Sirloin steak, 218*
Skim milk, 206*
Skin:
  acne, 108
  anemia, pernicious, 157
  asthma, 114

athlete's foot, 114–115
bedsores, 116
boil, 117
burns, 118–119
carbuncle, 121
copper, 68
dermatitis, 128–129
fats, 8
fever, 135
gallstones, 137
herpes zoster, 162
impetigo, 144
iron, 71–72
kwashiorkor, 147
lcukemia, 148
niacin, 36–37
protein, 9
psoriasis, 159–160
scurvy, 161
sulfur, 82–83
swollen glands, 164
vitamin A, 13–15, 17
vitamin B complex, 18–19, 21
vitamin B_2, 23–25
vitamin B_6, 26–27
vitamin C, 43–45, 47
vitamin D, 47–48, 50
Skullcap, 181
Smelt, 210*
Smoking:
  arteriosclerosis and atherosclerosis, 112
  bronchitis, 117
  cancer, 120
  cerebrovascular accident, 122
  dyspepsia, 145
  emphysema, 133
  halitosis, 139
  hypertension, 143
  sinusitis, 162
  vitamin C, 43, 45
Snails, 210*
Snapper, 212*
Soda crackers, 200*
Sodium, 81–82
  arteriosclerosis and atherosclerosis, 112
  burns, 119
  chloride, 65
  congestive heart failure, 126
  cystic fibrosis, 127–128
  diarrhea, 130–131
  edcma, 133
  fever, 135
  hypertension, 143
  leg cramp, 147–148
  nephritis, 154
  polio, 158–159
  potassium, 78–79
  seasonings, 191
  tooth and gum disorders, 165–166
Sodium chloride:
  chlorine, 65
  seasonings, 191
  (see also Sodium)
Sole, 210*
Sorbitol (sweeteners), 192

Sorrel, 228*
Soups, 222–224*
  crackers, 200*
Sour cream, 204*
Soybeans, 226*
  curd, 226*
  fermented, 226*
  flour, 202*
  granules, 226*
  lecithin, 195
  legumes, 189
  milk, 226*
  oil, 222*
  sprouts, 226*
Soy sauce, 222*
Spaghetti, 202*
Spareribs, pork, 218*
Spices, 191, 224–226*
Spinach, 232*
  New Zealand, 232*
Spleen:
  iron, 71
  vitamin D, 48
Sponge cake, 208*
Sprouts, 226*
Sprue, 32, 59
Squash, 232*
  seeds, 220*
  summer, 232*
  winter, 232*
Starch:
  carbohydrates, 7
  cystic fibrosis, 127
  kwashiorkor, 147
  tooth and gum disorders, 165
Steak, 216–218*
Stomach:
  anemia, pernicious, 157
  constipation, 126
  cystitis, 128
  digestion, 2
  drug abuse, 132
  dyspepsia, 145
  gallstones, 136–137
  gastritis, 137
  gastroenteritis, 138
  leukemia, 148
  menstruation, 171
  peptic ulcer, 163
  (see also Abdomen)
Strawberry, 181, 216*
Stress, 163–164
  alcoholism, 109
  anxiety, 163
  asthma, 114
  backache, 115–116
  canker sore, 120
  colitis, 124
  dermatitis, 128
  diabetes, 129
  diarrhea, 130
  epilepsy, 134
  folic acid, 32
  glaucoma, 138
  headache, 140

hypertension, 143
hyperthyroidism, 143
insomnia, 145–146
multiple sclerosis, 151
protein, 10
vitamin C, 43
Stretching, 4
Stroke, 141
  (see also Cerebrovascular accident)
Strontium, 85
Sugar, 208*
  beet (cane), 208*
  brown, 208*
  carbohydrates, 7–8
  cystic fibrosis, 127
  diabetes, 129
  fruits, 186–187
  hypoglycemia, 144
  myocardial infarction
  powdered, 208*
  sweeteners, 192–193
  syrup, 208*
  tooth and gum disorders, 165
Sulfur, 82–83
  "Available Forms of Nutrient
    Supplements," 105
  meats, 189
  "Rich Sources of Nutrients," 198
  "Summary Chart of Nutrients," 92
Sun:
  acne, 108
  hair problems, 139
  psoriasis, 159
  vitamin D, 47–48
Sunburn, 164
Sunflower seeds, 220*
  oil, 222*
Sweetbreads, 220*
Sweet potato, 232*
Sweeteners, 208*
  foods, 192–193
Swiss cheese, 204*
Swollen glands, 164–165
Swordfish, 212*
Syphilis:
  swollen glands, 164
  venereal disease, 168
Syrup, 208*

Tangelo, 216*
Tangerine, 216*
Tannic acid in tea, 194
Tapioca, 202*
  pudding, 208*
Tarragon, 226*
Tartar sauce, 222*
T-bone steak, 218*
Tea, 200*
  beverages, 193–194
  dyspepsia, 145
  glaucoma, 138
  hypertension, 143
  hyperthyroidism, 143
  hypoglycemia, 144
  insomnia, 145

Tetanus and epilepsy, 134
Tetany:
    calcium, 64–65
    rickets and osteomalacia, 161
    vitamin D, 48, 50
Theobromine in chocolate, 192
Thiamine (see Vitamin B₁)
Thomson seedless grapes, 214*
Thousand Island salad dressing, 222*
Throat:
    bronchitis, 117
    common cold, 125
    croup, 127
    ear infection, 132
    halitosis, 139
    headache, 140
    meningitis, 149
    mononucleosis, 151
    nephritis, 154
    rhinitis, 161
    sinusitis, 162
    swollen glands, 164
    tonsilitis, 165
    vitamin A, 143 .
Thrombophlebitis, 157–158
Thyme, 226*
Thyroid:
    cobalt, 67
    goiter, 138
    hyperthyroidism, 143
    iodine, 69–70
Thyroxine and iodine, 69–70
Tin, 85
Tinea pedis (athlete's foot), 114–115
Toasted bread, 200*
Tobacco:
    amblyopia, 28
    glaucoma, 138
    headache, 140
Tocopherol:
    "Available Forms of Nutrient
        Supplements," 103
    vitamin E, 50–55
Tofu, 226*
Tom Collins, 200*
Tomato, 232*
    catsup, 222*
    juice, 232*
    paste, 232*
    puree, 232*
    soup, 224*
Tongue, 218*
Tonsilitis, 165
Tooth and gum disorders, 165–166
    bone meal, 194
    calcium, 63–65
    childhood, 171
    fluorine, 68–69
    halitosis, 139–140
    phosphorus, 77–78
    rickets and osteomalacia, 161
    vitamin D, 48–50
Tooth-grinding (bruxism), 118
Tortilla, 202*
Tritium, 85

Trout, 212*
Tryptophan:
    niacin, 36
    protein, 235
Tuberculosis, 166
    alcoholism, 109
    swollen glands, 164
Tumor:
    backache, 115
    cancer, 120
    dizziness, 131
    fracture, 136
    glaucoma, 138
    hypoglycemia, 144
Tuna, 210*
Turkey, 220*
    soup, 224*
Turmeric, 226*
Turnips, 232*
    greens, 232*
Typhoid and chlorine, 65

Ulcer, 166–167
    (see also Peptic ulcer)
Umeboshi, 222*
Underweight, 167
Urinary tract:
    backache, 115
    cystitis, 128
    nephritis, 154
    prostatitis, 159
    renal calculi, 146–147

Vaginitis, 167
Vanadium, 83
Vanilla wafer, 208*
Varicose veins, 167–168
    phlebitis, 157–158
Veal, 220*
Vegetables, 226–232*
    beverages, 193
    cobalt, 67
    constipation, 126
    diabetes, 129
    folic acid, 32
    foods, 193
    iron, 70
    juice, 193, 232*
        diverticulitis, 131
    magnesium, 73
    manganese, 75
    oil, 222*
    peptic ulcer, 163
    potassium, 79
    protein, 10
    shortening, 222*
    soup, 224*
    tooth and gum disorders, 165
    vitamin A, 13–14
    vitamin B complex, 18
    vitamin C, 43
    vitamin E, 50–51
Vegetarianism, 102
    cobalt, 67
    vitamin B₁₂, 27

Venereal disease, 168
Venison, 220*
Vertigo (dizziness), 131
Vienna bread, 200*
Vienna sausage, 220*
Villi and absorption, 3
Vinegar, 222*
Virus:
    common cold, 125
    conjunctivitis, 126
    croup, 127
    herpes zoster, 162
    influenza, 145
    meningitis, 149
    mononucleosis, 151
    pneumonia, 158
    polio, 158–159
    tonsilitis, 165
Vision and focus disorders, 168–169
Vitamins, 11–12, 13–61
    alcoholism, 109
    "Available Forms of Nutrient
        Supplements," 100–105
    bedsores, 116
    carbohydrates, 8
    constipation, 126–127
    diabetes, 129–130
    diarrhea, 131–132
    fats, 8
    foods, 185
    fruits, 186–187
    kwashiorkor, 147
    meats, 189
    milk, 190
    nephritis, 154
    "Nutrients That Function Together," 93–99
    peptic ulcer, 163
    "Summary Chart of Nutrients," 86–92
    sweeteners, 192–193
    tonsilitis, 165
    tuberculosis, 166
    vegetables, 193
Vitamin A, 13–18
    abscess, 108
    acne, 108
    allergies, 110
    asthma, 114
    athlete's foot, 115
    "Available Forms of Nutrient
        Supplements," 102
    bedsores, 116
    boil, 117
    bronchitis, 117–118
    burns, 119
    bursitis, 119
    calcium, 63
    cancer, 120
    canker sore, 120–121
    carbuncle, 121
    celiac disease, 122
    chicken pox, 123
    cirrhosis of the liver, 124
    common cold, 125
    conjunctivitis, 126
    croup, 127

cystic fibrosis, 127–128
cystitis, 128
dermatitis, 128–129
diabetes, 129
eczema, 132
emphysema, 133
fats, 8–9
fever, 135
fish, 186
fruits, 186–187
gallstones, 137
gastroenteritis, 138
glaucoma, 138
hair problems, 139
halitosis, 140
hay fever, 140
headache, 140
hemorrhoids, 142
herpes zoster, 162
hyperthyroidism, 143
impetigo, 144
influenza, 145
measles, 149
meats, 189
meningitis, 149
mononucleosis, 151
nail problems, 153
nephritis, 154
night blindness, 155
"Nutrients That Function Together," 94–99
oils, 191
pneumonia, 158
polio, 158
prostatitis, 159
psoriasis, 159
renal calculi, 147
rhinitis, 161
"Rich Sources of Nutrients," 196
sinusitis, 162–163
"Summary Chart of Nutrients," 86
swollen glands, 164–165
tooth and gum disorders, 165
tuberculosis, 166
vaginitis, 167
vegetables, 193
vision and focus disorders, 168–169
vitamin D, 48
vitamin E, 50, 53
worms, 169
Vitamin B complex, 18–21
abscess, 108
aging, 173
anemia, 110
    pernicious, 157
arteriosclerosis and atherosclerosis, 112
arthritis, 113–114
asthma, 114
"Available Forms of Nutrient
    Supplements," 102
backache, 115–116
burns, 119
cancer, 120
carbohydrates, 8
celiac disease, 122
cerebrovascular accident, 122–123

cirrhosis of the liver, 124
common cold, 125
cystic fibrosis, 127–128
dermatitis, 128–129
diarrhea, 130
diverticulitis, 131
dyspepsia, 145
emphysema, 133
fatigue, 135
fever, 135
foods, 185
glaucoma, 138
gout, 139
grains, 187–188
hair problems, 139
headache, 140
heart disease, 141
herpes zoster, 162
hyperthyroidism, 143
influenza, 144
insomnia, 146
leukemia, 148
meats, 189
menopause, 172
mental illness, 149–150
milk, 191
mononucleosis, 151
multiple sclerosis, 151–152
neuritis, 154
"Nutrients That Function Together,"
    93–96, 98
nuts, 191
Parkinson's disease, 156
pellagra, 157–158
peptic ulcer, 163
phlebitis, 158
phosphorus, 77
pneumonia, 158
polio, 158
pregnancy, 170
prostatitis, 159
psoriasis, 159
seeds, 192
sulfur, 82
"Summary Chart of Nutrients," 86–87
supplements, 194–196
sweeteners, 192–193
vaginitis, 167
varicose veins, 168
vegetables, 193
worms, 169
Vitamin B$_1$, 21–23
"Available Forms of Nutrient
    Supplements," 102
beriberi, 117
constipation, 126–127
edema, 133
grains, 187–188
herpes zoster, 162
legumes, 188
manganese, 75
meats, 189
milk, 190
mononucleosis, 151
neuritis, 154

night blindness, 155
"Nutrients That Function Together,"
    94–96, 99
pellagra, 157–158
"Rich Sources of Nutrients," 196
"Summary Chart of Nutrients," 87
supplementary foods, 194–196
vitamin B complex, 18–21
worms, 169
Vitamin B$_2$, 23–25
acne, 108
"Available Forms of Nutrient
    Supplements," 102
cancer, 120
cataracts, 121
conjunctivitis, 126
grains, 187–188
legumes, 188
meats, 189
milk, 190
mononucleosis, 151
multiple sclerosis, 152
night blindness, 155
"Nutrients That Function Together," 94–95
pellagra, 157
pregnancy, 178
psoriasis, 159
"Rich Sources of Nutrients," 196
"Summary Chart of Nutrients," 87
supplementary foods, 194–196
vitamin B complex, 18–21
worms, 169
Vitamin B$_6$, 25–27
acne, 108
alcoholism, 109
anemia, 110
autism, 115
"Available Forms of Nutrient
    Supplements," 102
baldness, 116
common cold, 125
conjunctivitis, 126
dermatitis, 128–129
dizziness, 131
insomnia, 146
milk, 190
mononucleosis, 151
"Nutrients That Function Together,"
    94–96, 98
pregnancy, 170
renal calculi, 147
"Rich Sources of Nutrients," 196
"Summary Chart of Nutrients," 87
Vitamin B$_{12}$, 27–29
aging, 173
"Available Forms of Nutrient
    Supplements," 102
anemia, pernicious, 28, 157
celiac disease, 122
choline, 31
cobalt, 66
folic acid, 32
gastritis, 137
herpes zoster, 162
insomnia, 142

meats, 189
milk, 190
multiple sclerosis, 152
pellagra, 157
"Rich Sources of Nutrients," 196
"Summary Chart of Nutrients," 87
vitamin B$_6$, 25
worms, 169
Vitamin B$_{13}$, 29
"Available Forms of Nutrient
    Supplements," 102
multiple sclerosis, 152
"Rich Sources of Nutrients," 196
"Summary Chart of Nutrients," 87
Vitamin C, 43–47
abscess, 108
acne, 108
"Available Forms of Nutrient
    Supplements," 103
aging, 173
alcoholism, 109
allergies, 110
anemia, 110
    pernicious, 157
arteriosclerosis and atherosclerosis, 112
bedsores, 116
bioflavonoids, 59–61
boil, 117
bronchitis, 117–118
burns, 119
bursitis, 119
cancer, 120
carbuncle, 121
cataracts, 121
celiac disease, 122
cerebrovascular accident, 122–123
cirrhosis of the liver, 124
colitis, 125
common cold, 125
copper, 68
croup, 127
cystic fibrosis, 127–128
diabetes, 129–130
diarrhea, 130
ear infection, 132
emphysema, 133
fatigue, 135
fever, 135
food, 185
fracture, 136
fruits, 186
gastroenteritis, 138
glaucoma, 138
halitosis, 140
herpes zoster, 162
honey, 192–193
hypertension, 143
influenza, 145
insomnia, 146
iron, 71
leg cramp, 147–148
legumes, 188
leukemia, 148
meats, 189
meningitis, 149

menopause, 172
milk, 190
mononucleosis, 151
"Nutrients That Function Together," 93–98
peptic ulcer, 163
phlebitis, 158
pneumonia, 158
polio, 158
pregnancy, 170
prostatitis, 159
psoriasis, 159
rickets, 161
"Rich Sources of Nutrients," 197
scurvy, 161–162
sinusitis, 162–163
"Summary Chart of Nutrients," 89
supplementary foods, 195
sweeteners, 192–193
swollen glands, 164–165
tonsilitis, 165
tooth and gum disorders, 165
tuberculosis, 166
varicose veins, 168
vegetables, 193
vitamin A, 14–15
worms, 169
Vitamin D, 47–50
"Available Forms of Nutrient
    Supplements," 103
calcium, 63–64
canker sore, 121
celiac disease, 122
common cold, 125–126
cystic fibrosis, 127–128
eggs, 186
fats, 8
fatigue, 135
fish, 186
fracture, 136
gallstones, 137
lactation, 170–171
meats, 189
magnesium, 73–74
"Nutrients That Function Together,"
    93–94, 96–98
osteoporosis, 155
phosphorus, 77–78
pregnancy, 176
psoriasis, 159
renal calculi, 146–147
"Rich Sources of Nutrients," 197
rickets, 161
"Summary Chart of Nutrients," 89
tooth and gum disorders, 165
tuberculosis, 166
worms, 169
Vitamin E, 50–55
acne, 108
aging, 173
anemia, 110
    112
arteriosclerosis and atherosclerosis,
"Available Forms of Nutrient
    Supplements," 100, 103
bedsores, 116

burns, 119
cancer, 120
celiac disease, 122
cerebrovascular accident, 123
cystic fibrosis, 127–128
eggs, 186
emphysema, 133–134
fats, 8
gallstones, 137
gout, 139
honey, 192–193
intermittent claudication, 53
iron, 71
menopause, 172
"Nutrients That Function Together,"
    93–96, 98
nuts, 191
oils, 191
phlebitis, 158
pneumonia, 158
psoriasis, 159
"Rich Sources of Nutrients," 197
seeds, 192
sex, 172
soybeans, 189
"Summary Chart of Nutrients," 89
supplementary foods, 195
sweeteners, 192–193
Vitamin F, 55–58
"Available Forms of Nutrient
    Supplements," 104
"Rich Sources of Nutrients," 197
"Summary Chart of Nutrients," 89
Vitamin K, 58–59
anemia, 110
"Available Forms of Nutrient
    Supplements," 104
celiac disease, 122
cystic fibrosis, 127–128
fats, 8
gallstones, 137
"Nutrients That Function Together," 97
"Rich Sources of Nutrients," 197
"Summary Chart of Nutrients," 90
supplementary foods, 194–195
worms, 169
Vitamin P, 59–61
(see also Bioflavonoids)
Vitamin T, 61
Vitamin U, 61
Vitiligo and para-aminobenzoic acid, 38
Vision and focus disorders, 168–169
Vodka, 200*
Vomiting:
    alcoholism, 109
    beriberi, 117
    chlorine, 66
    dizziness, 131
    ear infection, 132
    fever, 135
    gallstones, 137
    gastritis, 137
    gastroenteritis, 138
    headache, 140
    magnesium, 74

meningitis, 149
nephritis, 154
potassium, 79
sodium, 81
tonsilitis, 165
worms, 169

Waffle, 204*
Wakame, 212*
Walking exercise, 4–5
Walnuts, 220*
Water, 85
 beverages, 193
 burns, 119
 chlorine, 65
 common cold, 125
 constipation, 126
 cystitis, 128
 diarrhea, 130
 digestion, 2
 diverticulitis, 131
 edema, 133
 fluorine, 69
 fruits, 186
 hemorrhoids, 142
 metabolism, 3
 nephritis, 154
 nutrients, 11
 osteoporosis, 155
 pneumonia, 158
 prostatitis, 159
 protein, 9
 sodium, 81
 tap water, 85
 vegetables, 193
 vitamin B complex, 18

 vitamin C, 43
 vitamins, 12
Water chestnuts, 232*
Watercress, 232*
Watermelon, 216*
Weight lifting, 5
Wheat:
 bran, 200*
 buckwheat flour, 202*
 bulgur, 200*
 celiac disease, 121–122
 cracked wheat bread, 200*
 crackers, 200*
 cream of, 200*
 flakes, 204*
 flour, 202*
 germ, 196, 204*
  oil, 222*
 gluten flour, 202*
 grains, 187–188
 pastry flour, 202*
 puffed, 204*
 shredded, 202*
 wheatmeal cereal, 204*
 whole wheat:
  bread, 200*
  muffins, 202*
  pancakes, 202*
  pasta, 202*
Whey, 206*
Whipping cream, 204*
Whiskey, 200*
White beans, 226*
White bread, 200*
White cake, 208*
Whitefish, 212*

Whiteheads (see Acne)
White sauce, 222*
Wild rice, 202*
Wilson's disease and copper, 68
Wine, 200*
Worcestershire sauce, 222*
Worms, 169
 vaginitis, 167

Xerosis and vitamin A, 15

Yams, 232*
Yarrow, 181–182
Yeast:
 Bakers', 232*
 brewer's, 232*
 folic acid, 32
 torula, 232*
 yogurt, 190
Yoga, 5
Yogurt, 190–191, 206*

Zinc, 82–84
 alcoholism, 109
 "Available Forms of Nutrient
  Supplements," 105
 cadmium, 62
 diabetes, 130
 fish, 186
 "Nutrients That Function Together," 94,
  97, 99
 "Rich Sources of Nutrients," 198
 sex, 172
 "Summary Chart of Nutrients," 92
Zucchini (see Squash)
Zwieback, 200*

Catalog

If you are interested in a list of fine Paperback
books, covering a wide range of subjects
and interests, send your name and address,
requesting your free catalog, to:

McGraw-Hill Paperbacks
1221 Avenue of Americas
New York, N.Y. 10020